LUNG CANCER THERAPY ANNUAL 5

LUNG
CANCER
THERAPY
ANNUAL 5

Edited by

Heine H Hansen MD FRCP

Professor of Medical Oncology
The Finsen Center, National University Hospital
Copenhagen, Denmark

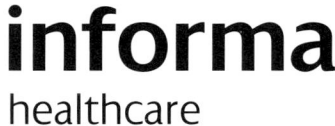

informa
healthcare

Contributors

Oliver Gautschi PhD
Division of Hematology/Oncology
Davis Cancer Center
University of California
Sacramento, CA, USA

Paul H Gumerlock PhD
Division of Hematology/Oncology
Davis Cancer Center
University of California
Sacramento, CA, USA

Heine H Hansen MD FRCP
Professor of Medical Oncology
The Finsen Center
National University Hospital
Copenhagen
Denmark

Rob J van Klaveren MD
Department of Pulmonology
Erasmus Medical Center
Rotterdam
The Netherlands

Jeroen S Kloover MD PhD
Department of Pulmonology
Erasmus Medical Center
Rotterdam
The Netherlands

Halla Skuladottir PhD
Department of Medical Oncology
Landspitali-University Hospital
Hringbraut
Reykjavik
Iceland

Morten Sørensen MD PhD
Department of Oncology
The Finsen Center
The National University Hospital
Copenhagen
Denmark

Rolf Stahel MD
Department of Medicine
Division of Oncology
University Hospital
Zürich
Switzerland

LUNG
CANCER
THERAPY
ANNUAL 5

Edited by

Heine H Hansen MD FRCP

Professor of Medical Oncology
The Finsen Center, National University Hospital
Copenhagen, Denmark

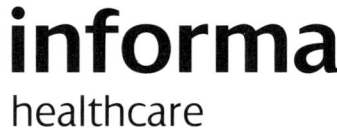

First published in the United Kingdom in 2006 by Informa Healthcare, 4 Park Square, Milton Park, Abingdon, Oxon OX14 4RN. Informa Healthcare is a trading division of Informa UK Ltd. Registered Office: 37/41 Mortimer Street, London W1T 3JH. Registered in England and Wales Number 1072954.

Tel: +44 (0)20 7017 6000
Fax: +44 (0)20 7017 6699
Email: info.medicine@tandf.co.uk
Website: www.tandf.co.uk/medicine

Second printing 2007

A CIP record for this book is available from the British Library.

Library of Congress Cataloging-in-Publication Data

Data available on application

ISBN-10: 0 415 38024 3
ISBN-13: 978 0 415 38024 9

Distributed in North and South America by

Taylor & Francis
6000 Broken Sound Parkway, NW, (Suite 300)
Boca Raton, FL 33487, USA

Within Continental USA	Distributed in the rest of the world by
Tel: 1 (800) 272 7737;	Thomson Publishing Services
Fax: 1 (800) 374 3401	Cheriton House
Outside Continental USA	North Way
Tel: (561) 994 0555;	Andover, Hampshire SP10 5BE, UK
Fax: (561) 361 6018	Tel: +44 (0)1264 332424
Email: orders@crcpress.com	Email: tps.tandfsalesorder@thomson.com

Composition by Wearset Ltd, Boldon, Tyne and Wear

Printed and bound in India by Replika Press Pvt. Ltd

Contents

Contributors

Oliver Gautschi PhD
Division of Hematology/Oncology
Davis Cancer Center
University of California
Sacramento, CA, USA

Paul H Gumerlock PhD
Division of Hematology/Oncology
Davis Cancer Center
University of California
Sacramento, CA, USA

Heine H Hansen MD FRCP
Professor of Medical Oncology
The Finsen Center
National University Hospital
Copenhagen
Denmark

Rob J van Klaveren MD
Department of Pulmonology
Erasmus Medical Center
Rotterdam
The Netherlands

Jeroen S Kloover MD PhD
Department of Pulmonology
Erasmus Medical Center
Rotterdam
The Netherlands

Halla Skuladottir PhD
Department of Medical Oncology
Landspitali-University Hospital
Hringbraut
Reykjavik
Iceland

Morten Sørensen MD PhD
Department of Oncology
The Finsen Center
The National University Hospital
Copenhagen
Denmark

Rolf Stahel MD
Department of Medicine
Division of Oncology
University Hospital
Zürich
Switzerland

Preface

The purpose of this fifth edition of the *Lung Cancer Therapy Annual* remains the same as that of the previous editions, namely to brief the oncology community about current developments in lung cancer by reviewing recent literature, with emphasis on therapeutic aspects, and to offer an update of the impact that this information will have on the day-to-day management of lung cancer patients.

Special thanks are due to my coauthors: Dr Halla Skulladottir (Chapter 2), Dr Oliver Gautschi and Dr Paul H Gumerlock (Chapter 3), Dr Rob van Klaveren (Chapters 4 and 6), Dr Jeroen S Kloover (Chapter 6), Dr Morten Sørensen (Chapter 7) and Dr Rolf Stahel (Chapter 9).

The authors also gratefully acknowledge the cooperation and help of Mr Robert Peden of Informa Healthcare. The interest and help of the publisher is greatly appreciated.

Heine H Hansen MD FRCP

1
Introduction

Heine H Hansen

Despite the very many efforts to reduce smoking rates around the world, lung cancer continues to be the leading worldwide cause of cancer death. In 2004 in Europe alone, 20% of all 1 711 000 cancer deaths were caused by lung cancer[1] and, in the USA lung cancer in women was responsible for as many deaths as breast cancer and as many deaths as all gynecologic cancers combined. Although it is encouraging to note that the incidence of lung cancer is decreasing among men (at least in some countries), it is alarming to see reports indicating the continuous rise in lung cancer in women in most countries, with the most recent reports coming from Europe and the Americas.[2–4] The gap between the incidence rates for the two genders is thus narrowing, with the male/female incidence ratio in the USA being 3.65 in 1975 and 1.56 in 1999.[5] In addition, women are relatively overrepresented among younger patients, raising the question of gender-specific differences in the susceptibility to lung cancer carcinogens.[6] Noteworthy also are the recent data demonstrating that women constitute 33.8% of the total group of patients with lung cancer, but that in the subgroup of non-smokers with lung cancer, 73.9% are women.

Among the epidemiologic changes, we also see a change in the histopathologic pattern, with a relative decrease in squamous cell carcinoma and a rise in adenocarcinoma. The dominant role of tobacco smoke as a causative factor in lung cancer is well established, and most studies report that more than 90% of patients with lung cancer are smokers, even though there is a trend towards an increase of lung cancers among non-smokers. Recent reports, e.g. from Iceland, have underscored the importance of genetic predisposition in the development of lung carcinoma, with its strongest effect in patients with early-onset disease. However, tobacco continues to play the dominant role in the pathogenesis of this disease, even among those individuals who are genetically predisposed to lung cancer.[7]

The fight against lung cancer continues all over the world, with more and more countries strengthening their efforts against tobacco smoking. It is thus noteworthy that as of January 1, 2006, smoking is prohibited in bars, restaurants, and public places in Ireland, Norway, Sweden, Spain, Italy, and parts of Australia – a dramatic change that originally was spearheaded by certain states in the USA and Canada.[8] At the same time, current health warnings against smoking are being enforced, and descriptions such as 'light' and 'mild' cigarettes have been banned (e.g. in the European Union), based on prior misleading figures for tar and nicotine on cigarette packets provided by the tobacco industry.[9] Fortunately, it is never too early or too late to stop smoking; there is always a health gain by quitting, as shown by Godtfredsen et al,[10] who observed that among individuals who smoke 15 or more cigarettes per day, a smoking reduction of 50% significantly reduces the risk of lung cancer.[11]

In the meantime, important new information as regards the biology of lung cancer is emerging, including new treatment approaches, resulting in a slow but steady improvement of the overall management, with increasing use of combined modality therapy consisting of surgery, chemotherapy and radiotherapy applied concurrently or sequentially in early-stage disease. Furthermore, new techniques are gaining ground, within both surgery and radiotherapy, and targeted medical therapy is being offered to more and more patients.

These developments have been presented in various oncology journals, with reviews on lung cancer covering epidemiology, cancer prevention, etiology, and multimodality therapy in cancer patients, including publications in connection with workshops on mesothelioma.[12–16] Also, consensus on medical treatment of non-small cell lung cancer has been reported from the Central Eastern Cooperative Oncology Group.[17] In addition, more than 1800 abstracts were presented at the 11th World Conference on Lung Cancer in Barcelona, July 3–6, 2005.[18]

REFERENCES

1. Boyle P, Ferleay J. Cancer incidence and mortality in Europe, 2004. Ann Oncol 2005; 16: 481–8.

2. Bosetti C, Malvezzi M, Chatenoud L et al. Trends in cancer mortality in the Americas, 1970–2000. Ann Oncol 2005; 16: 489–511.

3. O'Lorcain P, Comber H. Lung cancer mortality predictions for Ireland 2001–2015 and current trends in North Western Europe. Lung Cancer 2004; 46: 157–63.

4. Bosetti C, Levi F, Lucchini F et al. Lung cancer mortality in European women: recent trends and perspectives. Ann Oncol 2005; 16: 1597–604.

5. Fu JB, Kau TY, Severson RK et al. Lung cancer in women. Analysis of the national surveillance, epidemiology, and end results database. Chest 2005; 127: 768–77.

6. Thomas L, Doyle A, Edelman MJ. Lung cancer in women. Emerging differences in epidemiology, biology, and therapy. Chest 2005; 128: 370–81.

7. Jonsson S, Thorsteinsdottir U, Gudbjartsson DF et al. Familial risk of lung carcinoma in the Icelandic population. JAMA 2004; 292: 2977–83.

8. Boyle P, Dresler C. Preventing the lung cancer epidemic. Ann Oncol 2005; 16: 1565–6.

9. Gray N, Boyle P. Publishing tobacco tar measurements on packets. BMJ 2004; 329: 813–14.

10. Godtfredsen NS, Prescott E, Osler M. Effect of smoking reduction on lung cancer risk. JAMA 2005; 294: 1505–10.

11. Dacey LJ, Johnstone DW. Reducing the risk of lung cancer. JAMA 2005; 294: 1550–1.

12. Johnson D, Shepherd F, Bost G (eds). Lung cancer. Reviews. J Clin Oncol 2005; 23: 3173–93.

13. Lynch TJ, Boart JA, Curran WJ et al. Early stage lung cancer – new approaches to evaluation and treatment: conference summary statement. Clin Cancer Res 2005; 11: 4981s–83s.

14. Recent advances and continuing challenges in treating patients with lung cancer and poor performance status. Semin Oncol 2004; 31(6 Suppl 11): S1–530.

15. Invited papers from the IASLC Mesothelioma Workshop, September 29–October 2, 2004, Ermating, Switzerland. Lung Cancer 2005; 49(Suppl 1): S1–127.

16. Mornex F (ed). Non-small cell lung cancer. Semin Radiat Oncol 2004; 14: 277–347

17. Zielinski CC, Krainer M, Pirker R et al. Meeting report. Consensus on medical treatment of non-small-cell lung cancer – update 2004. Lung Cancer 2005; 50: 129–37.

18. Extended Abstracts of the 11th World Conference on Lung Cancer, 3–6 July 2005, Barcelona, Spain. Lung Cancer 2005; 49(Suppl 3).

2
Epidemiology

Halla Skuladottir

Lung cancer is the most common cancer in the world according to the most recent statistics of GLOBOCAN 2002, who estimated the occurrence of cancer worldwide for the year 2002. Approximately 970 000 men and 390 000 women were diagnosed with the disease, corresponding to 18% of all cancers in males in the more developed regions of the world (North America, Japan, Europe and Australia/New Zealand) and 16% in less-developed regions (rest of the world);[1,2] corresponding percentages for women were 8% and 7%, respectively. Lung cancer was the cause of death in 1.2 million individuals in the world in 2002: i.e. 18% of all cancer deaths were caused by the disease. Lung cancer incidence in different regions of the world is shown in Figure 2.1, and is generally higher in men than in women, the magnitude of the difference varying between two- and ninefold. Worldwide, lung cancer is the fifth most frequent cancer in women, but the occurrence has recently shown a steeper increase among women over time than among men. It is clear that the predominant risk factor is cigarette smoking. As industrial exposures also play an important role, lung cancer is largely a preventable disease.

GEOGRAPHICAL VARIATION

There is substantial geographical variation in the incidence of lung cancer among both men and women, reflecting the prevalence of the main cause of lung cancer, cigarette smoking. In populations that are not exposed to tobacco smoke or industrial lung carcinogens, the age-adjusted incidence rate (standardized to the World Standard Population) of lung cancer is generally below 5 per 100 000 per year.[2] The highest incidence rates of lung cancer among men were found in the industrialized world: African-American men and New Zealand Maoris had the highest incidences of all, at over 100 per 100 000 per year, and their lifetime risk for lung cancer was around 13%.[1] The highest incidence rates among women, around 34 per 100 000 per year, are observed in North America and north-western Europe, the latter including women in Denmark, Iceland and the United Kingdom.[1]

Most developing countries have still not experienced the worst consequences of the tobacco epidemic, as cigarette smoking has become

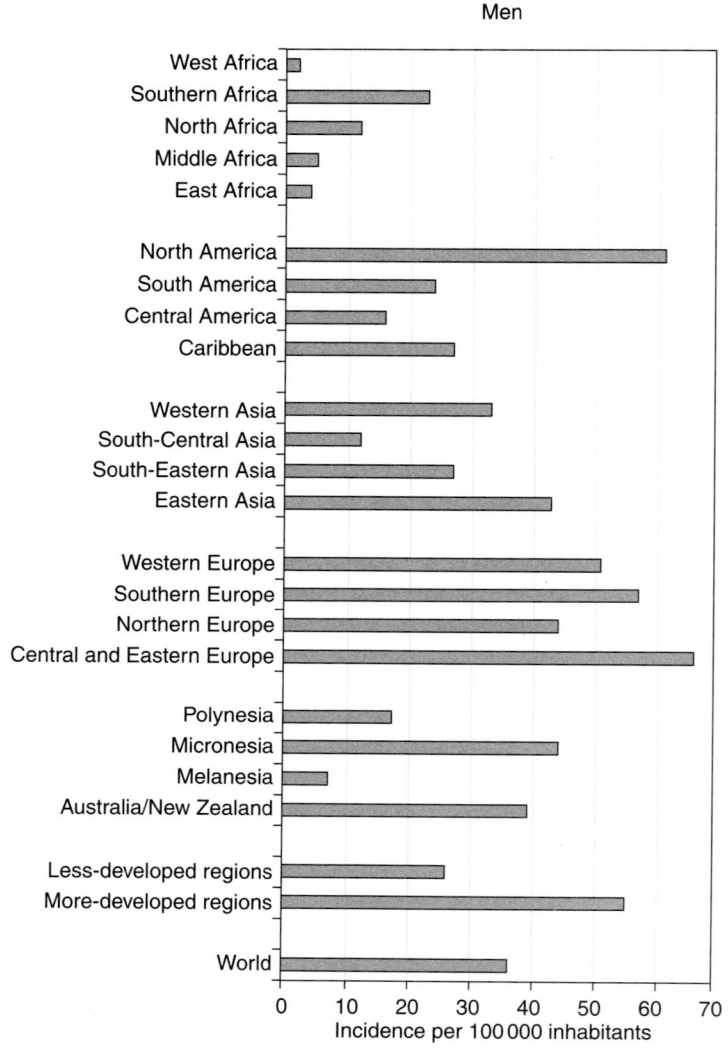

Figure 2.1

Age-standardized incidence rates by world region, standardized to the World Standard Population. (Based on data from The GLOBOCAN 2002 database.[1])

widespread only during the last 30 years. In China, inhabited by one-fifth of the world's population, and thus determining to a large scale the cancer burden at a global level, it has been estimated that lung cancer incidence will increase by 27% in men and 38% in women from year 2000 to 2005, mostly due to changes in cancer risk (cigarette smoking), but also to some degree due to population size and age structure.[3] The full effect of increased tobacco

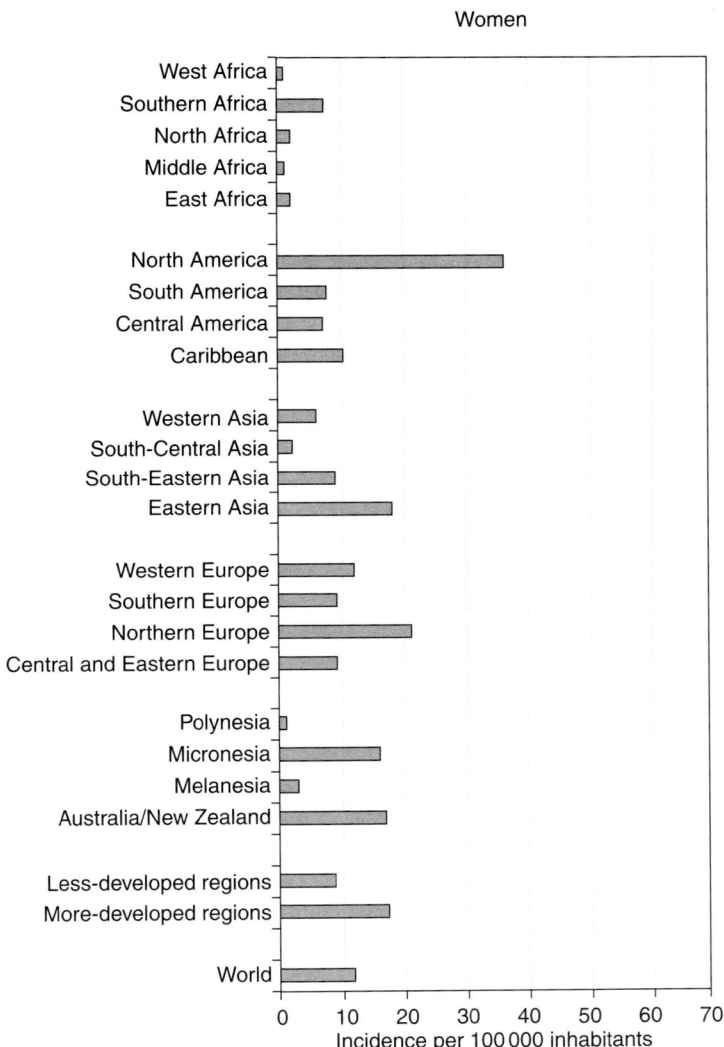

Figure 2.1
Continued

consumption will be expected to occur 20–30 years from now. It has been estimated that, worldwide, smoking caused 3 million deaths out of a total of 30 million adult deaths from all causes in 1990.[4] In 2030, this proportion will most likely increase to approximately 10 million out of about 60 million annual deaths. Most of the increase will probably take place in Asia, Africa, and South America.[4]

HISTOPATHOLOGY

Virtually all lung cancers arise from epithelial tissue. There are various sub-types of lung carcinoma, the commonest being squamous cell carcinoma, ade-nocarcinoma, small cell carcinoma and large cell carcinoma. These subtypes account for about 99% of all histologically verified lung cancers in a typical Western population of tobacco smokers; the remaining carcinomas are sarco-mas, lymphomas and some rare subgroups of neuroendocrine tumors of the lung. Smoking has been associated with all the major histologic subtypes of lung cancer, but the association has been weaker for adenocarcinoma.[5] Changes in the relative distribution of histologic subtypes have been observed, with recent increases in the incidence of adenocarcinoma. Rates of squamous and small cell carcinomas have decreased among males,[6] and adenocarcinoma has even surpassed squamous cell carcinoma in frequency among males in several populations in recent years: e.g. in the US population (Figure 2.2).[7] Among females, rates of all major histologic types have been rising, most rapidly for adenocarcinoma. The explanation for these observed changes in histology of lung cancer over time is probably due to changes in smoking habits, as originally proposed by Wynder and Hoffman,[8] with increasing con-sumption of low-yield filter-tipped cigarettes, previously believed to be less harmful than high-yield non-filter cigarettes. Smokers of low-yield filter-tipped cigarettes have to take both more frequent and larger puffs to fulfil their needs for nicotine, which allows the cigarette smoke to reach the distant branches of the bronchoalveolar tree where adenocarcinoma usually occurs.

RISK FACTORS

Age is a major determinant of risk for lung cancer, as it is closely correlated with duration of smoking. For example, there is a 30-fold increase in lung can-cer incidence in women and a 90-fold increase in men between the ages of 35 and 75 years.[5] This dependence on age means that it is important to adjust for differences in age composition when comparing the occurrence of lung cancer in different populations by calculating the age-adjusted (age-standardized) incidence rates using a standard population.

Since the early 1990s, it has been debated as to whether women are more susceptible to the carcinogenic effects of tobacco smoke than men. Some stud-ies, comparing the risk of lung cancer dose by dose in men and women, have found up to 50% higher risk in women compared with men, but not all studies were able to confirm these risk estimates. Recently, three large prospective studies have published their results on this issue: each study was unable to find a higher risk of lung cancer in female smokers compared with male smok-ers, bringing this debate largely to an end.[9–11]

Secondhand tobacco smoke, or environmental tobacco smoke (ETS), is the tobacco smoke that non-smokers are exposed to and consists of a sidestream

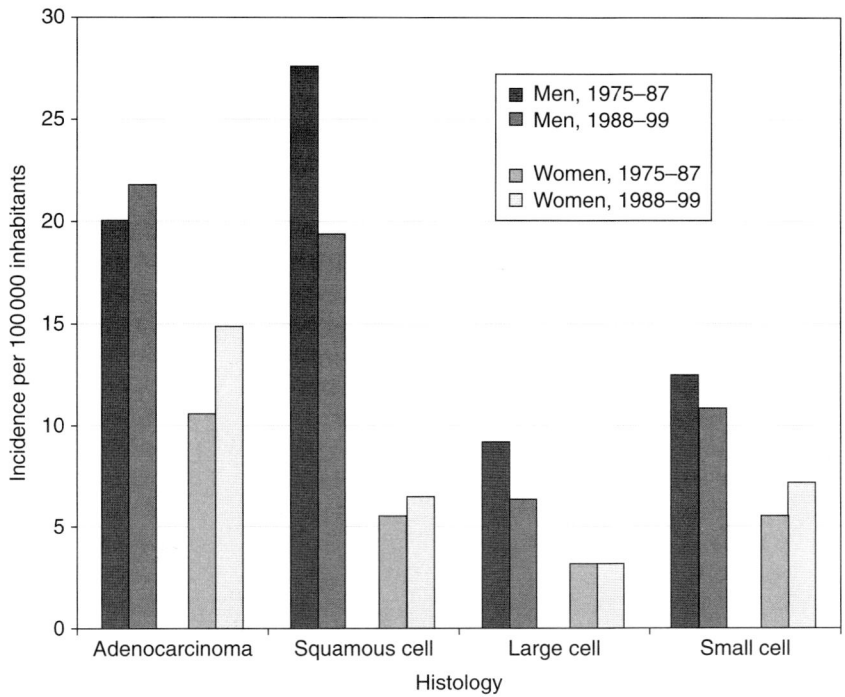

Figure 2.2

Incidence of the four major histologic subtypes of lung cancer among US men and women in two different time periods. (Data based on the SEER database.[7])

smoke that is not inhaled by the smoker together with the exhaled smoke.[5] Sidestream smoke contains the same numerous carcinogenic substances that are present in mainstream smoke. ETS diffuses into the peripheral parts of the lung and can cause peripheral lung cancers, particularly adenocarcinoma, among non-smokers. ETS is now classified as a group 1 carcinogen, with sufficient evidence for carcinogenicity in humans. Thus, secondhand tobacco smoke is a cause of lung cancer in non-smokers, increasing the risk of lung cancer by 20% when compared with non-exposed non-smokers.[5]

SURVIVAL

Many reports are available on the prognosis of patients with lung cancer in clinical trials whose main purpose was to test the impact of new treatments. The outcome, therefore, does not usually reflect the survival experience of patients with lung cancer in general, nor is it possible on the basis of trials to evaluate trends in survival over time. On the other hand, population-based cancer registries continuously collect information on the incidence and survival of malignant diseases over time in a defined population, on all individuals included in the population, regardless of prognostic factors.

The EUROCARE project was set up in 1989 to measure and explain international differences in cancer survival in Europe. It is a collaborative study on the survival of cancer patients in Europe. The first study covered the survival of 800 000 cancer patients who were diagnosed during 1978–1985 and followed up to the end of 1990 by 30 population-based cancer registries in 12 European countries. The most recent study, EUROCARE-3, involves 67 population-based cancer registries operating in 22 European countries and reports survival up to 5 years after diagnosis for 1.8 million adults who were diagnosed with cancer during the period 1990–1994 and followed up to the end of 1999.[12] The survival of lung cancer patients varies by more than twofold across Europe, but the highest 5-year survival rate for men diagnosed during the period 1990–1994 was under 15%, being highest in Austria, France and Spain (Figure 2.3). The survival of women is generally slightly better, and is highest among women in Switzerland, Austria and France. When the most recent results were compared with the two previous EUROCARE publications, a

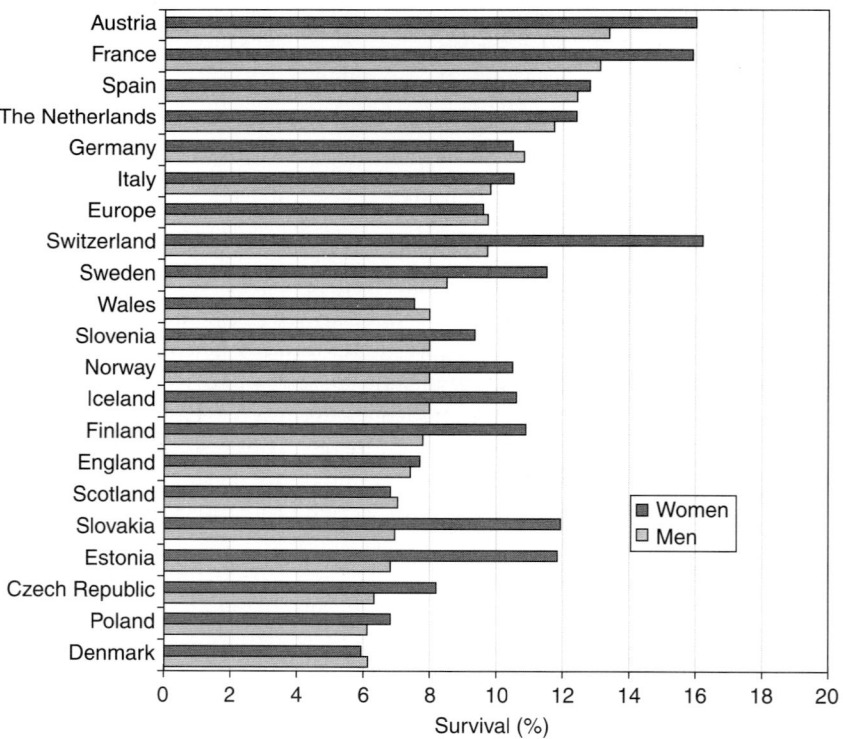

Figure 2.3

Five-year survival rate of lung cancer in Europe. (Based on data from the EUROCARE-3 study.[12])

modest improvement in 5-year survival rate over time was found, increasing from 7.5% to 9.2% among men and from 8.1% to 9.8% among women. The affluence of countries influenced survival, probably through the availability of adequate diagnostic and treatment procedures, suggesting that early diagnosis and treatment are extremely important for the treatment of lung cancer. The most recent report on lung cancer survival in the US population shows that the 5-year relative survival is still somewhat better than in Europe, being 13.6% for men and 17.2% for women, according to cancer registries participating in the National Cancer Institute (NCI') Surveillance, Epidemiology, and End Results (SEER) Program, which also showed a modest improvement over time[7,13]

REFERENCES

1. The GLOBOCAN 2002 database. http://www-dep.iarc.fr/globocan/database.htm.

2. Parkin DM. International variation. Oncogene 2004; 23: 6329–40.

3. Yang L, Parkin DM, Ferlay J et al. Estimates of cancer incidence in China for 2000 and projections for 2005. Cancer Epidemiol Biomarkers Prev 2005; 14: 243–50.

4. Peto R, Lopez AD, Boreham J et al. Mortality from Smoking in Developed Countries 1950–2000. Oxford: Oxford University Press, 1994.

5. International Agency for Research on Cancer. IARC Monographs on the Evaluation of Carcinogenic Risks of Chemicals to Humans. Vol 83: Tobacco Smoke and Involuntary Smoking. Lyon: IARC Press, 2004.

6. Devesa SS, Bray F, Vizcaino AP et al. International lung cancer trends by histologic type: male:female differences diminishing and adenocarcinoma rates rising. Int J Cancer 2005; 117: 294–9.

7. Fu JB, Kau TY Severson RK et al. Lung cancer in women. Analysis of the National Surveillance, Epidemiology, and End Results Database. Chest 2005; 127: 768–77.

8. Wynder EL, Hoffman D. Smoking and lung cancer: scientific challenges and opportunities. Cancer Res 1994; 54: 5284–95.

9. Bain C, Feskanich D, Speizer FE et al. Lung cancer rates in men and women with comparable histories of smoking. J Natl Cancer Inst 2004; 96: 826–34.

10. Thun MJ, Day-Lally CA, Calle EE et al. Excess mortality among cigarette smokers: changes in a 20-year interval. Am J Public Health 1995; 85: 1223–30.

11. Bach PB, Kattan MW, Thornquist MD et al. Variations in lung cancer risk among smokers. J Natl Cancer Inst 2003; 95: 470–8.

12. Sant M, Aareleid T, Berrino F et al. EUROCARE-3: survival of cancer patients diagnosed 1990–94 – results and commentary. Ann Oncol 2003; 14(Suppl 5): 61–118.

13. Jemal A, Clegg LX, Ward E et al. Annual report to the nation on the status of cancer, 1975–2001, with a special feature regarding survival. Cancer 2004; 101: 3–27.

3
Recent developments in the biology of lung cancer

Oliver Gautschi and Paul H Gumerlock

INTRODUCTION

Lung cancer is the leading cause of cancer mortality worldwide, and is responsible for 1 out of 3 cancer-related deaths in men and 1 out of 4 in women.[1] Over 70% of the patients will present with advanced disease at diagnosis, and fewer than 5% of those with metastatic disease will be alive at 5 years. Lung cancer is divided into two major histopathologic categories: small cell lung cancer (SCLC, 20–25%) and non-small cell lung cancer (NSCLC, 75–80%). NSCLC is further divided into adenocarcinoma, squamous cell carcinoma and large cell carcinoma. The epidemiology and histopathology of lung cancer are discussed in Chapters 2 and 5, respectively. Environmental risk factors for lung cancer are well known: an estimated 90–95% of lung cancers are caused by smoking and about 5% are associated with exposure to radon or asbestos. Cigarette smoke contains more than 60 different carcinogens, including polycyclic aromatic hydrocarbons and nicotine-derived nitrosamines.[2] Many of these carcinogens induce DNA mutations in alveolar and bronchial cells, some having preferred genetic sites for mutations of lung cancer-relevant genes, such as *TP53* and *KRAS*. The detailed biomolecular mechanisms of early lung carcinogenesis are not known, but multiple factors that are involved in the proliferation, survival, differentiation, invasion and motility of lung cancer cells have been elucidated. This chapter discusses some of the important findings, current approaches and technologies used to integrate the accumulating data into a comprehensive model. The discovery of molecular mechanisms involved in lung cancer has paved the way for the development of molecular-targeted anticancer agents. Some of these agents show activity in lung cancer patients in terms of survival, response or improvement of symptoms. Translational research, analyzing samples from patients treated with targeted agents, has dramatically improved our understanding of lung cancer in recent years. This fascinating process has revolutionized research in the field of lung cancer biology.

ACCUMULATING GENETIC DATA

Over the last three decades, a large number of biomolecular aberrations involved in lung cancer have been identified, leading to the proposal of a genetic multistep model for lung carcinogenesis[3] (Figure 3.1). Initially, cytogenetic studies, which have been refined and supplemented by comparative genomic hybridization (CGH), described frequent increases (1p, 1q, 3q, 5p, 6p, 8q, 12, 17q, 19p, 10q, 20p, 20q, X) and decreases (2q, 3p, 4p, 5p, 8p, 9p, 10p, 11p, 11q, 13q, 17p) in specific chromosomal copies or regions. Next,

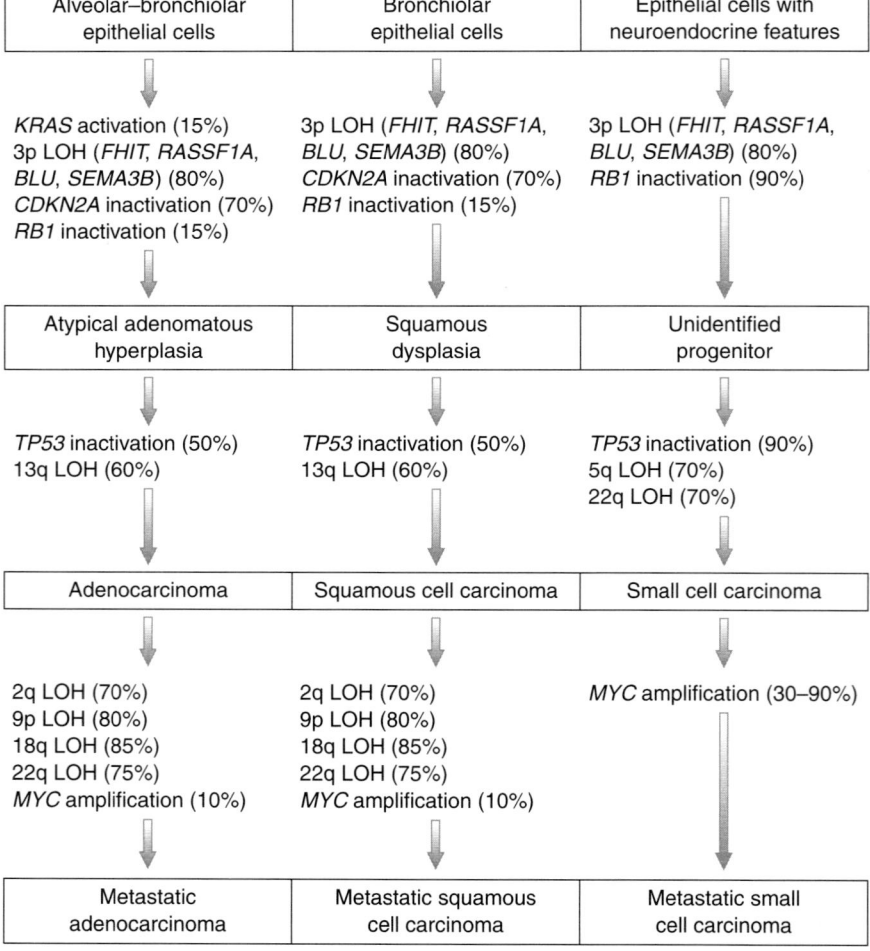

Figure 3.1

Multistep model of lung carcinogenesis. Genetic alterations in each proposed step of lung carcinogenesis are shown, with the frequencies of these alterations given in percentages. LOH, loss of heterozygosity. (Adapted from Yokota J and Kohno T.[5])

tumor-specific changes at the genetic level were described. Proto-oncogenes are normal human homologues of viral oncogenes, and play important roles in lung cancer.[4] Point mutations or amplification of a single allele are often sufficient for the conversion of proto-oncogenes to activated oncogenes. One of the first genetic changes found in lung cancer was amplification of the *MYC* proto-oncogene in SCLC. *MYC* is known to induce rapid growth and resistance to radiation in SCLC cells; however, its role in lung carcinogenesis requires further definition. The *KRAS* proto-oncogene (a homologue of a rat sarcoma virus oncogene) encodes for a protein with GTPase activity located in the inner leaflet of the cell membrane. *KRAS* is frequently activated by point mutations in NSCLC, leading to changes in the amino acid sequences of the encoded proteins that are associated with increased GTPase activity, promoting cell proliferation. The *HER2* (*ERBB2*) proto-oncogene, encoding for a growth factor receptor, is a homologue of the rat neuroblastoma oncogene *neu*. Alterations in these proto-oncogenes differ between histologic types of lung cancer, with *HER2* and *KRAS* activation being found in about 30% of NSCLC, but rarely in SCLC (Table 3.1). In contrast, *MYC* is frequently activated in SCLC but not in NSCLC.

Tumor suppressor genes (TSGs) lead to tumor growth when inactivated, and TSGs frequently involved in lung cancer include *CDKN2A* (p16^{INK4A}), *RB1* and *TP53* (p53).[5] TSGs control proliferation by regulating transcription and the cell cycle, and can be inactivated by homozygous loss-of-function mutations, deletion or both. Identification of new TSGs in lung cancer is a difficult process, and a significant portion of chromosomal deletions may simply be a consequence of genomic instability, not associated with inactivation of TSGs. There has been an intense hunt for candidate genes in chromosomal regions with a high frequency of loss of heterozygosity (LOH) where TSGs have not yet been identified. Especially interesting is the small arm of chromosome 3 (3p), where LOH occurs in up to 90% of all lung cancers.[6] The systematic

Table 3.1   Frequently activated proto-oncogenes in lung cancer[a]

Gene	Chromosome	Mode of activation	Frequency in SCLC (%)	Frequency in NSCLC (%)
MYC	8q24	Amplification	90	25
MYCN	2p24	Amplification	25	–
MYCL	1p34	Amplification	25	
KRAS	12p12	Mutation	<1	20–40
HRAS	11p15	Mutation	–	<10
NRAS	1p13	Mutation	–	<10
HER2 (*ERBB2*)	17q12	Amplification	<1	10–30

[a]Percentages of the most frequently activated proto-oncogens in small cell lung cancer (SCLC) and non-small cell lung cancer (NSCLC).

sequencing and mapping in the Human Genome Project was very important in this context, and genes mapped to 3p, including *RASSF1A*, *BLU* and *SEMA3B*, are found to be frequently downregulated in lung cancer.[7,8] Other than following the classical definition of a TSG, which implies that inactivation of both alleles of the gene contributes to a malignant phenotype, the three genes mapped to 3p appear to exert their effects in a coordinated way. This conclusion is based on experiments where inactivation of any one of these genes did not appear to contribute substantially to a cancer phenotype, but inactivation of all did. Again, inactivation of TSGs varies among the two major types of lung cancer histology (Table 3.2). For example, inactivation of *CDKN2A* is found in 20–70% of NSCLC, but rarely in SCLC, and inactivation of *RB1* is frequent in SCLC, but not in NSCLC.

The role of hereditary factors in lung cancer is controversial, but the fact that only 10–20% of all smokers develop lung cancer suggests that genetic predisposition may be important.[9] Results from segregation analysis have further supported the existence of heritable factors, particularly in patients where lung cancer was diagnosed before the age of 50 years.[10] Although lung cancer occasionally occurs in families with the Li–Fraumeni syndrome, which is characterized by inherited *TP53* mutations, no single high-penetrant, low-frequency lung cancer genes have been identified. On the other hand, several high-frequency, low-penetrant polymorphisms of genes involved in DNA repair and carcinogen detoxification have been suggested as modifiers of lung cancer risk. These include cytochrome P450 1A1 (*CYP1A1*), glutathione S-transferase M1 (*GSTM1*), myeloperoxidase (*MPO*) and NADH quinone oxidoreductase (*NQO1*). Today, because the results from different studies have not always

Table 3.2   Frequently inactivated tumor suppressor genes in lung cancer[a]

Gene	Chromosome	Mode of activation	Frequency in SCLC (%)	Frequency in NSCLC (%)
TP53	17p13	LOH, mutation	90	50
RB1	13q14	LOH, mutation	90	15
CDKN2A	9p21	Homozygous deletion, methylation, LOH, mutation	<10	20–70
SMAD2	18q21	LOH, mutation	<10	<10
SMAD4	18q21	LOH, mutation	<10	<10
PTEN	10q23	Homozygous deletion, LOH, mutation	10	<10
FHIT	3p14	Homozygous deletion, aberrant splicing	75	75
RASSF1	3p21	Methylation	80	30–40

[a]Percentages of the most frequently inactivated tumor suppressor genes in small cell lung cancer (SCLC) and non-small cell lung cancer (NSCLC). LOH, loss of heterozygosity.

been consistent, it appears that genotype may only moderately influence lung cancer risk.[11]

In addition to genetic alterations, epigenetic modifications such as DNA methylation and histone acetylation have been investigated in lung cancer.[12] Epigenetic modifications do not change the nucleotide sequence of DNA or the amino acid sequence of the protein, but can alter gene transcription (Figure 3.2). Aberrant methylation of gene promoter regions results in the inhibition of transcription of genes (silencing), including tumor suppressor genes, which appears to contribute to the pathogenesis of lung cancer.[13] Lung cancer-relevant genes modified by DNA methylation include *CDKN2A*, *RASSF1A*, *FHIT*, adenomatous polyposis coli (*APC*), and retinoic acid receptor 2-β (*RARB*). Methylation of the promoter region of *CDKN2A* has been reported to be associated with an unfavorable prognosis, and histopathologic lung cancer types

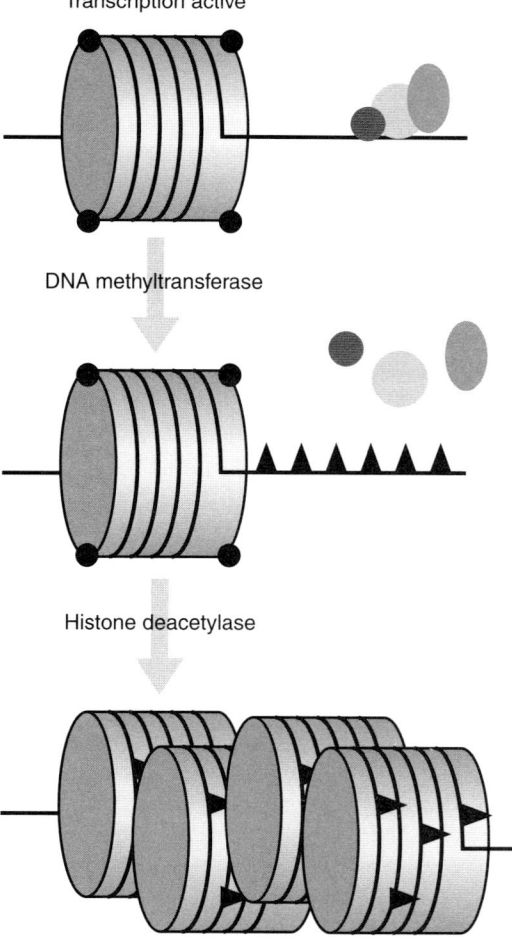

Transcription active

DNA methyltransferase

Histone deacetylase

Transcription blocked

Figure 3.2

Epigenetic alterations and gene transcription. In the nucleus, DNA is wound on histone octamers (represented by cylinders) to form nucleosomes. Only unwound DNA can be accessed by the transcription machinery. Two epigenetic modifications can block access of the transcription machinery to the DNA: (1) DNA methyltransferases add methyl groups (▲) to certain cytosines, preventing the binding of the transcription machinery; (2) histone deacetylases remove acetyl groups (●) from lysine residues of histones, leading to coiling of nucleosomes and formation of chromatin fibers. Both DNA methylation and histone deacetylation can be reversed by other enzymes.

have shown different methylation profiles of gene sets.[14,15] Based on these observations, inhibitors of DNA methyltransferase (DNMT), such as 5-azacytidine (5-AZA) and 5-aza-2-deoxycytidine (decitabine), have been developed and tested in clinical trials.[16] These agents showed limited activity in patients, which may be due to the global effects of turning on not only beneficial TSGs but also antiapoptotic or survival genes. Current approaches in epigenetic research include studies on DNA hypomethylation and development of new pharmacologic inhibitors of DNMT and histone deacetylase (HDAC).[17]

Thus, lung cancer is not only a multigenetic disease but also has the added complexity of epigenetic alterations, which demands new strategies to improve our still insufficient understanding of this disease.

LARGE-SCALE ANALYSES

The development of technologies for large-scale analyses of genes, gene products and epigenetic alterations has led to an accumulation of biomolecular data in cancer research.[18] Genomic profiling using mRNA microarray technology has revealed a large number of new genes being differentially expressed between lung cancer and normal lung tissue.[19] Results obtained with microarrays are highly reproducible,[20] but are limited to genes whose expression varies by two- to threefold or more. This may be more important than currently appreciated, because changes of only one- to twofold may have profound biologic effects. Nevertheless, microarrays have allowed identification of changes in gene expression in bronchial epithelium induced by cigarette smoking and by oncogenic *KRAS* mutation.[21,22] Using hierarchical and probabilistic clustering, different lung cancers have been classified according to their gene expression patterns, and groups of genes have been defined, separating patients by prognosis.[23] The US National Cancer Institute (NCI) initiated a study in early adenocarcinoma to prospectively test such approaches for multigenetic classification. Whereas it is anticipated that microarrays will be valuable to make individual treatment plans based on genetic profiles, the current high costs of these analyses limit their use.

Large-scale analysis has also become increasingly popular at the protein level, because mRNA and protein expression can be quite discordant in lung cancer.[24] Moreover, post-translational modifications are important for protein function, including protein phosphorylation, which plays a key role in intracellular signal transduction. Proteomic methods based on arrays, gels and mass spectrometry offer a broad range of interesting possibilities, including the identification of new tumor markers, antigens for vaccination strategies, drug targets and correlative markers for therapies with targeted agents. Reproductibility of proteomics is not as high as with genomics at the present time, which is partly explained by the lack of a specific amplification system similar to the polymerase chain reaction (PCR) for nucleic acids. These technical problems are being challenged now, with the hope that proteomics may soon become routinely applicable to lung cancer research. Analysis of pooled, robust genomic, epigenomic and proteomic data has tremendous potential to shed light on yet-unknown molecular mechanisms of lung cancer biology.

THE CANCER STEM CELL THEORY

It has been assumed for many years that lung cancer may arise from a component of the basal bronchial epithelium that is capable of differentiating into multiple histopathologic types. Transplant experiments in the 1970s had demonstrated that injection of autologous tumor cells in mice led to the growth of a new tumor only if more than a million cells were injected, and that only 1 out of 1000 tumor cells were found to form colonies in soft agar.[25] Although these surprising observations suggested the presence of a distinct group of progenitor cells in solid tumors, it was argued that many cells may not have survived the procedure. Two decades later, genetic data supported the stem cell origin of cancer in hematopoietic malignancies, and similar mechanisms have been suggested for solid cancers. In breast adenocarcinoma, two types of cancer cells have been identified: the vast majority comprise highly proliferative and partially differentiated cells, and there is also a small pool of slowly proliferating, self-renewing cells that can differentiate into the highly proliferating cells.[26] Only the slowly proliferating cells were able to form new tumors in vivo, which is consistent with the cancer stem cell theory. It has been speculated that conventional chemotherapy, while effectively killing the rapidly proliferating cancer cells, leaves untouched the cancer stem cells, which will then initiate tumor recurrence[27] (Figure 3.3). In mice, bronchioalveolar stem cells have been identified recently in normal lung and in lung adenocarcinoma, and expression of mutated oncogenic *KRAS* led to expansion of these stem cells.[28] There are now intensive studies ongoing to identify the genetic characteristics of normal and cancer stem cells in the human lung, with candidate genes being involved in the cell cycle, differentiation and mitosis. For example, overexpression of *CCND1* (cyclin D1), a cell cycle promoting gene, was reported in normal bronchial epithelia of patients with lung cancer, and was associated with smoking and survival.[29] The Wnt/Wingless signaling pathway plays an important role in human lung differentiation, and is altered in lung cancer.[30] Overexpression of *AURKB* (aurora B kinase), a mitotic kinase required for chromosome segregation, is associated with genetic instability in lung cancer.[31] Pharmaceutical inhibitors of aurora kinases are currently being studied in phase I and II therapeutic trials.[32] These compounds are likely to be very valuable reagents for stem cell research in the laboratory.

Stem cell research is currently moving rapidly, spurred by not only national funding but also state and private funding. Results of these studies are expected to provide new diagnostic and therapeutic options for all types of lung diseases, including cancer.

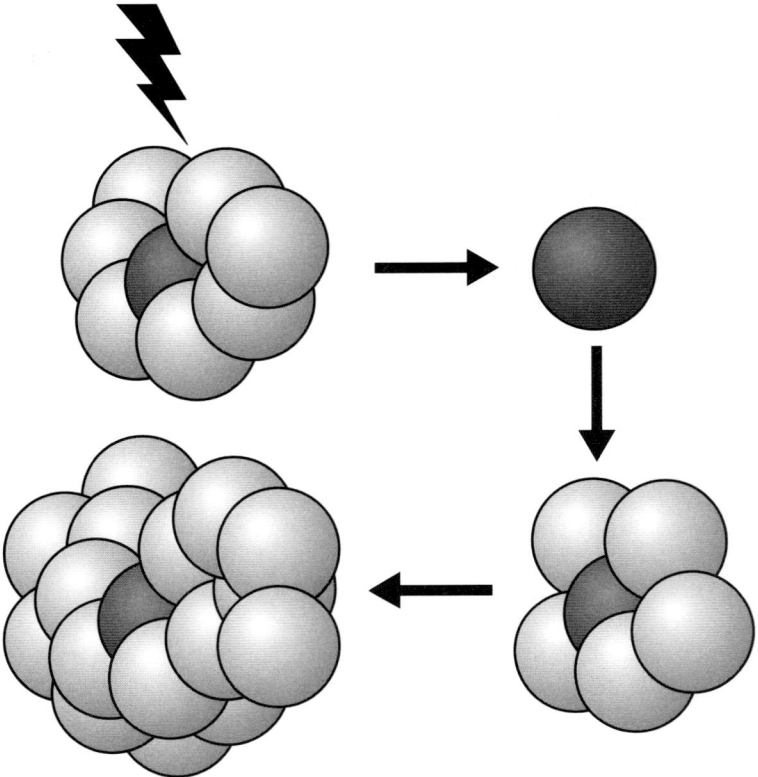

Figure 3.3

Therapeutic implications of the cancer stem cell model. Conventional
chemotherapy or radiation (lightning arrow) destroys the vast number of the
rapidly proliferating cancer cells. Because of slow proliferation, the cancer stem
cells are less sensitive to conventional therapy; they survive and induce tumor
recurrence. The risk of cancer recurrence may be reduced by new agents that
specifically target cancer stem cells.

TARGETING EGFR AS A ROLE MODEL FOR TRANSLATIONAL RESEARCH

The human epidermal growth factor receptor (HER) family of tyrosine kinases
plays a central role in epithelial cancers, including NSCLC.[33] Four family
members have been identified: HER1 (EGFR), HER2 (ERBB2/Neu), HER3
(ERBB3) and HER4 (ERBB4). These receptors contain an extracellular ligand-
binding domain, a transmembrane domain, an intracellular tyrosine kinase
domain and a regulatory region (Figure 3.4). Upon ligand binding, HER receptors dimerize with themselves or with other family members and undergo
cross-phosphorylation of several tyrosine residues within the regulatory

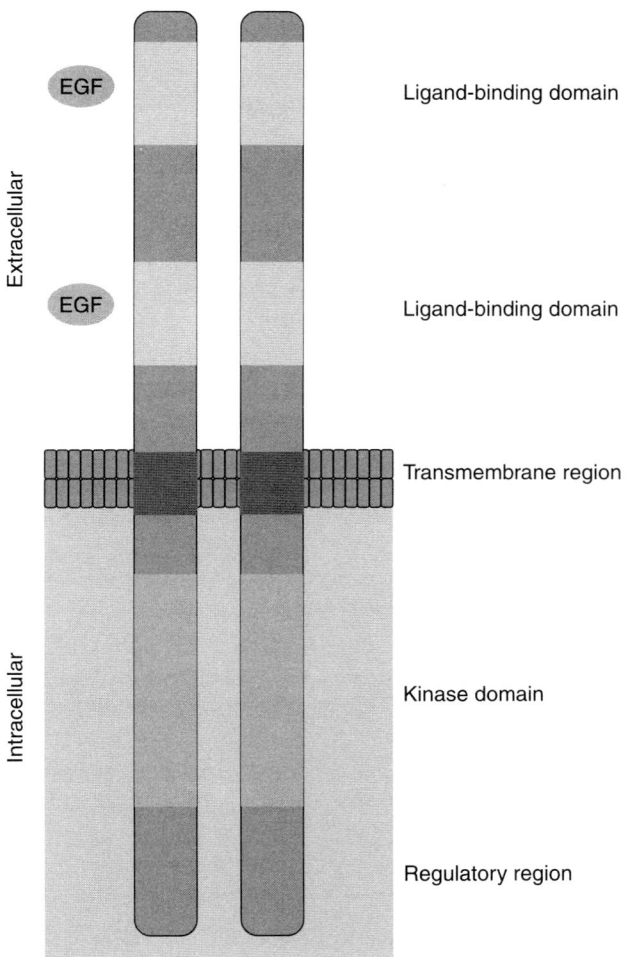

Figure 3.4

Schematic structure of the epidermal growth factor receptor (EGFR). EGFR contains two extracellular ligand-binding domains, a transmembrane region, an intracellular kinase domain and a regulatory region. EGF binding to EGFR leads to receptor dimerization, receptor tyrosine kinase activation and activation of a cascade of intracellular signaling pathways. Mutations involved in the sensitivity or resistance to tyrosine kinase inhibitors are located in the kinase domain.

region. The phosphorylated residues serve as docking sites for signaling molecules involved in intracellular signal transduction (Figure 3.5), controlling proliferation, survival, differentiation and motility. Although a ligand of HER2 has not been identified, this receptor is believed to be the preferred heterodimerization partner of other members of the HER family. In fact, EGFR:HER2 heterodimers have been shown to induce a very strong growth signal compared with other dimers in vitro.

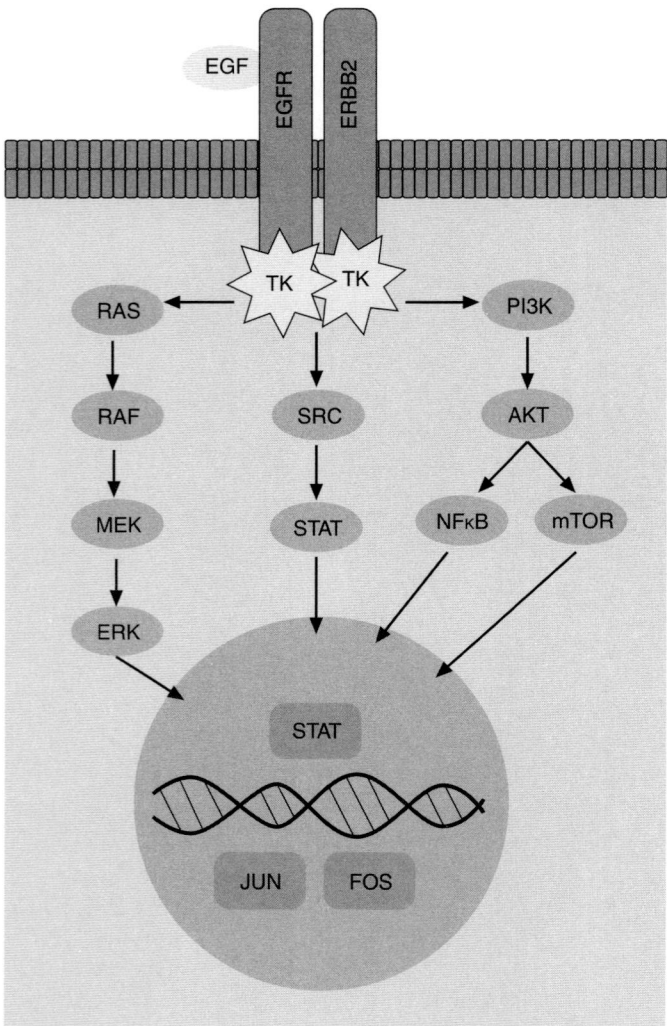

Figure 3.5

Intracellular signal transduction pathways. Proliferation is induced by binding of extracellular epidermal growth factor (EGF) to the EGF receptor (EGFR), which heterodimerizes with other members of the HER family, especially HER2 (ERBB2). This leads to increased receptor tyrosine kinase (TK) activity and activation of intracellular signaling pathways (RAS–RAF–MEK–ERK, SRC–STAT, PI3K–AKT–NFκB and mTOR). These pathways activate transcription factors in the nucleus (STAT, JUN, FOS), which regulate cell proliferation, survival, differentiation and motility.

EGFR is expressed in 40–80% of NSCLCs, as well as other cancers, which has prompted private industry to develop ATP-competitive anilinoquinazolines, selectively inhibiting EGFR and other tyrosine kinases.[34] In recent years, two such inhibitors have become the standard of care in second- and third-line treatment of NSCLC. Gefitinib (ZD1839) was the first oral EGFR inhibitor approved by the US Food and Drug Administration (FDA) in May 2003, after the phase II trials IDEAL1 and IDEAL2 reported responses in 18.4% and 11.8% of patients, respectively, with NSCLC previously treated with chemotherapy.[35,36] In November 2004, erlotinib (OSI-774), the second EGFR inhibitor, was approved by the FDA, based on the results from the randomized placebo-controlled phase III trial BR.21, which had shown a single-agent response rate of 8.9% and a significant improvement of median survival (6.7 vs 4.7 months; $p = 0.002$).[37] In June 2005, the FDA released restrictions, limiting gefitinib prescriptions to patients who currently or previously benefited from the drug. This decision was based on the results of ISEL, a placebo-controlled phase III study on gefitinib that showed increased response rate (8% vs 1%), but no significant difference in median survival (5.6 months vs 5.1 months; $p = 0.11$).[38] Altogether, clinical data suggested that erlotinib was more efficacious than gefitinib. One major factor that may explain this difference was that erlotinib was dosed at its maximum tolerated dose (MTD), whereas gefitinib was dosed at about one-third of its MTD, based on the idea that a molecular targeted therapy would not require the highest possible dose.[39] Additionally, erlotinib has an active metabolite, which has not been found from gefitinib.

Both gefitinib and erlotinib failed in combination with chemotherapy in the phase III trials INTACT1, INTACT2, TALENT and TRIBUTE.[40] Possible explanations for the disappointing results have been provided, the most likely being a lack of patient selection for target expression and antagonistic interactions between the targeted agent and chemotherapy.[41] The first point must certainly be considered in the planning of every new clinical trial with a molecular targeted agent. The second point shows the importance of careful preclinical experiments, which have indeed shown negative interactions between EGFR tyrosine kinase inhibitors and chemotherapy, but have also pointed towards new ways of combining targeted agents and chemotherapy.[42–44]

The clinical development of gefitinib and erlotinib has shed light on new biomolecular mechanisms of lung cancer.[45] The most frequent adverse effects of gefitinib and erlotinib were diarrhea and skin toxicity, and the severity of skin rash was associated with response in some studies,[46] as expected from the high expression of EGFR in skin and intestinal mucosa. Unexpectedly, the clinical trials consistently identified other predictive factors of response, including female gender, adenocarcinoma (especially the bronchioloalveolar subtype), being a never-smoker, and being of Asian ancestry, whereas expression of EGFR in the tumor was not always predictive. It has been shown that cytochrome P450-dependent metabolization of erlotinib is influenced by smoking, and this mechanism may also affect gender and ethnic differences.[47]

However, it did not appear to explain the dramatic responses seen in some of the patients treated with gefitinib or erlotinib.

In 2004, two groups simultaneously and independently reported mutations in the tyrosine kinase domain of the *EGFR* gene in gefitinib-sensitive NSCLC.[48,49] In analogy to the previous discovery of activating mutations in the *KIT* gene in imatinib-sensitive gastrointestinal stromal tumors (GISTs), it had been hypothesized that activating *EGFR* mutations may be found in NSCLC sensitive to tyrosine kinase inhibitors. The *EGFR* mutations discovered in NSCLC were located in exons 18–21, and were either small deletions affecting amino acids 747–750, or point mutations, most frequently leading to replacement of leucine by arginine at codon 858 (L858R). Evidence was generated that these mutations lead to increased binding of both ATP and of the inhibitor to the EGFR tyrosine kinase. Retrospective studies on a large number of tumor specimens confirmed that *EGFR* mutations were commonly found in NSCLC patients with dramatic responses to gefinib or erlotinib.[50]

EGFR mutations were found predominantly in Asian patients, consistent with the higher response rates to gefitinib and erlotinib seen in Japan compared with North America and Europe.[51] Lung cancers from patients with Asian ancestry, even when living outside of Asia, were found to have *EGFR* mutations in a higher frequency than patients of non-Asian ancestry, arguing against environmental exposure as the principal explanation for the ethnic difference.[52] *EGFR* mutations were associated with activated antiapoptotic pathways in vitro, irrespective of gefitinib treatment.[53] This led to the hypothesis that *EGFR* mutant tumors depend on the strong signal induced by their aberrant receptor tyrosine kinase (oncogene addiction). More recent investigations found that *EGFR* mutations can also be detected in histologically normal respiratory epithelium in lung cancer patients, in tumors that do not respond to gefitinib or erlotinib, and that other genetic alterations can be associated with gefitinib sensitivity, including multiple gene copies of *EGFR* and *HER2*,[54–57] again suggesting receptor heterodimerization as a relevant factor.

Mechanisms of resistance to EGFR tyrosine kinase inhibitors remained elusive until recently. In vitro modeling had predicted previously that a mutation at codon 766 of *EGFR* could interfere with the binding of a tyrosine kinase inhibitor.[58] Careful observation of a patient with NSCLC that was treated with gefitinib provided evidence for the presence of acquired resistance mutations in vivo.[59] The patient had a complete tumor remission with gefitinib, and the tumor carried a sensitivity mutation in *EGFR* (del747-S752). After 2 years of complete remission, the tumor progressed, and repeated biopsies revealed a new, second mutation in *EGFR*. This mutation was a C-to-T base-pair change at codon 790 in exon 20, predicted to change threonine to methionine (T790M), and to suppress the activity of gefitinib by steric hindrance. Cells transfected with the T790M mutant were less sensitive to tyrosine kinase inhibitors, and the T790M mutation was found in other NSCLCs resistant to EGFR tyrosine kinase inhibitors.[60] The relevance of the acquired T970M mutation has been questioned, because it was found only in a limited number of resistant tumors that had been treated with a tyrosine kinase inhibitor for a relatively long period of time, and has been found only in a small fraction of cancer cells extracted from recurrent NSCLC.[61] In contrast, increased internalization of ligand-activated EGFR was suggested as a major mechanism of primary resistance, and thus new irreversible EGFR inhibitors will be interesting to evaluate. More recently, mutations of KRAS were reported to be associated with resistance to gefitinib or erlotinib.[62] The types of KRAS mutations appear to be related with the history of smoking, with G–T or G–C transversions found in smokers and with G–A transitions present in never-smokers.[63] Regardless of the source, these mutations appear to confer distinct structural molecular changes, determining the sensitivity to EGFR tyrosine kinase inhibitors.

Thus, the studies on EGFR and its targeted agents have gone well beyond just a model, having opened multiple new doors on our understanding of lung cancer biology. It has become evident that a genetically more profound but also a more global view is required when studying new targeted agents in lung cancer.

LESSONS LEARNED FROM CLINICAL TRIALS WITH TARGETED AGENTS

Initially, targeted agents were clinically developed in the same way as conventional chemotherapy. However, several observations have raised fundamental questions on the practice of drug development. How to improve the testing of targeted agents and how to integrate biomolecular research best is currently being debated. Some of the most relevant aspects are discussed here.

How important is single-agent activity?

Cetuximab (C225), a monoclonal antibody targeting EGFR, was approved for patients with metastatic colon cancer by the FDA in February 2004. In NSCLC, cetuximab as a single agent showed a response rate of only 3.3%.[64] However, preclinical studies had suggested that cetuximab may have synergistic antitumor activity when combined with cytotoxic drugs, which led to the initiation of combination trials.[65] The results of the first phase II trials showed that cetuximab improved the response rate of chemotherapy in untreated NSCLC (53% vs 29%), and also in chemotherapy-refractory NSCLC.[66,67] Although these results need to be confirmed in phase III trials, they encourage preclinical testing of novel combinations despite the common reporting of apparently disappointing single-agent activities from early clinical trials. Moreover, these results support a general observation indicating that many targeted agents have cytostatic activity, rather than being cytotoxic. Therefore, disease stabilization and progression-free survival appear to be adequate endpoints for clinical trials, whereas the response rate may simply underestimate the efficacy of many targeted agents. These lessons learned with cetuximab will also support the development of other agents targeting EGFR, such as panitumumab (ABX-EGF).

Does the tumor type matter, or only the target?

Early excitement in the field of targeted agents led to the hypothesis that a targeted agent that is active in a certain tumor type will probably be active in another tumor type expressing the same target. Whereas this assumption was true for some new agents (e.g. cetuximab), it was wrong for others, reflecting the complexity of cancer biology. Interpretation of negative results from early clinical trials helped to improve the understanding of lung cancer biology. For example, trastuzumab has not shown activity in advanced NSCLC when given together with chemotherapy in randomized phase II studies, despite the frequent expression of *HER2* in NSCLC and the activity of trastuzumab in *HER2*-expressing breast cancer.[68,69] However, because receptors of the HER family can form heterodimers with different activity, it is important to assess if the composition of these dimers determines the activity of antibodies targeting receptors of the HER family in lung cancer.

Another example is the failure of imatinib in SCLC. Imatinib is a small-molecule inhibitor of the KIT receptor tyrosine kinase, which is expressed in up to 70% of SCLCs. Imatinib is active in GISTs expressing mutant KIT, but showed no clinical activity in SCLCs expressing wild-type KIT.[70] This observation led to the conclusion that the activity of a target, but not its expression alone, determines the success of a targeted agent. Measuring kinase activity and looking for specific mutations may help us to understand why some of the most promising kinase inhibitors such as imatinib have failed in lung cancer clinical trials and may allow us to identify patient subgroups that benefit from targeted therapy.

Where does gene therapy stand at the moment?

Gene therapy was among the earliest targeted strategies in lung cancer, and many gene therapy approaches were aimed at inducing apoptosis. Apoptosis (programmed cell death) is a physiologic mechanism in a multicellular organism that can be induced by extracellular and intracellular signals (Figure 3.6). Inactivation of *TP53* by mutation and overexpression of antiapoptotic proteins such as Bcl-2 are ways by which lung cancer cells can protect themselves from apoptosis to a certain degree.[71] Adenoviral vectors containing the wild-type *TP53* gene (Adv-p53) have been constructed and injected intratumorally to restore the function of *TP53*, and responses in NSCLC have been reported.[72] Further progress was slowed by the relatively low transfection rate of adenoviral vectors, concerns regarding the use of retroviral vectors and a fatal case in a gene therapy study on a metabolic disorder.[73] Non-viral approaches with antisense oligonucleotides, short interfering RNA (siRNA), short hairpin RNA

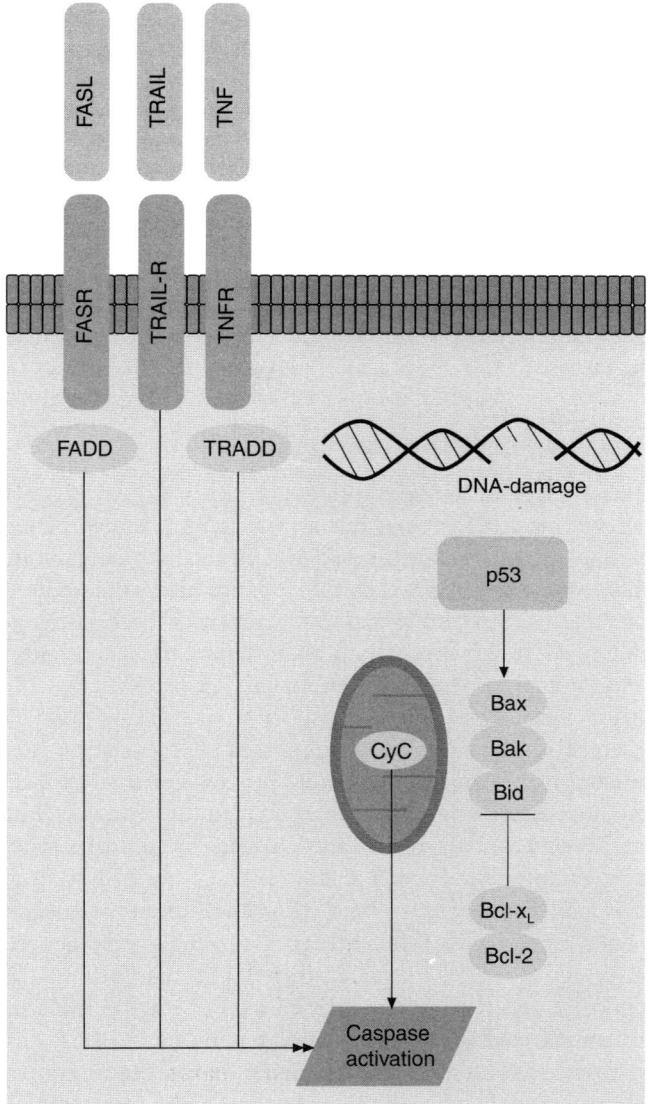

Figure 3.6

Apoptosis signaling pathways. Extrinsic induction of apoptosis occurs upon binding of death ligands (FASL, TNF, TRAIL) with death receptors (FASR, TNFR, TRAIL-R). This activates the receptor-associated death domains (FADD, TRADD), leading to activation of caspases and apoptosis. Intrinsic induction of apoptosis occurs when DNA damage is recognized by p53. p53 recruits Bid, Bax and Bak to the mitochondrial membrane, which leads to release of cytochrome c (CyC) from mitochondria and activation of caspases. Bcl-2/Bcl-x_L inhibit Bax/Bak/Bid.

(shRNA) and ribozymes were also developed.[74] Oblimersen (G3139) is an anti-sense oligonucleotide, binding mRNA and inhibiting translation of the Bcl-2 protein, which is overexpressed in about 25% of lung cancers. G3139 was tested in combination with carboplatin and etoposide in a phase I study in SCLC,[75] with an encouraging response rate (86%) and time to progression. The results from a randomized phase II study in NSCLC are awaited. Negative results of a phase III trial with a protein kinase C (PKC) antisense oligonu-cleotide in combination with chemotherapy in NSCLC were reported recently.[76] These results again raised issues, including possible antagonistic effects, the importance of PKC in lung cancer, the necessity of combined tar-geted approaches and the development of novel, efficient transfection systems for nucleotide-based therapies.

How selective must targeted therapy be?

Tumor selectivity has been claimed as an advantage of novel targeted agents over chemotherapy. Indeed, many targeted agents appear to be tolerated better than conventional cytotoxic drugs, but antitumor activity remains a concern in many cases. This weakness may be explained by the large number of biomolec-ular factors involved in lung cancer, and several strategies have been pursued to overcome this problem. First, novel targeted agents have been combined with conventional chemotherapy, a strategy that appears to be efficient with agents such as cetuximab, as discussed above. Secondly, an increasing number of agents targeting different mechanisms are being tested. For example, AE-941, a compound extracted from cartilage, was initially developed as an oral inhibitor of matrix metalloproteinases (MMPs) to inhibit tumor invasion, but was later shown to also have antiangiogenic activity, because it competes with the binding of vascular endothelial growth factor (VEGF) to its receptor (VEGFR), stimulates tissue plasminogen activator (tPA) and induces apoptosis in endothelial cells.[77] Lung cancer cells frequently produce angiogenic factors such as VEGF, which binds to VEGFR on endothelial cells and stimulates angiogenesis. The prognostic and therapeutic implications of angiogenesis in lung cancer have been summarized elsewhere.[78] Similar to EGFR, VEGFR has an intracellular tail with tyrosine kinase activity, which makes the design of multiply targeted inhibitors feasible. ZD6474, an orally available inhibitor of VEGF receptor-2 tyrosine kinase and EGFR tyrosine kinase, is another exam-ple of a multitargeted agent in recent development.[79] Dual-receptor tyrosine kinase inhibitors such as ZD6474 are expected to have a strong therapeutic potential in lung cancer. ZD6474 in combination with docetaxel has showed prolongation of time to progression compared with docetaxel alone in a phase II study in NSCLC, and a phase III study is planned.[80]

Another strategy is to combine different targeted agents. For example, the monoclonal anti-VEGF antibody bevacizumab is being tested in combination with erlotinib. Bevacizumab in combination with chemotherapy has been shown to improve response rate (27% vs 10%; $p < 0.0001$), progression-free survival (6.5 vs 4.5 months; $p < 0.0001$) and median survival time (12.5 vs 10.2 months; $p < 0.0075$) compared with chemotherapy alone in a phase III study in non-squamous cell NSCLC.[81] A previous phase II study including all histopathologic types of NSCLC had showed that bevacizumab was associated with life-threatening hemoptysis in 6 patients, and that hemoptysis was fatal in 4 patients who all had squamous cell NSCLC.[82] As expected from the mechanism of action, other adverse events were hypertension, thrombosis, proteinuria and minor bleeding, including epistaxis. Encouraging preliminary results have now been reported from a phase I/II combination study on bevacizumab and erlotinib in NSCLC.[83] Preclinical data had shown greater growth inhibition with the combination than with either agent alone. Forty patients with non-squamous cell advanced NSCLC were treated with bevacizumab and erlotinib at the full doses. Responses were reported in 8 patients (20%), with no pharmacokinetic interaction or enhanced toxicity. Although these data are limited, they strongly support the combination of molecular agents targeting different biomolecular mechanisms, which appears key in genetically complex NSCLC, which constitute the majority of lung cancers.

OTHER PERSPECTIVES

Non-receptor kinases are intracellular, cytoplasmatic proteins that transduce extracellular signals from receptors to transcription factors in the nucleus. These transcription factors, through the genes they regulate, then control proliferation, survival, differentiation and motility. Non-receptor kinases act in cascades, and are activated by receptor tyrosine kinases such as EGFR[84] (see Figure 3.5). KRAS was one of the first molecules in this system to be targeted in lung cancer, because it is activated in 30% of NSCLCs. Post-translational farnesylation is required to enable binding of KRAS to the inner cell membrane, where it can interact with the EGFR. Although this process can be blocked with farnesyl transferase inhibitors (FTIs), the FTI ionafarnib has shown low clinical activity in NSCLC.[85,86] It is known that KRAS can also be activated by other post-translational modifications such as geranylgeranylation, but the toxicity of pharmacologic inhibitors of geranylgeranylation has prevented further development of these compounds so far. Instead, multiple other non-receptor kinases downstream of *EGFR*, including *AKT*, *MEK* and *SRC*, are currently being evaluated as potential drug targets in lung cancer.

The *SRC* proto-oncogene encodes for a tyrosine kinase that is activated in many lung cancer cells. The viral homologue v-*SRC* was the first oncogene discovered, based on the work of Peyton Rous with chicken sarcoma, described in the seminal articles in the *Journal of Experimental Medicine* in 1910 and 1911.[87] It was more than 50 years later that the causative gene was identified, and found to have a cellular homologue in the human genome.[88] This led to the Nobel Prize in Physiology or Medicine being awarded to Rous in 1966 and to J Michael Bishop and Harold E Varmus in 1989. SRC tyrosine kinases are activated by different growth receptors, including EGFR, and despite their apparently low oncogenic potential in lung cancer, their central position in multiple signaling pathways has made them attractive targets for drug development. Several pharmacologic approaches are now pursued to disrupt the function of SRC kinases in lung cancer: interference with protein binding, inhibition of protective factors (chaperones) or inhibition of kinase activity by the small-molecule inhibitors dasatinib and AZDO530.

Apart from non-receptor kinases, several other new promising targets and targeted agents are currently being studied in lung cancer, including the proteasome inhibitor bortezomib (PS-341), the retinoic acid receptor agonist bexarotene, cyclooxygenase inhibitors and autologous tumor vaccines[89–93] (Table 3.3). The reader is also encouraged to study the recent advances in the development of circulating biomarkers.[94] Circulating biomarkers are increasingly studied in trials with targeted agents in lung cancer, because they are easily obtained, accepted by patients and allow sequential evaluation.

CONCLUSIONS

We have entered an extremely exciting period in lung cancer research in recent years. The biology of lung cancer is genetically complex, and our understanding needs to be improved. However, research is advancing rapidly in this field, mostly as a consequence of emerging high-throughput technologies and a growing number of pharmacologic agents targeting different molecular mechanisms of lung cancer. These agents offer great opportunities for translational research, which is expected to shed light not only on new mechanisms involved in advanced lung cancer, but also on those involved in early carcinogenesis. Targeted agents as monotherapy have now become a part of the standard treatment in advanced lung cancer. The combination of different targeted agents, and the combination of targeted agents with conventional therapeutic modalities, has the potential to improve the prognosis of lung cancer patients in the near future.

ACKNOWLEDGMENTS

We thank Nichole Farneth for valuable comments. Oliver Gautschi is supported by the Swiss National Science Foundation and the Swiss Cancer League.

Table 3.3   Targeted agents in lung cancer trials[a]

Target	Agent	Important side effects (if known)	Clinical activity
Receptor ligand			
VEGF	Bevacizumab*	Hypertension, bleeding	+ (phase II/III)
Receptor extracellular domain			
EGFR (ERBB1)	Cetuximab* (C225)	Skin rash, chills, nausea	+ (phase II/III)
	Panitumumab (ABX-EGF)	Skin rash	?
HER2 (ERBB2/Neu)	Trastuzumab*	Fever, chills, cardiotoxicity	−? (phase II/III)
	Pertuzumab	Diarrhea, skin rash	?
VEGFR	1C11	—	?
TRAIL-R (TR)	Mapatumumab	—	?
Receptor tyrosine kinase			
EGFR-TK	Gefitinib* (ZD1839)	Skin rash, diarrhea	+ (phase II)
	Erlotinib* (OSI-774)	Skin rash, diarrhea	+ (phase II/III)
VEGFR-TK	ZD6474*	Rash, diarrhea, QT prolongation	+? (phase II)
	Vatalanib (PKT787)	Fatigue	?
	SU011248	—	?
PDGFR-TK			
KIT	Imatinib* (STI-571)	Hematotoxicity	−? (phase II)
Signal transduction			
RAS	Ionafarnib* (SCH66336)	Hematotoxicity, diarrhea	−? (phase III)
	Tipifarnib (R115777)	—	?
RAF	Sorafenib (BAY43-9006)	Hematotoxicity, skin reaction	?
MEK	CI-1040	Skin rash, diarrhea, fatigue	?
AKT	Perifosine	Nausea, fatigue	?
SRC	SKI-606	—	?
	AZD0530	—	?
	AP23464	—	?

continued

Table 3.3   continued

mTOR	Temsirolimus (CCI-779)	Skin rash, stomatitis	?
	Everolimus (RAD001)	Rash, anemia, mucositis	?
	AP23573	–	?
PKC	Aprinocarsen	Thrombopenia	–/? (phase III)
CDK	Flavopiridol	Diarrhea, hyperglycemia	+/? (phase I/II)
	7-Hydroxystaurosporin (UCN-01)	Hyperglycemia, arrhythmia	?
Aurora A, B, C	VX-680*	–	? (phase I)
Other targets			
Bcl-2	G3139*	Fever, nausea	+/? (phase I)
MMP	BMS 275291	Musculoskeletal toxicity	–/? (phase III)
TP53	Adenovirus p53 (Adv-p53)*	Local inflammation	+/? (phase I/II)
Proteasome	Bortezomib (PS-341)	Thrombopenia, neurotoxicity	+/? (phase I/II)
Retinoic acid receptor (RAR)	Bexarotene	Hyperlipidemia, hypothyreosis	–/? (phase III)
Cyclooxygenase (COX-2)	Celecoxib	Nephrotoxicity	?
Hsp90	17-DMAG	–	?
	17-AAG	–	?
Tumor antigen	Vaccination (GVAX)	–	+/? (phase I)

aA limited selection of targets and targeted agents that are currently being evaluated in lung cancer studies are shown. Agents marked * are discussed in this chapter.

REFERENCES

1. Alberg AJ, Brock MV, Samet JM. Epidemiology of lung cancer: looking to the future. J Clin Oncol 2005; 23: 3175–85.

2. Pfeifer GP, Denissenko MF, Olivier M et al. Tobacco smoke carcinogens, DNA damage and p53 mutations in smoking-associated cancers. Oncogene 2002; 21: 7435–51.

3. Minna JD, Fong K, Zochbauer-Muller S et al. Molecular pathogenesis of lung cancer and potential translational applications. Cancer J 2002; 8(Suppl 1): S41–6.

4. Fong KM, Sekido Y, Gazdar AF et al. Lung cancer. 9: Molecular biology of lung cancer: clinical implications. Thorax 2003; 58: 892–900..

5. Yokota J, Kohno T. Molecular footprints of human lung cancer progression. Cancer Sci 2004; 95: 197–204.

6. Janne PA, Li C, Zhao X, Girard L et al. High-resolution single-nucleotide polymorphism array and clustering analysis of loss of heterozygosity in human lung cancer cell lines. Oncogene 2004; 23: 2716–26.

7. Cavalli-Sforza LL. The Human Genome Diversity Project: past, present and future. Nat Rev Genet 2005; 6: 333–40.

8. Ito M, Ito G, Kondo M et al. Frequent inactivation of RASSF1A, BLU, and SEMA3B on 3p21.3 by promoter hypermethylation and allele loss in non-small cell lung cancer. Cancer Lett 2005; 225: 131–9.

9. Schwartz AG. Genetic predisposition to lung cancer. Chest 2004; 125(5 Suppl): 86–9S.

10. Matakidou A, Eisen T, Houlston RS. Systematic review of the relationship between family history and lung cancer risk. Br J Cancer 2005; 93: 825–33.

11. Wenzlaff AS, Cote ML, Bock CH et al. GSTM1, GSTT1 and GSTP1 polymorphisms, environmental tobacco smoke exposure and risk of lung cancer among never smokers: a population-based study. Carcinogenesis 2005; 26: 395–401.

12. Herman JG. Epigenetics in lung cancer: focus on progression and early lesions. Chest 2004; 125(5 Suppl): 119–22S.

13. Das PM, Singal R. DNA methylation and cancer. J Clin Oncol 2004; 22: 4632–42.

14. Toyooka S, Suzuki M, Maruyama R et al. The relationship between aberrant methylation and survival in non-small-cell lung cancers. Br J Cancer 2004; 91: 771–4.

15. Toyooka S, Toyooka KO, Maruyama R et al. DNA methylation profiles of lung tumors. Mol Cancer Ther 2001; 1: 61–7.

16. Digel W, Lubbert M. DNA methylation disturbances as novel therapeutic target in lung cancer: preclinical and clinical results. Crit Rev Oncol Hematol 2005; 55: 1–11.

17. Hoffmann MJ, Schulz WA. Causes and consequences of DNA hypomethylation in human cancer. Biochem Cell Biol 2005; 83: 296–321.

18. Meyerson M, Carbone D. Genomic and proteomic profiling of lung cancers: lung cancer classification in the age of targeted therapy. J Clin Oncol 2005; 23: 3219–26.

19. Kaminski N, Krupsky M. Gene expression patterns, prognostic and diagnostic markers, and lung cancer biology. Chest 2004; 125(5 Suppl): 111–15S.

20. Parmigiani G, Garrett-Mayer ES, Anbazhagan R et al. A cross-study comparison of gene expression studies for the molecular classification of lung cancer. Clin Cancer Res 2004; 10: 2922–7.

21. Spira A, Beane J, Shah V et al. Effects of cigarette smoke on the human

airway epithelial cell transcriptome. Proc Natl Acad Sci USA 2004; 101: 10143–8.

22. Sweet-Cordero A, Mukherjee S, Subramanian A et al. An oncogenic KRAS2 expression signature identified by cross-species gene-expression analysis. Nat Genet. 2005; 37: 48–55.

23. Beer DG, Kardia SL, Huang CC et al. Gene-expression profiles predict survival of patients with lung adenocarcinoma. Nat Med 2002: 8: 816–24.

24. Granville CA, Dennis PA. An overview of lung cancer genomics and proteomics. Am J Respir Cell Mol Biol 2005; 32: 169–76.

25. Betticher DC, Heighway J. The investigation of bronchial epithelia from lung cancer patients: a better way of understanding lung cancer biology. Lung Cancer 2005; 49(Suppl 2): ES16.

26. Al-Hajj M, Wicha MS, Benito-Hernandez A et al. Prospective identification of tumorigenic breast cancer cells. Proc Natl Acad Sci USA 2003; 100: 3983–8.

27. Dick JE. Breast cancer stem cells revealed. Proc Natl Acad Sci USA 2003; 100: 3547–9.

28. Kim CF, Jackson EL, Woolfenden AE et al. Identification of bronchioalveolar stem cells in normal lung and lung cancer. Cell 2005; 121: 823–35.

29. Ratschiller D, Heighway J, Gugger M et al. Cyclin D1 overexpression in bronchial epithelia of patients with lung cancer is associated with smoking and predicts survival. J Clin Oncol 2003; 21: 2085–93.

30. He B, Barg RN, You L et al. Wnt signaling in stem cells and non-small-cell lung cancer. Clin Lung Cancer 2005; 7: 54–60.

31. Smith SL, Bowers NL, Betticher DC et al. Overexpression of aurora B kinase (AURKB) in primary non-small cell lung carcinoma is frequent, generally driven from one allele, and correlates with the level of genetic instability. Br J Cancer 2005; 93: 719–29.

32. Andrews PD. Aurora kinases: shining lights on the therapeutic horizon? Oncogene 2005; 24: 5005–15.

33. Rabindran SK. Antitumor activity of HER-2 inhibitors. Cancer Lett 2005; 227: 9–23.

34. Sridhar SS, Seymour L, Shepherd FA. Inhibitors of epidermal-growth-factor receptors: a review of clinical research with a focus on non-small-cell lung cancer. Lancet Oncol 2003; 4: 397–406.

35. Fukuoka M, Yano S, Giaccone G et al. Multi-institutional randomized phase II trial of gefitinib for previously treated patients with advanced non-small-cell lung cancer. J Clin Oncol 2003; 21: 2237–46.

36. Kris MG, Natale RB, Herbst RS et al. Efficacy of gefitinib, an inhibitor of the epidermal growth factor receptor tyrosine kinase, in symptomatic patients with non-small cell lung cancer: a randomized trial. JAMA 2003; 290: 2149–58.

37. Shepherd FA, Rodrigues Pereira J, Ciuleanu T et al. National Cancer Institute of Canada Clinical Trials Group. Erlotinib in previously treated non-small-cell lung cancer. N Engl J Med 2005; 353: 123–32.

38. Thatcher N, Chang A, Parikh P et al. ISEL: a phase III survival study comparing gefitinib (Iressa) plus best supportive care with placebo plus BSC in patients with advanced NSCLC who had received one or two prior chemotherapy regimens. Lung Cancer 2005; 49(Suppl 2): S4(Abst PR4).

39. Siegel-Lakhai WS, Beijnen JH, Schellens JH. Current knowledge and future directions of the selective epidermal growth factor receptor inhibitors erlotinib (Tarceva) and gefitinib (Iressa). Oncologist 2005; 10: 579–89.

40. Herbst RS, Prager D, Hermann R et al. TRIBUTE Investigator Group. TRIBUTE: a phase III trial of erlotinib hydrochloride (OSI-774)

combined with carboplatin and paclitaxel chemotherapy in advanced
non-small-cell lung cancer. J Clin
Oncol 2005; 23: 5892–9.

41. Gandara DR, Gumerlock PH. Epidermal growth factor receptor tyrosine
kinase inhibitors plus chemotherapy:
case closed or is the jury still out? J
Clin Oncol 2005; 23: 5856–8.

42. Solit DB, She Y, Lobo J, Kris MG et
al. Pulsatile administration of the
epidermal growth factor receptor
inhibitor gefitinib is significantly
more effective than continuous dosing for sensitizing tumors to paclitaxel. Clin Cancer Res 2005; 11:
1983–9.

43. Gumerlock PH, Pryde BJ, Kimura T
et al. Enhanced cytotoxicity of docetaxel OSI-774 combination in non-
small cell lung carcinoma (NSCLC).
Proc Am Soc Clin Oncol 2003; 22:
662(Abst 2661).

44. Davies AM, Lara PN, Lau DH et al.
Intermittent erlotinib in combination
with docetaxel (DOC): phase I
schedules designed to achieve phar-
macodynamic separation. Proc Am
Soc Clin Oncol 2005; 24: Abst 7038.

45. Janne PA, Engelman JA, Johnson BE.
Epidermal growth factor receptor
mutations in non-small-cell lung
cancer: implications for treatment
and tumor biology. J Clin Oncol
2005; 23: 3227–34.

46. Perez-Soler R, Saltz L. Cutaneous
adverse effects with HER1/EGFR-tar-
geted agents: is there a silver lining? J
Clin Oncol 2005; 23: 5235–46.

47. Hamilton M, Wolf JL, Zoborowski D
et al. Tarceva (erlotinib) exposure
effects (EE) analysis from a phase III
study in advanced NSCLC: effect of
smoking on the PK of erlotinib. Proc
Am Assoc Cancer Res 2005; 46: 56.

48. Paez JG, Janne PA, Lee JC et al.
EGFR mutations in lung cancer: correlation with clinical response to
gefitinib therapy. Science 2004; 304:
1497–500.

49. Lynch TJ, Bell DW, Sordella R et al.

Activating mutations in the epidermal growth factor receptor underlying responsiveness of non-small-cell
lung cancer to gefitinib. N Engl J
Med 2004; 350: 2129–39.

50. Pao W, Miller VA. Epidermal growth
factor receptor mutations, small-molecule kinase inhibitors, and non-
small-cell lung cancer: current
knowledge and future directions. J
Clin Oncol 2005; 23: 2556–68.

51. Shigematsu H, Lin L, Takahashi T et
al. Clinical and biological features
associated with epidermal growth
factor receptor gene mutations in
lung cancers. J Natl Cancer Inst
2005; 97: 339–46.

52. Sellers WR, Meyerson M. EGFR gene
mutations: a call for global x global
views of cancer. J Natl Cancer Inst
2005; 97: 326–8.

53. Sordella R, Bell DW, Haber DA, Set-
tleman J. Gefitinib-sensitizing EGFR
mutations in lung cancer activate
anti-apoptotic pathways. Science
2004; 305: 1163–7.

54. Tang X, Shigematsu H, Bekele BN et
al. EGFR tyrosine kinase domain
mutations are detected in histologically normal respiratory epithelium
in lung cancer patients. Cancer Res
2005; 65: 7568–72.

55. Takano T, Ohe Y, Sakamoto H et al.
Epidermal growth factor receptor
gene mutations and increased copy
numbers predict gefitinib sensitivity
in patients with recurrent non-small-
cell lung cancer. J Clin Oncol 2005;
23: 6829–37.

56. Hirsch FR, Varella-Garcia M, McCoy
J et al. Increased epidermal growth
factor receptor gene copy number
detected by fluorescence in situ
hybridization associates with
increased sensitivity to gefitinib in
patients with bronchioloalveolar
carcinoma subtypes: a Southwest
Oncology Group Study. J Clin Oncol
2005; 23: 6838–45.

57. Cappuzzo F, Varella-Garcia M,
Shigematsu H et al. Increased *HER2*

gene copy number is associated with response to gefitinib therapy in epidermal growth factor receptor-positive non-small-cell lung cancer patients. J Clin Oncol 2005; 23: 5007–18.

58. Blencke S, Ullrich A, Daub H. Mutation of threonine 766 in the epidermal growth factor receptor reveals a hotspot for resistance formation against selective tyrosine kinase inhibitors. J Biol Chem 2003; 278: 15435–40.

59. Kobayashi S, Boggon TJ, Dayaram T et al. EGFR mutation and resistance of non-small-cell lung cancer to gefitinib. N Engl J Med 2005; 352: 786–92.

60. Pao W, Miller VA, Politi KA et al. Acquired resistance of lung adenocarcinomas to gefitinib or erlotinib is associated with a second mutation in the EGFR kinase domain. PLoS Med 2005; 2: e73.

61. Kwak EL, Sordella R, Bell DW et al. Irreversible inhibitors of the EGF receptor may circumvent acquired resistance to gefitinib. Proc Natl Acad Sci USA 2005; 102: 7665–70.

62. Eberhard DA, Johnson BE, Amler LC et al. Mutations in the epidermal growth factor receptor and in KRAS are predictive and prognostic indicators in patients with non-small-cell lung cancer treated with chemotherapy alone and in combination with erlotinib. J Clin Oncol 2005; 23: 5900–9.

63. Gumerlock PH, Holland WS, Chen H et al. Mutational analysis of K-RAS and EGFR implicates K-RAS as a resistance marker in the Southwest Oncology Group (SWOG) trial S0126 of bronchioalveolar carcinoma (BAC) patients (pts) with gefitinib. Proc Am Soc Clin Oncol 2005; 24: Abstract 7008.

64. Lynch TJ, Lilenbaum R, Bonomi P et al. A phase II trial of cetuximab as therapy for recurrent non-small cell lung cancer (NSCLC): final results.

Proc Am Soc Clin Oncol 2005; 24: Abstract 7036.

65. Giaccone G. Epidermal growth factor receptor inhibitors in the treatment of non-small-cell lung cancer. J Clin Oncol 2005; 23: 3235–42.

66. Rosell R, Daniel C, Ramlau R et al. Randomized phase II study of cetuximab in combination with cisplatin and vinorelbine (CV) vs. CV alone in the first-line treatment of patients with epidermal growth factor receptor expressing advanced non-small-cell lung cancer. Proc Am Soc Clin Oncol 2004; 23: 618.

67. Kim ES, Maurer AM, Fossella F et al. A phase II study of Erbitux (IMC-C225), an epidermal growth factor receptor (EGFR) blocking antibody, in combination with docetaxel in chemotherapy refractory/resistant patients with advanced non-small cell lung cancer (NSCLC). Proc Am Soc Clin Oncol 2002; 21: Abstract 1168.

68. Gatzemeier U, Groth G, Butts C et al. Randomized phase II trial of gemcitabine–cisplatin with or without trastuzumab in HER2-positive non-small-cell lung cancer. Ann Oncol 2004; 15: 19–27.

69. Langer CJ, Stephenson P, Thor A et al. Trastuzumab in the treatment of advanced non-small-cell lung cancer: is there a role? Focus on Eastern Cooperative Oncology Group Study 2598. J Clin Oncol 2004; 22: 1180–7.

70. Dy GK, Miller AA, Mandrekar S et al. CALGB, NCCTG. A phase II NCCTG/CALGB trial of imatinib (STI571) in patients (pts) with c-kit-expressing relapsed small cell lung cancer (SCLC). Proc Am Soc Clin Oncol 2005; 24: Abstract 7048.

71. Viktorsson K, Lewensohn R, Zhivotovsky B. Apoptotic pathways and therapy resistance in human malignancies. Adv Cancer Res 2005; 94: 143–96.

72. Poulsen TT, Pedersen N, Poulsen HS. Replacement and suicide gene

therapy for targeted treatment of lung cancer. Clin Lung Cancer 2005; 6: 227–36.

73. Wade N. Death leads to concerns for future of gene therapy. NY Times September 30, 1999: A22.

74. Stein CA, Benimetskaya L, Mani S. Antisense strategies for oncogene inactivation. Semin Oncol 2005; 326: 563–72.

75. Rudin CM, Kozloff M, Hoffman PC et al. Phase I study of G3139, a *bcl-2* antisense oligonucleotide, combined with carboplatin and etoposide in patients with small-cell lung cancer. J Clin Oncol 2004; 22: 1110–17.

76. Gandara D, Douillard J, Koralewski P et al. Phase III trial of the protein kinase C alpha antisense oligonucleotide Aprinocarsen plus gemcitabine/cisplatin versus gemcitabine/cisplatin alone in advanced stage nonsmall cell lung cancer: updated results of a randomized phase III trial. Lung Cancer 2005; 49(Suppl 2): S31 (abstract O-085).

77. Latreille J, Batist G, Laberge F et al. Phase I/II trial of the safety and efficacy of AE-941 (Neovastat) in the treatment of non-small-cell lung cancer. Clin Lung Cancer 2003; 4: 231–6.

78. Herbst RS, Onn A, Sandler A. Angiogenesis and lung cancer: prognostic and therapeutic implications. J Clin Oncol 2005; 23: 3243–56.

79. Ryan AJ, Wedge SR. ZD6474 – a novel inhibitor of VEGFR and EGFR tyrosine kinase activity. Br J Cancer 2005; 92(Suppl 1): S6–13.

80. Herbst R, Johnson B, Rowbottom J et al. ZD6474 plus docetaxel in patients with previously treated NSCLC: results of a randomized, placebo controlled phase II trial. Lung Cancer 2005; 49(Suppl 2): S35 (abstract O-100).

81. Sandler AB, Gray R, Brahmer J et al. Randomized phase II/III trial of paclitaxel plus carboplatin with or without bevacizumab in patients with advanced non-squamous non-small cell lung cancer. Lung Cancer 2005; 49(Suppl 2): S31 (abstract O-086a).

82. Johnson DH, Fehrenbacher L, Novotny WF et al. Randomized phase II trial comparing bevacizumab plus carboplatin and paclitaxel with carboplatin and paclitaxel alone in previously untreated locally advanced or metastatic non-small-cell lung cancer. J Clin Oncol 2004; 22: 2184–91.

83. Herbst RS, Johnson DH, Mininberg E et al. Phase I/II trial evaluating the anti-vascular endothelial growth factor monoclonal antibody bevacizumab in combination with the HER-1/epidermal growth factor receptor tyrosine kinase inhibitor erlotinib for patients with recurrent non-small-cell lung cancer. J Clin Oncol 2005; 23: 2544–55.

84. Adjei AA, Hidalgo M. Intracellular signal transduction pathway proteins as targets for cancer therapy. J Clin Oncol 2005; 23: 5386–403.

85. Johnson BE, Heymach JV. Farnesyl transferase inhibitors for patients with lung cancer. Clin Cancer Res 2004; 10: 4254–7s.

86. Blumenschein G, Ludwig C, Thomas G et al. A randomized phase III trial comparing ionafarnib/carboplatin/paclitaxel versus carboplatin/paclitaxel in chemotherapy naive patients with advanced or metastatic non small cell lung cancer. Lung Cancer 2005; 49(Suppl 2): S30 (abstract O-082).

87. Peyton Rous. A sarcoma of the fowl transmissible by an agent separable from the tumor cells. J Exp Med 1911; 13: 397–411.

88. Martin GS. The road to Src. Oncogene 2004; 23: 7910–17.

89. Lara PN Jr, Bold JR, Mack PC et al. Proteasome inhibition in small-cell lung cancer: preclinical rationale and clinical applications. Clin Lung Cancer 2005; 7: 567–71.

90. Davies AM, Lara PN, Mack PC et al.

Bortezomib-based combinations in the treatment of non-small cell lung cancer. Clin Lung Cancer 2005; 7(Suppl 2): S59–63.

91. Gatzemeier U, Blumenschein G, Jotte R et al. A phase III randomized trial of carboplatin/paclitaxel with or without bexarotene (Targretin) in chemotherapy naive patients with advanced or metastatic non-small cell lung cancer. Lung Cancer 2005; 49(Suppl 2): S31 (abstract O-086).

92. Brown JR, DuBois RN. Cyclooxygenase as a target in lung cancer. Clin Cancer Res 2004; 10: 4266–9s.

93. Raez LE, Santos ES, Mudad R et al. Clinical trials targeting lung cancer with active immunotherapy: the scope of vaccines. Expert Rev Anticancer Ther 2005; 5: 635–44.

94. Bremnes RM, Sirera R, Camps C. Circulating tumour-derived DNA and RNA markers in blood: a tool for early detection, diagnostics, and follow-up? Lung Cancer 2005; 49: 1–12.

4
Prevention, early detection and screening

Rob J van Klaveren

CHEMOPREVENTION

The topic of chemoprevention was the subject of several review articles in 2004 and 2005.[1-6] Chemoprevention builds on the concept of field cancerization and multistep carcinogenesis, and can be defined as the use of natural or chemical compounds to prevent, inhibit or reverse the process of carcinogenesis. Apart from reviewing the results of the large randomized and non-randomized chemoprevention trials that have been undertaken, these review articles also address future directions of research. Today's efforts are particularly focusing on the identification of new biomarkers as surrogate or intermediate endpoints for chemoprevention trials, the identification of the optimal target population for chemoprevention studies and the identification of new classes of chemopreventive agents.[2]

Identification and validation of indeterminate biomarkers would allow smaller trials of shorter duration than when overt cancer is used as a primary endpoint. However, before a surrogate marker can be used in clinical practice, the marker needs to be validated in prospective clinical trials. The marker should be involved in the process of carcinogenesis, so that modulation of expression correlates with the course of the disease. It should also have different expression levels in normal versus preneoplastic tissue, and expression/evaluation should be easily reproducible. Promising markers include morphologic changes of the bronchial epithelium, especially moderate dysplasia or worse, as well as cytogenetic and molecular changes. Ki67, MCM2, p53, epidermal growth factor receptor (EGFR) and HER2 have been studied, but still need to be validated before they can be used as indeterminate endpoints. Merrick et al[7] investigated 264 bronchoscopically obtained biopsies from 132 patients for EGFR, HER2, Ki67, MCM2 and p53 expression and correlated them with the histologic grade ranging from normal to invasive carcinoma. They demonstrated a progressive increase in EGFR expression in association with increasing severity of bronchial dysplasia, which suggests that expression of this receptor may be important in the development and progression of lung cancer, and could be an effective target for chemopreventive strategies. Furthermore, a dual EGFR and HER2 overexpression was associated with Ki67, MCM2 and p53 expression, suggesting a central role for this pathway in the control of proliferation and other cellular processes involved in the development of lung cancer.[7] Also, pathway-specific downstream proteins are studied as surrogate markers for the biologic effect of the different chemopreventive agents. Actually, all molecular markers involved in the multistep process of lung cancer development – characterized by the accumulation of numerous cytogenetic imbalances and molecular genetic and epigenetic changes – could potentially be used for risk assessment, early detection and surrogate markers for chemoprevention trials[8]. New markers are under development from microchip gene arrays and proteomic evaluation of multiple proteins, but so far only limited data have become available.[6,9]

Another challenge for future chemoprevention studies is the identification of the optimal target population. In most trials, people have been selected based on smoking history, but radon exposure, chronic obstructive pulmonary disease (COPD), prior resected stage I cancer and family history of lung cancer have also been used to select participants. In the ongoing Colorado high-risk study, the lung cancer detection rate was 7.9% in the screened high-risk cohort with airflow obstruction ($n = 88$), 5.2% in the high-risk cohort with airflow obstruction but without screening ($n = 38$) and 1.0% in the high-risk cohort without airflow obstruction and without screening ($n = 304$).[10] From this study, we can conclude that airflow obstruction appears to be an important and easy method to identify risk factors for lung cancer. Although usually the number of pack-years smoked is used to identify the high-risk population, there is strong evidence that smoking duration and the age at which smoking is begun are much more important than the number of cigarettes smoked per day.[6] The role of sputum cytology as a risk factor for the detection of bronchial preneoplasia and overt lung cancer is still under investigation, but moderate or worse atypia seems to increase the likelihood for developing lung cancer. In the Colorado high-risk study of participants with a smoking history of 30 pack-years and COPD, those moderate or worse atypia on sputum cytology had an increased risk for developing lung cancer of 3.2, and on adding DNA methylation the risk increased to 10.2.[6] From a clinical point of view, there is no controversy that sputum cytology leading to either invasive cancer or carcinoma in situ mandates further investigation and, eventually, also intervention. The usual work-up in these patients includes bronchoscopy and computed tomography (CT) scan. In the presence of severe sputum atypia, there is a high likelihood that lung cancer will be imminently diagnosed; in two studies, approximately 45% of the subjects with severe atypia developed lung cancer within 2 years. The Colorado high-risk study (Table 4.1) supports the proposition that for patients with severe sputum atypia or worse, further investigation and intervention are warranted. It is still debatable, however, what the clinical consequences of moderate sputum atypia should be, and very sparse data are available in the literature. In a recently published study from the University of Colorado Cancer Center, of 79 patients with moderate sputum atypia and normal chest radiographs, 5 patients (6.3%) were found to have either invasive cancer (3 patients) or carcinoma in situ (2 patients) at follow-up bronchoscopy.[11] This surprisingly high fraction might justify further investigation in this particular subgroup as well. Ongoing studies include biomarkers, and results from these studies might further refine the group with moderate sputum atypia who will benefit from early bronchoscopy and, eventually, early intervention. In a nested case–control study of the same high-risk cohort of patients followed at the University of Colorado, DNA methylation of certain genes was studied in sputum as a risk marker for developing lung cancer.[12] Preliminary analysis has been performed based on 57 cases and matched controls, and it was found that DNA methylation of a panel of 7 genes added significantly to the odds ratio (OR) for sputum atypia. Combined with sputum atypia (moderate or worse), the risk of developing lung cancer increased, with an OR of 7.9 (see Table 4.1). This study is currently being enlarged and includes about 120 cases and controls. Currently, it is too early to make any conclusions whether DNA methylation in sputum can be used as a marker for selection of patients to screening or chemoprevention studies, and prospective validation studies are needed. In a pilot study of 33 cases and controls with COPD and with a history of at least 30 pack-years, sputum aneusomy was tested by multitarget DNA fluorescent in situ hybridization (FISH) assay.[13] In the sputum cytology specimens collected within 12 months preceding the diagnosis of lung cancer, the abnormality was more frequent among the 18 lung cancer cases (41%) than in the 17 controls (6%, $p < 0.05$). Aneusomy had no significant association with cytologic atypia, suggesting that molecular and morphologic changes could be independent markers of tumorigenesis, and that a combination of both tests may improve the sensitivity of sputum cytology as a predictive marker of lung cancer.

Table 4.1 DNA methylation and sputum cytology as risk markers for lung cancer development

Marker positive	Odds ratio	
	All samples	Sample closest to diagnosis
Gene 1	1.9	2.2[a]
Gene 2	1.3	1.3
Gene 3	1.1	1.7
Gene 5	1.5	2.0
Gene 6	1.8	1.8
Gene 7	1.9	1.7
Gene 8	2.8	3.8[a]
Moderate cytologic atypia or worse	1.8	2.6[a]
Any methylation marker	3.0[a]	3.9[a]
Any biomarker, cytologic or methylated	5.9[a]	7.7[a]

[a] $p < 0.05$.

Advances in molecular biology have led to a better understanding of the different pathways for lung cancer development, and antibodies and small molecules targeting these specific proteins lead to blockage of these important signaling pathways. As a result, there is increasing acceptance of the use of the same molecular-targeted approaches for both cancer therapy and cancer prevention in high-risk subjects, and thus potential new classes of chemopreventive agents have become available (Table 4.2).[14,15] In this regard, the reviews of Hirsch and Lippman[1] and Vignot et al[2] are of particular interest.

There is growing evidence that there is a dynamic balance between enzymes involved in the metabolism of linoleic acid and arachidonic acid. Both the linoleic acid and arachidonic fatty acid metabolic pathways play a key role in tumorigenesis,[16] and it appears that the profile of downstream cyclooxygenase (COX) metabolites and targets is more relevant to tumorigenesis than is COX-2 protein or activity itself.[16] Increased COX-2 leads to elevated prostaglandin E_2 (PGE$_2$) levels, and the PGE$_2$ receptor type 3 seems to be involved in the appearance of the malignant phenotype in lung cells.[17] On the other hand, prostacyclin (PGI$_2$) is antineoplastic, and normal lung contains high levels of PGI$_2$, and relatively low levels of PGE$_2$, suggesting that high levels of PGI$_2$ may protect against lung tumor formation.[18] Preclinical studies have also shown that selective pulmonary overexpression of prostacyclin synthase successfully chemoprevents lung cancer in a variety of lung carcinogenesis models, including cigarette smoke exposure.[19] These findings support the rationale for the ongoing randomized control trial of the oral PGI$_2$ analogue iloprost in a dose-escalating fashion versus placebo for 6 months.[19] The primary endpoint is bronchial histology. To date, 45 subjects have been enrolled in several institutions.[19] Also, 15-hydroxyprostaglandin dehydrogenase (15-PGDH), which degrades PGE$_2$, has tumor suppressor activity, and induction of 15-PGDH may reverse carcinogenesis.[20] EGFR is upstream of several important lung cancer prevention targets, including COX-2. Tobacco carcinogens activate EGFR signaling, which increases PGE$_2$ by inducing COX-2 and by downregulating 15-PGDH, which degrades PGE$_2$.[21] PGE$_2$ in turn further activates EGFR signaling. As PGE$_2$-stimulated non-small cell lung cancer (NSCLC) cell growth is resistant to EGFR inhibition, the combined targeting of COX-2 and the EGFR might be more effective in preventing lung cancer, as has been shown already in preclinical studies in head and neck cancer.[22]

Table 4.2   List of possible new chemopreventive agents

EGFR inhibitors	Angiogenesis inhibitors
COX-2 inhibitors	Cell cycle inhibitors
Lipoxygenase inhibitors	Proteasome inhibitors
Prostacyclin analogues	mTOR inhibitors
Farnestyltransferase inhibitors	Protein kinase C inhibitors
Ras inhibitors	Demethylation agents
Rexinoids	DMFO combination
PPARγ agonists	Budesodine

Another important pathway for chemoprevention is insulin-like growth factor (IGF)-mediated signaling. IGF-1 increases COX-2 expression and PGE_2 production. Celecoxib has been shown to downregulate the IGF-I receptor and suppress IGF-II-related tumor growth.[23] Inhibition of Akt, a downstream kinase of P13K, induces apoptosis of premalignant and malignant human lung cells and is preventive in an animal model of lung carcinogenesis.[24]

Recent studies have reported the presence of DNA markers in the serum, plasma, saliva, bronchoalveolar lavage (BAL) fluid and urine of patients with a variety of cancers, including lung cancers.[25–27] Tests for DNA (polymorphisms, mutations and abnormal DNA methylation) and RNA alterations in plasma and BAL fluid supernatants have great potential for early detection and follow-up, but much needs to be done to validate this technique in much larger series.[28,29] So far, there are 22 clinical studies available evaluating the role of circulating nucleic acids in blood as possible markers in lung cancer patients, including total DNA levels, gene expression levels, mutations in specific oncogenes, tumor suppressor genes, microsatellite alterations, promotor methylation of various suppressor genes and tumor-related RNAs. As circulating DNA and RNA are easily accessible in the blood and appear to be relevant surrogate markers for genetic alterations present in the primary tumor, tests for DNA and RNA in the plasma may have great potential for early detection, diagnosis and relapse during follow-up. Of all the 22 repeated studies, in which in total of 1618 patients and 595 control cases are enrolled, plasma and serum abnormalities were found in 43% (range 0–78%) and in 9.9% among control cases.[27] The tests obviously need to be validated in large prospective clinical trials.

One approach for the early detection of lung cancer is the detection of de-novo methylation of CpG islands within the promoters of tumor suppressor genes that lead to gene inactivation, which could serve as a biomarker for lung cancer development. Kim et al[30] investigated aberrant methylation by methylation-specific polymerase chain reaction (PCR) in tumor tissue and BAL samples of NSCLC patients and compared them with the same genes in BAL samples of cancer-free individuals to discriminate between age- or smoking-related methylation and tumor-specific methylation. They found that hypermethylation of p16, RARb, H-cadherin and *RASSF1A* promoters was not related to age and smoking and thus may be a valuable biomarker for the early detection of lung cancer.

Very similar results were found by another group of investigators,[31] who found at least one promoter-hypermethylated gene in all 31 lung cancer tumors studied, and that aberrant methylation in BAL DNA was accompanied by methylation in the matched tumor samples, whereas BAL samples from 10 controls without cancer revealed no or very low levels of methylation in the investigated genes. Choi et al[32] investigated retrospectively whether RASSF1A is an appropriate early detection marker for NSCLC. In 116 tumor tissue samples and 60 corresponding non-malignant lung tissue specimens collected in the period 1994–2001, 41% of all tumors showed hypermethylation of *RASSF1A*: 49% for adenocarcinomas and 37% for squamous cell carcinomas.

They also found that stage I tumors had a low methylation ratio of 30% for all stage I tumors: 45% for adenocarcinomas and 31% for squamous cell carcinomas. They concluded that because of the low incidence of *RASSF1A* methylation, inactivation of one single tumor suppressor gene (*RASSF1A*) is not useful in the early detection of lung cancer.[32] However, when the methylation status of a panel of five tumor suppressor genes is used, 77% of the tumor tissues obtained from lung cancer patients showed methylation of at least one gene, and 89% of the tissues from patients with serum DNA methylation also had methylated genes. When serum methylation of at least one gene was considered as positive, sensitivity, specificity and predictive values of methylation were 49.5%, 85% and 75%, respectively. When adjusted for age, smoking status, gender and protein markers, results of methylation in at least one gene and two of more genes showed a 5.28 (confidence interval (CI) 2.39–11.7, $p < 0.001$) and 5.89 (CI 1.53–22.7, $p = 0.01$) times higher probability of having lung cancer, respectively.[1] Also, in early-stage disease in 50.9% of patients, serum DNA methylation was found. In 1–8% of the patients with nonmalignant disease, DNA methylation was also detected, probably caused by smoking, occult malignancies or precancerous lesions, or age-related DNA methylation.[1] The limitation of serum DNA methylation as a screening tool for lung cancer is its low sensitivity, which could be improved by using larger numbers of genes or by applying quantitative methylation assays. The strength of the test is in its high specificity, which makes a combination with a highly sensitive screening tool such a spiral CT screening very attractive, but further studies are warranted to confirm the efficiency of the test. The sensitivity and specificity of serum tumor markers range from 50% to 90%, depending on the study and the stage of disease. In early stages, sensitivity is between 0% and 33% for carcinoembryonic antigen (CEA), Cyfta 21-1 and the cancer antigens CA125 and CA19.9, but the specificity is 100%.

Tumor-associated changes were detected in DNA samples from BAL fluid in 47% of the 30 patients with lung cancer and RNA in all patients analyzed.[28] This study demonstrates that it is possible to isolate DNA and RNA in sufficient quantities to be amplified in PCR and reverse transcription (RT)–PCR analyses, respectively, and that it is possible to detect tumor-associated alterations in cell-free DNA and RNA from cell-free BAL supernatants. Also the detection of tumor-associated genetic alterations in plasma DNA has been proposed as a simple method for the early diagnosis of lung cancer and for identifying individuals at high risk of lung cancer who might be included in screening or chemoprevention trials. Khan et al[33] selected 3 primer pairs targeting common deletions in lung cancer on chromosomes 3p and 8p in a large cohort of lung cancer patients and patients with other respiratory diseases such as COPD and bronchiectasis. They found that the genetic alterations occurred in 69% of the 120 lung cancer patients, results comparable with other studies, but the same alterations were also found in 42% of the plasma of the 86 patients attending general pulmonary clinics with common respiratory diseases; 8 of these patients subsequently developed lung cancer. Khan et al conclude that this panel of primer pairs is not suitable as a diagnostic test for lung cancer, but may identify a high-risk group of individuals suitable for screening or chemoprevention.

Breath analysis is another new technique for biomarker screening that may help in the early detection of roentgenographically occult lung cancer. For the first time, it was demonstrated that in a group of 30 patients with proven NSCLC the exhaled endothelin-1 (ET-1) concentrations in breath condensate were significantly higher than in a healthy control group of 15 subjects ($p < 0.0001$), that the ET-1 concentrations were higher in stage IV than in earlier-stage disease and that the ET-1 levels decreased after surgical removal of the tumor.[34] On the basis of these results, the potent growth factor ET-1 in exhaled breath condensate could be used as a marker for early detection of lung cancer and for monitoring the evolution of the tumor.[34]

SCREENING

Based on the results of several completed and ongoing lung cancer screening trials in different parts of the world, several new position statements from professional organizations were released in 2004 and 2005. In 1998, the International Conference on Prevention and Early Diagnosis of Lung Cancer was held in Varese, Italy. The consensus statement recognized 'the potential of early detection to improve outcome in lung cancer', but no consensus was reached at that time that screening should be offered outside experimental trials. The Varese Conference was an important catalytic event that helped to reawaken interest in lung cancer screening. At the conference, it was also concluded that the existing scientific evidence from the screening trials conducted in the 1970s was not solid enough to conclude that lung cancer screening is ineffective. Based on the recommendations from the Varese Conference, the American Cancer Society (ACS) modified its recommendation not to screen into a recommendation where individuals at high risk for lung cancer should be informed about their risk, and that those who seek testing for early lung cancer detection should be informed about options for testing for early detection and about the risks and benefits, so that they can make an informed decision. In 2003, the Como Conference was held to consider whether there was sufficient basis to go beyond the 1998 Varese consensus statement and to recommend lung cancer screening of asymptomatic individuals outside clinical trials.[35] The recommendations of the Como Conference include, again, an informed decision-making for – more specified now – high-risk individuals aged above 45 or 50 years who are current or former smokers with at least 20 to 30 pack-years of cumulative exposure and without life-limiting comorbidities. The issues that should be addressed during the discussion with the physician are summarized in Table 4.3.[35,36] In an recently updated statement, the ACS continues to recommend that CT screening should not be performed in asymptomatic at-risk persons, but, recognizing that many heavy smokers choose on their own to be

Table 4.3   Topics to be discussed with the screenee to enable informed decision-making for lung cancer screening with spiral computed tomography (CT)
• The most effective way for patients to improve their health is to stop smoking • Assistance for smoking cessation should be provided • Former smokers and those who underwent curative resection should be informed about their continuing risk of lung cancer • Available imaging methods for early detection of lung cancer are spiral CT and chest X-ray • There are no data available from randomized CT screening trials, but results are expected in 4–5 years • Results from observational CT screening studies show a high rate of stage I lung cancer, and as such probably a better chance for a successful outcome • CT screening will reveal many non-calcified lung nodules, but only a small fraction represents lung cancer • Evaluation of indeterminate lung nodules may require invasive procedures with associated risks • Diagnostic work-up should be done by physicians experienced in such evaluations • Critical for an optimal outcome is to choose a screening facility where a multidisciplinary team of physicians is available for work-up, diagnosis and treatment

screened, the ACS recommend informed decision-making, and performance of the CT screening test in experienced centers that are linked to multidisciplinary specialty groups for diagnosis and follow-up.[37] In contrast, the US Preventive Services Task Force makes no recommendation for or against the use of CT screening in their latest updated recommendations on lung cancer screening, and also advises discussion of the pros and cons with the screenee.[38] They conclude also that (from the available data) spiral CT screening can diagnose lung cancer at a significantly earlier stage than by current clinical practice.[38]

Not only the renewed interest in screening but also the rapidly expanding literature on lung cancer screening has led to several review articles in this field.[39–48] Apart from placing lung cancer screening in a historical perspective by summarizing the results of the screening trials with plain chest radiography that were published between 1960 and 1980, these review articles summarize the advances in new imaging technology with spiral CT, the potential screening biases, the continuing debate on the potential overdiagnosis as a result of lung cancer screening, the cost-effectiveness of spiral CT screening and alternative approaches for early detection such as automated quantitative cytometry (Perceptronics Medical, Vancouver, Canada) and autofluorescence bronchoscopy. With regard to the cost-effectiveness issue, it is important to realize that the cost-effectiveness of a screening program cannot be assessed before its effectiveness is established.[39] Although the papers published between 2002 and 2003 on the cost-effectiveness of lung cancer screening are instructive in exploring cost-effectiveness in early studies,[49] only large randomized clinical trials such as the US National Lung Screening Trial and the Dutch NELSON trial can answer these questions. An important review on this topic has recently been published.[50]

Currently, a large number of non-randomized cohort studies on lung cancer spiral CT screening have been completed, whereas several randomized trials are still ongoing. A selection of the most important trials are presented in Table 4.4.

In the cohort studies completed so far, 55–85% of the cancers detected at baseline and 60–100% of the cancers detected at annual repeat are stage I tumors.[36] This is markedly better than the current state of practice, where only 15–20% of all newly diagnosed lung cancer cases are in stage I disease. Since the introduction of spiral CT screening in the 1990s in Japan, the 5-year survival rate of all stages of lung cancer has improved from 48.8% to 80.4%.[51] Although these data are very promising, they do not prove that lung cancer screening improves lung cancer survival, because it might be possible that, by screening, people know their diagnosis earlier, without living any longer (lead time bias). However, the fall in advanced cancers detected is of interest: in the old Mayo Clinic study with chest X-ray screening, there were 3.2 advanced-stage lung cancers per 1000 person-years, whereas in the Mayo Clinic CT screening trial and the ELCAP trial this number is 1.1 and 0.9 per 1000 person-years, respectively.[52,53] However, in the Mayo Clinic spiral CT screening trial, Swensen et al[54] compared the lung cancer mortality with the lung cancer mortality of the Mayo Clinic Lung Project with chest X-ray screening, and found no difference (2.8 vs 2.0 per 1000 person-years). The authors recognize that there is inadequate power for such comparison, but the goal of the analysis was exploratory and hypothesis-generating rather than definitive. Henschke et al[55] found a clear relationship between tumor size and lymph node status. The percentages of cases with no lymph node metastases were 91%, 85%, 63% and 61% for tumor size categories of <15 mm, 16–25 mm, 26–35 mm and >35 mm, respectively. The percentages are much higher than previously reported in the US National Cancer Institute (NCI) SEER (Surveillance, Epidemiology, and End Results) registry, and confirms the usefulness of detecting asymptomatic lung cancer at small sizes, thereby supporting the hypothesis that the smaller the cancer detected, the better is the prognosis.

Invasive procedures for benign lesions have been performed in 4–22% of patients at baseline and 14–55% during incidence screening,[56,57] and the percentage of interval cancers varied between 0 and 33%[57] (Table 4.5). In the NCI Lung Screening Study[58] the rate of detection of cancer in stage I was only 40% for baseline screening and only 25% for annual follow-up. Factors that potentially contributed to the disparity between these rates and those reported in other series include the small number of subjects, the composition of the cohort and variations in test performance among the different institutes. The vast majority of the interval cancers are symptomatic and in an advanced stage and with a poor prognosis. The only study published so far with a consistent

Table 4.4 Selection of the most important completed and ongoing lung cancer screening studies with low-dose spiral computed tomography

First author	Year	Country	Design	N	Ps1	Control group 'intervention'	Selection criteria	
							Lower age	Upper age
Sone[66]	2001	Japan	Cohort	5 483	0.80	NA	40	74
Nawa[67]	2002	Japan	Cohort	7 956	0.70	NA	50	69
Sobue[68]	2002	Japan	Cohort	1 611	0.73	NA	40	79
Nakagawa[69]	2005	Japan	Cohort	12 645	NR	NA	50	69
Seki[70]	2005	Japan	Cohort	2 889	NR	NA	NR	NR
Henschke[55]	Ongoing	USA	Cohort	26 557	NR	NA	40	
Henschke[71]	1999	USA	Cohort	1 000	0.84	NA	60	NR
Diederich[57]	2004	Germany	Cohort	817	0.81	NA	40	78
Swensen[54]	2002	USA	Cohort	1 520	NA	NA	50	85
Pastorino[62]	2003	Italy	Cohort	1 035	NR	NA	50	84
McRedmond[72]	2004	Ireland	Cohort	449	NR	NA	50	74
Belani[73]	2005	USA	Cohort	902	0.98	NA	50	79
Brechot[74]	2005	France	RCT	$N_s = 284$ $N_c = 237$	NR	X-ray	50	75
Pedersen[75]	Ongoing	Denmark	RCT	$N_s = 2000$ $N_c = 2000$	NA	None	50	65
Infante[76]	Ongoing	Italy	RCT	$N_s = 1200$ $N_c = 1200$	NR	None	60	75
Ronchi[77]	Ongoing	Italy	RCT	$N_s = 1500$ $N_c = 1500$	NR	None	55	69
Van Klaveren[78]	Ongoing	Holland/ Belgium	RCT	$N_s = 8000$ $N_c = 8000$	NR	None	50	74
Gohagan[79]	2005	USA	RCT (pilot)	$N_s = 1660$ $N_c = 1658$	0.86	X-ray	55	74
Gohagan[79]	Ongoing	USA	RCT	$N_s = 25\ 000$ $N_c = 25\ 000$		X-ray	55	74

N_c, number of participants in the control group; N_s, number of participants in the screengroup or, in the case of cohort, number of participants in the cohort; Ps1, compliance in the screengroup or, in case of cohort study, compliance in the cohort at the first incidence screen; NA, not applicable; NR, not reported; PY, pack-years (number of packs of cigarettes a day multiplied by the number of years of smoking); RCT, randomized controlled trial.

...oking ...tory	Former smokers	Detection rate 1st screen: N (%)	Mean/ median age	Mean/ median pack-years	Percent current smokers	Percent male	Percent stage 1
. PY, and ...ver-smokers	Yes	22 (0.4%)	64	NR	46	55	91
. PY, and ...ver-smokers	Yes	41 (0.5%)	NR[b]	NR	62	79	85
. PY, and ...ver-smokers	Yes	14 (0.9%)	NR[c]	NR	86	88	71
. PY, and ...ver-smokers	Yes	60 (0.5%)	57		64 current or former smoker	82	90
. PY, and ...ver-smokers	Yes	19 (0.7%)	63	NR	92	87	79
. PY	Yes	NR	NA	NA	NA	NA	NR
0 PY	No	27 (2.7%)	67	45	100	54	81
0 PY	No	12 (1.5%)	53	45	100	72	58
0 PY	Yes, quit <10 years	31 (2.0%)	59	51	61	52	63
0 PY	Yes	11 (1.1%)	58	40	86	71	55
0 PY	No	2 (0.5%)	55	53	100	50	50
2.5 PY	Yes, quit <10 years	20 (2.3%)	NR	46	62	48	33
2 PY	Yes	6 (2.1%) 1 (0.4%)	58	NR	68	69	50
0 PY	Yes, quit <10 years	NA	NA	NA	NA	NA	NA
0 PY	Yes, quit <10 years	21 (2.8%)	NA	NA	NA	100	48
0 PY	Yes	6 (1.9%)	NA	NA	NA	55	33
7 PY	Yes, quit <10 years	NA	NA	NA	NA	NA	NA
0 PY	Yes, quit <10 years	30 (1.9%)	NR[a]	54	58	59	53 (stage Ia)
0 PY	Yes, quit <15 years	NA	NA	NA	NA	NA	NA

[a] Age distribution: 55–64 year olds = 68% and 65–74 year olds = 32%.
[b] Age distribution: 50–59 year olds = 76% and 60–69 year olds = 24%.
[c] Age distribution: 40–59 year olds = 48% and 60–79 year olds = 52%.

Table 4.5   Comparison of screening results at baseline and annual follow-up in five large selected screening cohorts

	Baseline screening ($n = 13\ 122$)	Annual follow-up ($n = 10\ 245$)
Total number of tumors detected	112	55
Stage I (%)	55–85	60–100
Stage III, IV (%)	3–36	0–36
Rate of cancer (%)	0.4–2.7	0.07–1.1
Mean diameter of nodule (mm)	14–21	10–16
Invasive procedure for benign lesions (%)	4–22	14–55
Interval cancers (%)	NA	0–22

Data from the Anti-Lung Cancer Association (ALCA), Japan; Early Lung Cancer Action Project (ELCAP), USA; the Mayo Clinic Study, USA; the Lung Cancer Screening Study Milan, Italy; and Hitachi Health Center, Japan.

high participation rate during five consecutive annual screening rounds (98% in the second year to 80% in the fifth year) is the Mayo Clinic study.[54] Because of its high attendance rate and the availability of reliable follow-up data, this study is very useful for analysis of the performance of spiral CT as a screening tool. Of the 68 lung cancers detected over the 5-year period, only 3 interval cancers were detected, 2 of them by sputum cytology. This means that the sensitivity of spiral CT scanning in detecting lung cancer is 93% (63/68), the specificity 99% and the positive predictive value 84%. Although these figures are excellent, confirmation from large ongoing randomized trials is needed.

An important question is whether the cancer cases detected by spiral CT screening are a true representation of the spectrum of lung cancers present in the population, or whether a certain subgroup of slowly growing tumors is detected. Recent estimates from the SEER database are that 14% of all new lung cancers in the USA are of small cell histology. Even though small cell lung cancer has a rapid doubling time, both in the Mayo Clinic,[54] and in the screening trial in Münster, Germany,[59] 12% of the screen-detected lung cancer cases were of small cell histology.

Overdiagnosis – the detection of lung cancer cases that would not lead to an individual's death because of slow growth rate or competing age-related risks for death remains an important theoretical concern, as CT resolution continues to find ever-smaller primary lung cancers.[60] So far, no firm evidence exists that allows a reliable estimate of its influence in lung cancer screening trials. Review of the lung cancer cases detected in the ELCAP trial revealed that the histopathology was consistent with the invasive characteristics of conventionally detected lung cancers.[61] In addition, the gene expression profile of lung cancer cases detected in the Milan trial by cDNA microarray analyses were compared with matched series of symptom-detected lung cancers in addition to quantitative real-time PCR and immunohistochemistry, and suggest that the aggressive biologic behaviour of CT-detected cancers is similar to that of symptom-detected ones.[62,63] In current clinical practice, approximately 30–40% of lung cancer deaths are expected to be associated with histologic findings of adenocarcinoma. One could speculate that the higher rate of adenocarcinoma (especially bronchoalveolar carcinoma) observed in the Mayo Clinic trial (74% prevalence, 37% incidence),[54] is due to overdiagnosis in this high-risk cohort. This higher than expected rate of adenocarcinoma indicates that slower-growing adenocarcinomas (especially bronchoalveolar carcinomas) are predominantly identified by screening and probably represent overdiagnosed cases. Also, tumor doubling time might be a marker for overdiagnosis. For tumors with a doubling time of >400 days on a chest X-ray, it would take at least 7.7 years for a 3 mm lesion to grow to a diameter of 15 mm, which is, according to some authors, consistent with overdiagnosis. Of the 82 cancers detected in a CT screening trial, Hasegawa et al[64] noted that 27 (33%) had a mean doubling time of >400 days, or, according to this definition, represent overdiagnosed cases.

Features of nodules may help to discriminate between benign and malignant processes, but suggested criteria such as spiculated distribution of calcium are not sufficiently informative.[36] Henschke et al[55] retrospectively reviewed whether non-calcified nodules <5 mm in diameter identified on initial CT at baseline screening might not justify immediate further work-up, but merely the first annual repeat screening to determine whether the nodule has grown. A work-up after 1 year decreased further immediate work-up by 54%, without missing any malignancy. However, this implies that even the smallest nodule detected at baseline needs re-examination at first annual repeat scan to determine whether interim growth has occurred.[55] Growth of nodules, defined as at least 8–10% increase in volume per month, led to a recall rate of 12% at baseline and 6% at follow-up scanning after 1 year. Based on nodule growth and needle biopsy, the rate of diagnosis of cancer was 90% in the ELCAP study.[36] However, some nodules decrease in size over time or even resolve, probably due to focal inflammation, mucoid impaction or intermittent enlargement of benign intrapulmonary lesions. In a retrospective study, Diederich et al[65] could not demonstrate specific features of resolving nodules, but resolving nodules were mostly <10 mm, peripherally located, solid, well defined and non-lobulated. Most nodules resolved within a variable time interval, ranging from several days to years. Demographic or morphologic features that allow differentiation between nodules that will or will not resolve during follow-up were not identified.[65] The role of [18F]fluorodeoxyglucose positron emission tomography (FDG-PET) in the evaluation of screen-detected nodules is retrospectively reviewed in participants of the NCI-sponsored spiral CT screening trial.[40] The false-negative rate of PET was 32% in this population, much higher than the 5% in the general population, due to the smaller size of the screen-detected nodules and a higher rate of bronchoalveolar carcinomas. Also, for staging purposes, the PET scan is less helpful in a screening population. PET accurately staged 86% (12/14) of the 14 PET-positive tumors and CT scanning 86% (18/21) of the CT-detected tumors. Because bronchoalveolar cell carcinomas are usually PET-negative, and have a high rate of ground-glass attenuation, the use of PET scans should be discouraged in the evaluation of nodules with ground glass attenuation.[40]

REFERENCES

1. Hirsch FR, Lippman SM. Advances in the biology of lung cancer chemoprevention. J Clin Oncol 2005; 23: 3186–97.

2. Vignot S, Spano JP, Lantuejoul S et al. Chemoprevention of lung cancer. Recent Results Cancer Res 2005; 166: 145–65.

3. Saba N, Jain S, Khuri F. Chemoprevention in lung cancer. Curr Probl Cancer 2004; 28: 287–306.

4. Chanin TD, Merrick DT, Franklin WA et al. Recent developments in biomarkers for the early detection of lung cancer: perspectives based on publications 2003 to present. Curr Opin Pulm Med 2004; 10: 242–7.

5. Cohen V, Khuri FR. Chemoprevention of lung cancer: concepts and strategies. Expert Rev Anticancer Ther 2005; 5: 549–65.

6. Winterhalder RC, Hirsch FR, Kotantoulas GK et al. Chemoprevention of lung cancer – from biology to clinical reality. Ann Oncol 2004; 15: 185–96.

7. Merrick DT, Winterhalder RC, Kittelson J et al. Increased expression of C-erb-B1 (EGF-R) but not C-erb-B2 (HER2) is associated with dysplastic change in bronchial airways: correlation with increased K167, MCM2 and P53 expression. Lung Cancer 2005; 49(Suppl 2): S83.

8. Mitsuuchi Y, Testa JR. Cytogenetics and molecular genetics of lung cancer. Am J Med Genet 2002; 115: 183–8.

9. Hirano T, Ohira T, Suga Y et al. Quantitative proteomic exploration of biomarkers for early detection of adenocarcinoma of the lung. Lung Cancer 2005; 49(Suppl 2): S179.

10. Bechtel J, Kelley W, Coons T et al. Lung cancer detection in high risk patients with airflow obstruction: an ongoing study. Lung Cancer 2005; 49(Suppl 2): S177.

11. Kennedy TC, Franklin WA, Prindiville SA et al. High prevalence of occult endobronchial malignancy in high risk patients with moderate sputum atypia. Lung Cancer 2005; 49: 187–91.

12. Prindiville SA, Byers T, Hirsch FR et al. Sputum cytological atypia as a predictor of incident lung cancer in a cohort of heavy smokers with airflow obstruction. Cancer Epidemiol Biomarkers Prev 2003; 12: 987–93.

13. Varella-Garcia M, Kittelson J, Schulte AP et al. Multi-target interphase fluorescence in situ hybridization assay increases sensitivity of sputum cytology as a predictor of lung cancer. Cancer Detect Prev 2004; 28: 244–51.

14. Abbruzzese JL, Lippman SM. The convergence of cancer prevention and therapy in early-phase clinical drug development. Cancer Cell 2004; 6: 321–6.

15. Lippman SM, Levin B. Cancer prevention: strong science and real medicine. J Clin Oncol 2005; 23: 249–53.

16. Muller R. Crosstalk of oncogenic and prostanoid signaling pathways. J Cancer Res Clin Oncol 2004; 130: 429–44.

17. Yamaki T, Endoh K, Miyahara M et al. Prostaglandin E2 activates Src signaling in lung adenocarcinoma cell via EP3. Cancer Lett 2004; 214: 115–20.

18. Keith RL, Miller YE, Hudish TM et al.

Pulmonary prostacyclin synthase overexpression chemoprevents tobacco smoke lung carcinogenesis in mice. Cancer Res 2004; 64: 5897–904.

19. Keith RL, Miller YE, Kelly K et al. Clinical update on the phase II trial of oral iloprost in the chemoprevention of lung cancer in high risk patients. Lung Cancer 2005; 49(Suppl 2): S83.

20. Ding Y, Tong M, Liu S et al. NAD$^+$-linked 15-hydroxyprostaglandin dehydrogenase (15-PGDH) behaves as a tumor suppressor in lung cancer. Carcinogenesis 2005; 26: 65–72.

21. Backlund MG, Mann JR, Holla VR et al. 15-Hydroxyprostaglandin dehydrogenase is down-regulated in colorectal cancer. J Biol Chem 2005; 280: 3217–23.

22. Chen Z, Zhang X, Li M et al. Simultaneously targeting epidermal growth factor receptor tyrosine kinase and cyclooxygenase-2, an efficient approach to inhibition of squamous cell carcinoma of the head and neck. Clin Cancer Res 2004; 10: 5930–9.

23. Pold M, Krysan K, Pold A et al. Cyclooxygenase-2 modulates the insulin-like growth factor axis in non-small-cell lung cancer. Cancer Res 2004; 64: 6549–55.

24. Chun KH, Kosmeder JW 2nd, Sun S et al. Effects of deguelin on the phosphatidylinositol 3-kinase/Akt pathway and apoptosis in premalignant human bronchial epithelial cells. J Natl Cancer Inst 2003; 95: 291–302.

25. Sozzi G, Conte D, Leon M et al. Quantification of free circulating DNA as a diagnostic marker in lung cancer. J Clin Oncol 2003; 21: 3902–8.

26. Kennedy TC, Hirsch FR. Using molecular markers in sputum for the early detection of lung cancer: a review. Lung Cancer 2004; 45(Suppl 2): S21–7.

27. Bremnes RM, Sirera R, Camps C. Circulating tumour-derived DNA and RNA markers in blood: a tool for

early detection, diagnostics, and follow-up? Lung Cancer 2005; 49: 1–12.

28. Schmidt B, Carstensen T, Engel E et al. Detection of cell-free nucleic acids in bronchial lavage fluid supernatants from patients with lung cancer. Eur J Cancer 2004; 40: 452–60.

29. Bunn PJ Jr. Early detection of lung cancer using serum RNA or DNA markers: ready for 'prime time' or for validation? J Clin Oncol 2003; 21: 3891–3.

30. Kim H, Kwon YM, Kim JS et al. Tumor-specific methylation in bronchial lavage for the early detection of non-small-cell lung cancer. J Clin Oncol 2004; 22: 2363–70.

31. Topaloglu O, Hoque MO, Tokumaru Y et al. Detection of promoter hypermethylation of multiple genes in the tumor and bronchoalveolar lavage of patients with lung cancer. Clin Cancer Res 2004; 10: 2284–8.

32. Choi N, Son DS, Song I et al. RASSF1A is not appropriate as an early detection marker or a prognostic marker for non-small cell lung cancer. Int J Cancer 2005; 115: 575–81.

33. Khan S, Coulson JM, Woll PJ. Genetic abnormalities in plasma DNA of patients with lung cancer and other respiratory diseases. Int J Cancer 2004; 110: 891–5.

34. Carpagnano GE, Foschino-Barbaro MP, Resta O et al. Endothelin-1 is increased in the breath condensate of patients with non-small-cell lung cancer. Oncology 2004; 66: 180–4.

35. Strauss GM, Dominioni L, Jett JR et al. Como International Conference Position Statement: lung cancer screening for early diagnosis 5 years after the 1998 Varese Conference. Chest 2005; 127: 1146–51.

36. Mulshine JL, Sullivan DC. Clinical practice. Lung cancer screening. N Engl J Med 2005; 352: 2714–20.

37. Smith RA, Cokkinides V, Eyre HJ. American Cancer Society guidelines

for the early detection of cancer, 2004. CA Cancer J Clin 2004; 54: 41–52.

38. Humphrey LL, Teutsch S, Johnson M. Lung cancer screening with sputum cytologic examination, chest radiography, and computed tomography: an update for the U.S. Preventive Services Task Force. Ann Intern Med 2004; 140: 740–53.

39. Mulshine JL. New developments in lung cancer screening. J Clin Oncol 2005; 23: 3198–202.

40. Lindell RM, Hartman TE, Swensen SJ et al. Lung cancer screening experience: a retrospective review of PET in 22 non-small cell lung carcinomas detected on screening chest CT in a high-risk population. AJR Am J Roentgenol 2005; 185: 126–31.

41. Rossi A, Maione P, Colantuoni G et al. Screening for lung cancer: new horizons? Crit Rev Oncol Hematol 2005; 56: 311–20.

42. Kuzniar T, Masters GA, Ray DW. Screening for lung cancer – a review. Med Sci Monit 2004; 10: RA21–30.

43. Ashton RW, Jett JR. Screening for non-small cell lung cancer. Semin Oncol 2005; 32: 253–8.

44. Manser R. Screening for lung cancer: a review. Curr Opin Pulm Med 2004; 10: 266–71.

45. Ganti AK, Mulshine JL. Lung cancer screening: panacea or pipe dream? Ann Oncol 2005; 16(Suppl 2): ii215–19.

46. Kawahara M. Screening for lung cancer. Curr Opin Oncol 2004; 16: 141–5.

47. van Meerbeeck JP, Tournoy KG. Screening and diagnosis of NSCLC. Ann Oncol 2004; 15(Suppl 4): iv65–70.

48. Lenox RJ. To screen or not to screen. Chest 2005; 127: 1091–2.

49. Wisnivesky JP, Mushlin AI, Sicherman N et al. The cost-effectiveness of low-dose CT screening for lung cancer: preliminary results of baseline screening. Chest 2003; 124: 614–21.

50. Marshall D, Long K. Economic Evaluation of Lung Cancer Screening. London: Martin Dunitz, 2005.

51. Ohmatsu H, Kaneko M, Kakinuma R et al. Lung cancer screening using low-dose helical CT over 10 years. Lung Cancer 2005; 49(Suppl 2): S20.

52. Patz EF Jr, Swensen SJ, Herndon JE 2nd. Estimate of lung cancer mortality from low-dose spiral computed tomography screening trials: implications for current mass screening recommendations. J Clin Oncol 2004; 22: 2202–6.

53. Tockman MS. Improbable estimate of lung cancer mortality from screening trials. J Clin Oncol 2005; 23: 2106–7; author reply 2107–8.

54. Swensen SJ, Jett JR, Hartman TE et al. CT screening for lung cancer: five-year prospective experience. Radiology 2005; 235: 259–65.

55. Henschke C, Sone S, Markowitz S et al. CT screening for lung cancer: the relationship of disease stage to tumor size. Lung Cancer 2005; 49(Suppl 2): S18.

56. Jett JR. Limitations of screening for lung cancer with low-dose spiral computed tomography. Clin Cancer Res 2005; 11: 4988–92S.

57. Diederich S, Wormanns D. Impact of low-dose CT on lung cancer screening. Lung Cancer 2004; 45(Suppl 2): S13–19.

58. Gohagan J, Marcus P, Fagerstrom R et al. Baseline findings of a randomized feasibility trial of lung cancer screening with spiral CT scan vs chest radiograph: the Lung Screening Study of the National Cancer Institute. Chest 2004; 126: 114–21.

59. Diederich S, Thomas M, Semik M et al. Screening for early lung cancer with low-dose spiral computed tomography: results of annual follow-up examinations in asymptomatic smokers. Eur Radiol 2004; 14: 691–702.

60. Mulshine JL. Clinical issues in the

management of early lung cancer. Clin Cancer Res 2005; 11: 4993–8S.

61. Henschke CI, Wisnivesky JP, Yankelevitz DF et al. Small stage I cancers of the lung: genuineness and curability. Lung Cancer 2003; 39: 327–30.

62. Pastorino U, Bellomi M, Landoni C et al. Early lung-cancer detection with spiral CT and positron emission tomography in heavy smokers: 2-year results. Lancet 2003; 362: 593–7.

63. Mulshine JL, Weinstein JN. Is the gene expression pattern of lung cancer detected by screening with spiral computed tomography different from that of symptom-detected lung cancer? Clin Cancer Res 2004; 10: 5973–4.

64. Hasegawa M, Sone S, Takashima S et al. Growth rate of small lung cancers detected on mass CT screening. Br J Radiol 2000; 73: 1252–9.

65. Diederich S, Hansen J, Wormanns D. Resolving small pulmonary nodules: CT features. Eur Radiol 2005; 15: 2064–9.

66. Sone S, Li F, Yang ZG et al. Results of three-year mass screening programme for lung cancer using mobile low-dose spiral computed tomography scanner. Br J Cancer 2001; 84: 25–32.

67. Nawa T, Nakagawa T, Kusano S et al. Lung cancer screening using low-dose spiral CT: results of baseline and 1-year follow-up studies. Chest 2002; 122: 15–20.

68. Sobue T, Moriyama N, Kaneko M et al. Screening for lung cancer with low-dose helical computed tomography: Anti-Lung Cancer Association Project. J Clin Oncol 2002; 20: 911–20.

69. Nakagawa T, Kusano S, Yamamoto S et al. CT screening for lung cancer in health examination. Lung Cancer 2005; 49(Suppl 2): S84.

70. Seki N, Eguchi K, Kaneko M et al. The decreased detection rate and the stage shift in lung adenocarcinoma during long-term repeat low-dose helical CT screening. Lung Cancer 2005; 49(Suppl 2): S186.

71. Henschke CI, McCauley DI, Yankelevitz DF et al. Early Lung Cancer Action Project: overall design and findings from baseline screening. Lancet 1999; 354: 99–105.

72. MacRedmond R, Logan PM, Lee M et al. Screening for lung cancer using low dose CT scanning. Thorax 2004; 59: 237–41.

73. Belani C, Fuhrman C, Wilson D et al. Two-year outcomes from lung cancer screening with low-dose helical computed tomography. Lung Cancer 2005; 49(Suppl 2): S177.

74. Brechot J, Blanchon T, Lemairie E et al. A French pilot lung cancer screening trial randomizing multi-slice-spiral CT scan (MSCT) vs chest X-ray (CXR): prevalence results. Lung Cancer 2005; 49(Suppl 2): S178.

75. Pedersen JH, Dirksen A, Olsen JH. [Screening for lung cancer with low-dosage CT]. Ugeskr Laeger 2002; 164: 167–70.

76. Infante M, Lutman F, Brambilla G et al. Dante: a randomized study on lung cancer screening with spiral CT. Work in progress. Lung Cancer 2005; 49(Suppl 2): S180.

77. Ronchi M, Cordopatri G, De Francisci A et al. ITALUNG – CT screening for lung cancer: preliminary results. Lung Cancer 2005; 49(Suppl 2): S185.

78. van Klaveren, van Iersel C, de Koning H et al. Recruitment and first screening results of the Dutch–Belgian lung cancer screening trial (NELSON). Lung Cancer 2005; 49(Suppl 2): S188.

79. Gohagan JK, Marcus PM, Fagerstrom RM et al. Final results of the Lung Screening Study, a randomized feasibility study of spiral CT versus chest X-ray screening for lung cancer. Lung Cancer 2005; 47: 9–15.

5
Histopathology

Heine H Hansen

The 1999 histologic classification of malignant lung and pleural tumors published by the World Health Organization (WHO) on the basis of recommendations by the Pathology Panel of the International Association for the Study of Lung Cancer (IASLC) is listed in Table 5.1. It contains the morphologic codes of the International Classification of Disease for Oncology (ICD-O) and the Systematized Nomenclature of Medicine (SNOMED).[1]

Inaccuracy in reporting the histologic type of lung cancer can affect estimates of (1) histologic type-specific incidence trends, (2) survivorship by histologic type and (3) risk estimates associated with various etiologic factors. Surprisingly few studies have been performed comparing the agreement between registry and independently reviewed lung cancer histologic types, but an article by Field et al[2] sheds further light on this topic. They examined whether the Iowa Surveillance, Epidemiology, and End Results (SEER) Cancer Registry reported lung cancer histologic diagnoses were reliable, investigating agreement between lung cancer histologic types for 413 patients with lung cancer reported by the Iowa Cancer Registry and those obtained through an independent review of diagnostic slides. Among lung cancer histologic types, small cell lung carcinoma (SCLC) had the highest sensitivity (94.1%; 95% confidence interval (CI) 85.6–98.4), positive prediction value (94.1%; 95% CI 85.6–98.4), negative predictive value (98.8%; 95% CI 96.9–99.7), and highest percent exact agreement (98.0%; 95% CI 96.6–99.4). The lowest sensitivity (21.9%; 95% CI 9.3–40.0) and positive predictive value (23.3%; 95% CI 9.9–42.3) were noted for large cell carcinoma, probably because other more specific features of adenocarcinoma or squamous carcinoma were absent. Adenocarcinoma had the lowest specificity (84.4%; 95% CI 79–88.9), negative predictive value (85.2%; 95% CI 79.9–89.6) and percent exact agreement (82.9%; 95% CI 79.2–86.6). Samples collected by cytologic examination (odds ratio (OR) = 2.4; 95% CI 1.1–5.2) or biopsy examination (OR = 2.2; 95% CI 1.1–4.2) were more likely to be misclassified than samples obtained by resection.

Overall, the histologic results of the classification by the registry were reasonably reliable, but independent slide review is obviously needed for precise histologic typing of lung cancer.

With respect to the WHO classification, in 1999, a major change from the 1981 classification was the introduction of the concept of neuroendocrine

Table 5.1   Histologic classification of lung and pleural tumors [a]

1. Epithelial tumors
   1.3 Malignant
   1.3.1 Squamous cell carcinoma   8070/3
          Variants:
          1.3.1.1 Papillary   8052/3
          1.3.1.2 Clear cell   8084/3
          1.3.1.3 Small cell   8073/3
          1.3.1.4 Basaloid   8083/3
   1.3.2 Small cell carcinoma   8041/3
          Variant:
          1.3.2.1 Combined   8045/3
   1.3.3 Adenocarcinoma   8140/3
          1.3.3.1 Acinar   8550/3
          1.3.3.2 Papillary   8260/3
          1.3.3.3 Bronchioloalveolar carcinoma   8250/3
               1.3.3.3.1 Non-mucinous   8252/3
               1.3.3.3.2 Mucinous   8253/3
               1.3.3.3.3 Mixed mucinous and non-mucinous or
                   indeterminate cell type   8254/3
          1.3.3.4 Solid adenocarcinoma with mucin   8230/3
          1.3.3.5 Adenocarcinoma with mixed subtypes   8255/3
          1.3.3.6 Variants:
               1.3.3.6.1 Well-differentiated fetal adenocarcinoma   8333/3
               1.3.3.6.2 Mucinous ('colloid') adenocarcinoma   8480/3
               1.3.3.6.3 Mucinous cystadenocarcinoma   8470/3
               1.3.3.6.4 Signet ring adenocarcinoma   8490/3
               1.3.3.6.5 Clear cell adenocarcinoma   8310/3
   1.3.4 Large cell carcinoma   8012/3
          Variants:
          1.3.4.1 Large cell neuroendocrine carcinoma   8013/3
               1.3.4.1.1 Combined large cell neuroendocrine
                   carcinoma
          1.3.4.2 Basaloid carcinoma   8123/3
          1.3.4.3 Lymphoepithelioma-like carcinoma   8082/3
          1.3.4.4 Clear cell carcinoma   8310/3
          1.3.4.5 Large cell carcinoma with rhabdoid phenotype   8014/3
   1.3.5 Adenosquamous carcinoma   8560/3
   1.3.6 Carcinomas with pleomorphic, sarcomatoid or sarcomatous
          elements
          1.3.6.1 Carcinomas with spindle and/or giant cells   8030/3
               1.3.6.1.1 Pleomorphic carcinoma   8022/3
               1.3.6.1.2 Spindle cell carcinoma   8032/3
               1.3.6.1.3 Giant cell carcinoma   8031/3
          1.3.6.2 Carcinosarcoma   8980/3
          1.3.6.3 Pulmonary blastoma   8972/3
          1.3.6.4 Others
   1.3.7 Carcinoid tumor   8240/3
          1.3.7.1 Typical carcinoid   8240/3
          1.3.7.2 Atypical carcinoid   8249/3

Table 5.1 continued	
1.3.8 Carcinomas of salivary gland type	
1.3.8.1 Mucoepidermoid carcinoma	8430/3
1.3.8.2 Adenoid cystic carcinoma	8200/3
1.3.8.3 Others	
1.3.9 Unclassified carcinoma	8010/3

[a] Modified from Travis WD, Colby TV, Corrin B et al (eds). Histological Typing of Lung and Pleural Tumours. WHO International Histological Classification of Tumours. Berlin: Springer-Verlag, 1999: 22–3.

tumors of the lung, which has been refined by recognition of large neuroendocrine carcinomas and modification of the criteria for atypical carcinoids. Neuroendocrine tumors are defined as a distinct subset of tumors that share certain morphologic, ultrastructural and immunohistochemical characteristics. The major categories of morphologically identifiable neuroendocrine tumors are small cell carcinoma, large cell neuroendocrine carcinoma, typical carcinoids and atypical carcinoids. The criteria for diagnosis of these tumors are given in Table 5.2.

Since the reclassification, the literature has been rich in publications on this topic, and 2004–5 was no exception. Mezzetti et al[3] reviewed the original histologic diagnosis using the 1999 WHO criteria and identified 88 patients with typical carcinoids (TC) and 10 with atypical carcinoids (AC) among 98 pulmonary resections that had been performed from 1980 to 2001 for primary bronchial carcinoid tumors. The 5-year overall survival rate was 91.9% for TC and 71% for AC, while the 10-year overall survival rate was 89.7% for TC and 60% for AC.

As for other histologic types of lung cancer, the survival rate was clearly related to the TNM stage. Overall, the prognosis is thus rather favorable for both subtypes in the early stage.

Histologic differentiation between SCLC and large cell neuroendocrine carcinoma (LCNEC) can be very difficult in some cases, and Hiroshima et al[4] studied the genetic alterations found in LCNEC and compared these with those of SCLC and classic large cell carcinoma (CLCC).

Twenty-two patients with LCNEC, 12 patients with CLCC and 11 patients with SCLC were studied. The tissue was obtained at primary resection of the tumor. Loss of hyterozygosity (LOH) of the tumor cells was detected using fluorescent primers. Methylation status of the *p16* gene and expression of the p53 protein, retinoblastoma protein and p16 protein were evaluated immunohistochemically. The genetic alterations of LCNEC were akin to those of SCLC. However, allelic losses at 5q and abnormalities in the *p16* gene may differentiate LCNEC from SCLC.

Other immunohistochemistry studies in pulmonary neuroendocrine tumors included the E-cadherin and β-catenin cell adhesion systems, which were found to be abnormal in all subtypes of the 210 neuroendocrine tumors studied, as

Table 5.2   Criteria for diagnosis of neuroendocrine (NE) tumors[a]

Tumor	Description[b]
Typical carcinoid	A tumor with carcinoid morphology and <2 mitoses per 2 mm² (10 HPF), lacking necrosis and 0.5 cm or larger
Atypical carcinoid	A tumor with carcinoid morphology with 2–10 mitoses per 2 mm² (10 HPF) or necrosis (often punctate)
Large cell neuroendocrine carcinoma	1. A tumor with a neuroendocrine morphology (organoid nesting, palisading, rosettes, trabeculae) 2. High mitotic rate; ≥11 per 2 mm² (10 HPF), median of 70 per 2 mm² (10 HPF) 3. Necrosis (often large zones) 4. Cytologic features of a non-small cell lung cancer (NSCLC): large cell size, low nuclear-to-cytoplasmic ratio, vesicular or fine chromatin, and/or frequent nucleoli. Some tumors have fine nuclear chromatin and lack nucleoli, but qualify as NSCLC because of large cell size and abundant cytoplasm 5. Positive immunohistochemical staining for one or more neuroendocrine markers (other than neuron-specific enolase) and/or neuroendocrine granules by electron microscopy
Small cell carcinoma	1. Small size (generally less than the diameter of three small resting lymphocytes) 2. Scant cytoplasm 3. Nuclei: finely granular nuclear chromatin, absent or faint nucleoli 4. High mitotic rate (≥11 per 2 mm²) (10 HPF), median of 80 per 2 mm² (10 HPF) 5. Frequent necrosis, often in large zones

[a] Modified from Travis WD, Colby TV, Corrin B et al (eds). Histological Typing of Lung and Pleural Tumours. WHO International Histological Classification of Tumours. Berlin: Springer-Verlag, 1999.
[b] For an explanation of HPF (high-power field) and mitosis counting, see page 10 of Travis et al.

β-catenin expression was retained in all tumors; furthermore, a disarrayed E-adherin distribution pattern was associated with the pathologic lymph node classification and the number of involved lymph nodes based on multivariate analysis.[5]

Immunohistochemical investigations have also been performed to detect occult lymph node metastases in non-small cell lung cancer (NSCLC) using staining for cytokeratin.[6] The Cancer and Leukemia Group B (CLGB) examined 825 lymph nodes from 193 patients entered into one of the CLGB protocols. All patients had clinically staged T12N0M0 NSCLC and underwent curative resections of their primary tumors. Samples of the primary tumor and lymph nodes were taken from lymph node stations 2–12 and stained with hematoxylin and eosin (H&E) as well as with immunohistochemical stain using antibodies to cytokeratin.

Altogether, 825 lymph nodes were examined, and H&E staining allowed the investigators to detect 18 positive lymph nodes, whereas immunohistochemical staining detected 45 positive lymph nodes ($p < 0.0001$). There were 28 detected only by immunohistochemistry compared with 1 metastasis detected only by H&E staining. For the probability of detecting metastases by H&E to exceed 0.50, the maximum diameter of the metastasis must be greater than 0.23 mm.

Thus, immunohistochemical staining detects more than twice as many positive regional lymph nodes as does H&E staining, but whether these findings will have an impact on prognosis and on treatment strategy and how the results compare with other immunohistochemical markers await further investigation.

Immunohistochemical analysis may include expression of Bcl-2 family protein, which in a pilot study has shown to differ significantly between squamous cell carcinoma and adenocarcinoma.[7] These differences will require verification in a larger series of samples according to disease stage and degree of differentiation in order to confirm the findings and to investigate the basis of this difference.

REFERENCES

1. Travis WD, Colby TV, Corrin B et al. Histological Typing of Lung and Pleural Tumors. WHO International Histological Classification of Tumours, 3rd edn. Berlin: Springer-Verlag, 1999.

2. Field RW, Smith BJ, Platz CE et al. Lung cancer histologic type in the Surveillance Epidemiology, and End Results registry versus independent review. J Natl Cancer Inst 2004; 96: 1105–7.

3. Mezzetti M, Raveglia F, Panigalli T et al. Assessment of outcomes in typical and atypical carcinoids according to latest WHO classification. Ann Thorac Surg 2003; 76: 1832–42.

4. Hiroshima K, Lyoda A, Shibuya K et al. Genetic alterations in early-stage pulmonary large cell neuroendocrine carcinoma. Cancer 2004; 100: 1190–8.

5. Pelosi G, Scarpa A, Puppa G et al. Alteration of the E-cadherin/

β-catenin cell adhesion system is common in pulmonary neuroendocrine tumors and is an independent predictor of lymph node metastasis in atypical carcinoids. Cancer 2005; 103: 1154–64.

6. Vollmer RT, Herndon JE 2nd, D'Cunha J et al. Immunohistochemical detection of occult lymph node metastases in non-small cell lung cancer: anatomical pathology results from Cancer and Leukemia Group B Trial 9761. Clin Cancer Res 2003; 9: 5630–6.

7. Berrieman, HK, Smith L, O'Kane SL et al. The expression of Bcl-2 family proteins differs between nonsmall cell lung carcinoma subtypes. Cancer 2005; 103: 1415–19.

6
Staging, staging procedures and prognostic factors

Rob J van Klaveren and Jeroen S Kloover

NON-SMALL CELL LUNG CANCER

Staging

Preoperative tumor staging in patients with non-small cell lung cancer (NSCLC) is important in order to identify those patients with localized disease who are likely to benefit from surgical resection. The TNM staging system, revised in 1997, is the most widely accepted classification system for pre- and postoperative staging. The American Thoracic Society and the European Respiratory Society advocate no preoperative imaging of the skeleton and brain in patients with NSCLC who have no symptoms or other evidence of metastases, because most skeletal metastases in lung cancer are clinically symptomatic and the incidence of bone metastases in early-stage disease is low. Papers on staging in the last 2 years have dealt with the question of whether a routine bone scan and head computed tomography (CT) should be performed in asymptomatic potentially resectable NSCLC patients. Hetzel et al[1] investigated the impact of symptoms, serum calcium and alkaline phosphatase levels on the sensitivity of the bone scan in 153 consecutive NSCLC and small cell lung cancer (SCLC) patients. In this study population, skeletal metastases were found in 33%. All of them had normal serum calcium and alkaline phosphatase, 75% had symptoms, but in only 19% did the localization of the metastases correspond to the localization of the symptoms. The sensitivity of routine bone scans was 73% (95% confidence interval (CI) 56–85%) and the specificity 99% (95% CI 93–100%), but if bone scans had been done only on patients with complaints, the sensitivity would have dropped to 53%, and if they had been restricted to those with suspicious complaints, it would have dropped to 20%. The authors recommend a routine bone scan for all patients with lung cancer, independent of complaints or serum calcium or alkaline phosphatase levels.[1] A similar conclusion is made by other investigators.[2–4] Failure to perform a bone scan in asymptomatic patients reduced the sensitivity to 19–39%, and 14–22% of the patients would have undergone unnecessary surgery.[3] For operable NSCLC patients, bone scanning could prevent futile thoracotomies in 8%.[4]

Another important issue is the performance of a standard head CT in screening for cerebral metastases for patients with potentially resectable

NSCLC. In a prospective study of 105 NSCLC patients, cerebral metastases were identified by CT (sensitivity = 83%), which led to a saving of £45 000 (US$74 600) by avoiding thoracotomies, whereas the cost of 105 CTs was £16 000 (US$26 000). The authors conclude that screening for asymptomic cerebral metastases is both worthwhile and cost-effective. Magnetic resonance imaging (MRI) has been found to be even more sensitive (100%) in a series of 134 asymptomatic lung cancer patients.[5] In the UK, the National Institute for Clinical Excellence (NICE) guidelines also advised the use of MRI as the method of choice for detecting brain metastases; however, they stated that screening was not clinically or financially worthwhile.[6]

In 101 lung cancer patients, ultrasound of the neck was performed with fine-needle aspiration (FNA) if CT staging showed suspected N2 or N3 disease.[7] In those with enlarged nodules on CT, the yield of malignancy was 75% and in a further 43% invasive procedures were avoided, but ultrasound of the neck led to upstaging in only 10%;[7] and therefore, it is unclear whether this technique should be employed routinely in the staging of lung cancer patients.

Staging procedures

Positron emission tomography

Positron emission tomography (PET) technology has enabled a functional approach complementary to the anatomic assessment by CT and MRI in the evaluation and staging of lung cancer, but PET also provides information additional to CT in the evaluation and management of persistent and recurrent disease, and responses measured on PET might help to predict survival.[8–14] The role of PET in the diagnosis of solitary pulmonary nodules, (re)-staging, response to therapy and prognosis is reviewed in several excellent papers.[8–14] Accurate mediastinal staging is crucial in the management of patients with NSCLC. The CT scan has a poor sensitivity and specificity for identifying mediastinal metastases.

In the past decade several studies on PET imaging for mediastinal staging have been published. In a meta-analysis of 39 studies, it was concluded that for [18F]fluorodeoxyglucose (FDG)-PET) the median sensitivity and specificity are 85% and 90%, and for CT 61% and 79%, respectively.[15] It was also demonstrated – based on 14 studies – that FDG-PET was more sensitive but less specific when the CT scan already showed enlarged mediastinal lymph nodes (median sensitivity 100%, specificity 78%) than when the CT scan showed no lymph node enlargement (median sensitivity 82%, specificity 93%). This implies that in patients with enlarged lymph nodes on CT, the PET scan is more often a false-positive test, and in this situation biopsy confirmation by cervical mediastinoscopy is warranted.[15] A similar conclusion was made by Gonzalez-Stawinski et al[16] in a study of 202 NSCLC patients who underwent prospectively both mediastinoscopy and PET. A positive PET scan does not necessarily represent malignant disease and histologic confirmation is always needed; although a negative PET scan is relatively powerful (negative predictive value = 88.3%), N2 and N3 disease could be missed, and mediastinoscopy remains the gold standard.[16]

Kelly et al[17] investigated the cost-effectiveness of FDG-PET scanning in potentially resectable NSCLC patients. They also concluded that selective PET imaging may improve the sensitivity of non-invasive staging for patients without enlarged mediastinal lymph nodes on CT, but that PET may understage patients with adenocarcinoma and mediastinal lymph nodes <1 cm on CT. PET scanning in stage I and II NSCLC also has a large impact on subsequent clinical management.[18] In 20% of the patients, PET scanning led to a change in stage, mostly due to the identification of ipsilateral mediastinal lymph node involvement (N2 disease). This study was conducted in Australia, where mediastinoscopy is not routinely performed in patients with clinical stage I or II disease. In 13/18 patients (72%), the change in stage occurred in patients without enlarged mediastinal lymph nodes on CT. The sensitivity and specificity for detecting mediastinal disease were 73% and 90%, respectively, which are lower than reported previously. The authors attribute this to the lower volume of mediastinal disease in this population of stage I and II disease, which increases the likelihood of false-positive and false-negative findings.[18]

An important question is whether the accuracy of an integrated PET–CT is higher than for a dedicated PET alone in the staging of patients with NSCLC.[19] In a prospectively blinded trial, 129 consecutive NSCLC patients underwent an integrated PET–CT scan. First, the PET–CT images were read; then, within 2 weeks, the PET images without the CT images. The conclusions of this study are that integrated PET–CT is a significantly better predictor for stage I (52% vs 33%) and for stage II (70% vs 36%). It was also more sensitive and specific and had a higher positive predictive value for both N2 and N1 nodes ($p < 0.05$ for all), but still only achieved an accuracy of 96% and 90% for N2 and N1 nodes, respectively.[19]

Kahn et al[20] investigated the diagnostic accuracy of FDG-PET and technetium-99m (^{99m}Tc) depreotide, a somatostatin analogue, for the diagnosis and staging of patients with NSCLC.[20] ^{99m}Tc depreotide uses standard nuclear medicine gamma cameras, which are more widely available at lower costs. The two techniques turned out to be comparable with regard to the sensitivity of detecting lung cancer in the primary lesion, but the specificity is superior for FDG-PET. The accuracy to stage the mediastinum was also found to be similar.[20]

One of the limitations of FDG-PET is that the technique is sometimes false-negative for the primary tumor. Cheran et al[21] investigated, retrospectively, the natural history of a series of 20 false-negative malignant lung cancers between 1994 and 2002. Most of the cases had a favorable outcome, which might (according to the authors) suggest that PET-negative indeterminate pulmonary nodules can be managed conservatively with careful follow-up to monitor growth. Although bronchioloalveolar carcinoma (BAC) is usually reported to be PET-negative, this appeared only be true for pure BAC without invasive component, according to the new WHO classification.[22] PET was as sensitive for tumors with BAC components as for other NSCLC types. Of interest is the study by Duysinx et al.[23] They evaluated the role of FDG-PET in the discrimination between benign and malignant pleural disease in 98 consecutive patients presenting with either pleural thickening or an exudative pleural effusion. Before the diagnosis was made by an invasive procedure, all patients underwent an FDG-PET scan. The sensitivity, specificity and negative predictive value were 96.8%, 88.5% and 93.8%, respectively, and the authors conclude that FDG-PET is an effective tool to differentiate between benign and malignant pleural disease. The discriminating value was weaker when the uptake was only moderate, but this occurred in <15% of the cases. Because of this high negative predictive value, invasive diagnostic evaluation could be avoided in cases where a benign lesion is suspected. However, in some cases (mesothelioma, tuberculosis), thoracoscopy or closed biopsy may still be indicated for accurate diagnosis or culture.[23]

PET might seem to be an ideal tool to restage patients after induction therapy, and to identify downstaged patients who might benefit from subsequent surgery, but the available data so far are conflicting and the role of PET in restaging is yet unclear. Despite initial very promising results, more recent data suggest that FDG-PET has only poor specificity (55%) in predicting the response of the primary tumor to induction chemotherapy and, even more important, the positive predictive value for N2 disease was less than 20%.[24] Even when the subset of patients with peripheral tumors was considered separately, the overall accuracy of nodal staging improved to only 66%. The authors conclude that the PET scan does not perform better than the CT scan in restaging of the mediastinum. All PET scans were made 2 weeks after the last chemotherapy to allow patients to undergo a resection in a timely manner.[24] Delaying the PET scan for an additional 2–4 weeks might have increased the accuracy, but the clinical utility of this approach is questionable.[24] Hellwig et al[25] performed the PET scan 2–11 weeks (median 5 weeks) after completion of the induction therapy and obtained higher sensitivity rates (81%), but this was probably due to regrowth of micrometastatic mediastinal lymph node metastases.

Endoesophageal ultrasonography and endobronchial ultrasonography

During the past few years, several new staging procedures have been developed for the mediastinum. In patients with suspected lymphatic disseminated malignancy, assessment of mediastinal lymph nodes through the esophagus (endoesophageal ultrasonography, EUS) and trachea (endobroncheal ultrasonography, EBUS) provides the clinician with real-time images and the possibility of acquiring samples via FNA for assessment by a pathologist. An overview of the available tools is shown in Table 6.1.

Although several studies have shown EUS–FNA to be equal or superior to PET and CT in diagnostic accuracy (Table 6.2), it is as yet unclear what the place of EUS should be in the diagnostic approach to patients with possible locally advanced NSCLC.[26] The technique has only been studied in expert

Table 6.1   Overview of diagnostic tools for establishing tissue diagnosis and staging in non-small cell lung cancer

Technique	Target areas	Advantages	Limitations
Mediastinoscopy: Parasternal Cervical	5, 6 1, 2L, 2R, 3, 4L, 4R, 7	Histologic sampling	Complication rate 2.5%; requires general anesthesia and hospitalization
EUS–FNA	4L, 5, 7, 8, 9; retroperitoneal; left adrenal gland; left lobe of liver	Outpatient procedure; no general anesthesia; low complication rate; only minor complications	Only cytologic assessment; cartilage rings
EBUS–FNA	2, 3, 4, 7, 10, 11	Outpatient procedure; no general anesthesia; low complication rate; only minor complications	Only cytologic assessment; cartilage
PTNB	Peripheral intrapulmonary lesions; mediastinal and pleural tumors	High rate of success (76–97%)	Pneumothorax; systemic arterial air embolism
TBNA (blind)	7	See EBUS–FNA	Minor bleeding; pneumothorax; pneumomediastinum
VATS	Left or right hemithorax	Histologic sampling	Only unilateral assessment; requires general anesthesia and hospitalization

EUS, endoscopic ultrasound; FNA, fine-needle aspiration; EBUS, endobronchial ultrasound; PTNB, percutaneous transthoracic needle biopsy; TBNA, transbronchial needle aspiration; VATS, video-assisted thoracoscopic surgery.

centers and in highly selected patients. However, as was concluded by Fritscher-Ravens et al,[27] EUS is the most powerful tool to identify patients who are inoperable. Given the relatively low complication rate and the potential huge impact on clinical management, EUS–FNA should be used as a first-line diagnostic tool besides bronchoscopy, CT and PET.

During the EUS procedure, the shape, size, boundary and core structure of the lymph nodes can be assessed, but only the size of the lymph nodes appears to be a significant predictor of malignancy.[28,29]

The use of minimally invasive techniques such as EUS and EBUS is steadily increasing and it has been demonstrated that the use of these techniques influences clinical management. Whereas, for example, lung cancer invasion into the aortic wall (T4, stage IIIb) assessed with CT or MRI has only limited predictive value[30] and may lead to unnecessary thoracotomies or inadequately treated patients, EUS may help to provide a better identification of resectable patients with aortic wall involvement. The sensitivity of EUS was shown to be as high as 83.3% and 92.9% for pT4 and pT2 tumors, respectively. In comparison, the sensitivity of CT for pT4 was 16.7% and for pT2 4.7%.[30] Additionally, surgical interventions could be avoided in 57% of studied patients with enlarged and/or PET-positive mediastinal lymph nodes based on the results of EUS–FNA.[31]

LeBlanc et al[32] investigated the accuracy of EUS in patients with a negative mediastinum on CT. Seventy-two patients were enrolled in this study, of whom were found to be inoperable (mostly pN3) by EUS–FNA. Stage IV disease could be excluded in 9 other patients after assessment of suspicious lesions in the left adrenal gland and left lobe of the liver by EUS–FNA. Consequently, management was altered by EUS in 18 out of 72 patients (25%). All patients with a surgically proven negative mediastinum were correctly staged with EUS–FNA, whereas 5 out of 12 patients with pN2 disease were correctly identified as malignant by the same technique. A major limitation of this study is that PET was not routinely performed in all enrolled patients.

The diagnostic performance of EUS–FNA in the detection of mediastinal lymph node involvement was also investigated by Kramer et al,[29] although only patients with enlarged and/or PET-positive lymph nodes in mediastinum or upper retroperitoneum ($n = 81$) were enrolled in this study. Malignant cells were found in 62% (50/81) of the patients. EUS–FNA was negative or inconclusive in 31 patients (38%), and 19 (61%) of them were eventually found to have lymphatic disseminated disease, either by surgery ($n = 14$) or follow-up ($n = 5$). Therefore, a negative or inconclusive EUS–FNA does not reliably prove the absence of mediastinal metastasis when the pre-test probability based on enlarged lymph nodes on CT is high, although, to a lesser extent, false-negative results have also been reported by others, ranging between 4%[31] and 15%.[33] However, this lower rate of false-negative results could have been biased, because in these series only patients with EUS-accessible lymph nodes have been selected. In conclusion, the negative predictive value (NPV) of EUS–FNA in a patient with a negative mediastinum on CT is high, but the

Table 6.2 Overview of the literature on the diagnostic power of different non-small cell lung cancer (NSCLC) staging procedures of 2004 and 2005

Technique	References (main author)	Sensitivity	Specificity	PPV	NPV	Accuracy
CT	Eloubeidi[31]	NA[e]	NA	NA	NA	40 (31–51)
	Fritscher-Ravens[27]	43 (27–59)	91 (75–98)	85 (62–97)	56 (41–70)	NA
PET	Eloubeidi[31]	NA	NA	NA	NA	50 (37–61)
	Kramer[29]	68 (50–81)	72 (53–86)	75 (58–88)	64 (46–79)	NA
EUS	Eloubeidi[31,a]	80 (64–90)	63 (50–74)	57 (43–70)	83 (70–93)	69 (59–77)
EUS–FNA	Eloubeidi[31,a,b]	93 (80–98)	100 (94–100)	100 (90–100)	95 (88–99)	97 (92–99)
		NA	NA	NA	NA	77 (68–86)
	Caddy:[33,a]					
	Overall	93 (77–99)	100 (78–100)	100 (87–100)	88 (63–99)	95 (84–99)
	NSCLC	92 (73–99)	100 (69–100)	100 (85–100)	83 (51–98)	94 (80–99)
	LeBlanc:[32,c]					
	Overall	NA	90 (76–97)	NA	NA	NA
	N0	NA	100 (91–100)	NA	NA	NA
	N2	29 (10–56)	NA	NA	NA	NA
	Fritscher-Ravens[27,d]	63 (46–77)	100 (89–100)	100 (86–100)	68 (53–81)	NA
EBUS–FNA	Yasufuku[37]	96 (NA)	100 (NA)	NA	NA	97 (NA)
	Rintoul[35]	85 (NA)	100 (NA)	NA	NA	89 (NA)
	Hsu[38]	75[f]–81[g] (NA)	NA	NA	NA	76 (NA)

CT, computed tomography; PET, positron emission tomography; EUS, endoscopic ultrasound; FNA, fine-needle aspiration; EBUS, endobronchial ultrasound; NA, not given; PPV, positive predictive value; NPV, negative predictive value.
Numbers were rounded to whole numbers and expressed as % (95% confidence interval in parentheses).

a Selection of patients was based on CT- and/or PET-positive mediastinum.
b Only patients with EUS-accessible lymph nodes on CT.
c Only patients with a negative mediastinum on CT were studied.
d Only resectable NSCLC cases.
f Hilar mediastinal.
g Submucosal–peribronchial.

positive predictive value (PPV) of EUS–FNA in patients with enlarged and/or PET-positive lymph nodes is low and needs additional investigation.

EUS–FNA significantly increases accuracy when compared with EUS alone (see Table 6.2). This additional affect of FNA on EUS is based on assessment of cytologic tissue samples. Interestingly, the recent development of an EUS-guided FNA/reverse transcription polymerase chain reaction (RT–PCR) could further enhance the diagnostic yield of EUS–FNA.[34] This technique is based on the detection of lung cancer-associated genes such as *CEA*, *CK19*, *KS1/4*, *lunx*, *muc1* and *PDEF* in tissue obtained with EUS–FNA, with *KS1/4* being the most sensitive marker for metastatic disease (93% of cytology-positive samples).[34] Of special interest is a subgroup of patients (approx 30%) in whom a negative cytology was accompanied by KS1/4 positivity. Future studies will have to address whether these patients are at increased risk for recurrence of malignancy after surgical treatment and whether they should be treated with neoadjuvant chemotherapy.

Like EUS–FNA, real-time EBUS-guided transbronchial needle aspiration (TBNA) is an elegant technique for the assessment of mediastinal lymph nodes. Used together with EUS–FNA, almost all mediastinal lymph node stations (Table 6.1) can be reached and sampled.[35] The indications for EBUS include (1) determination of the depth of invasion of tracheobronchial tumors, (2) assessment of tumor invasion into mediastinal blood vessels, (3) visualization and acquiring samples of peritracheal and peribroncheal lymph nodes, and (4) localization and qualitative diagnosis of peripheral pulmonary lesions.[36] Yasufuku et al[37] studied the accuracy of EBUS–FNA in a study comprising 70 patients, in which adequate samples were obtained in 68 patients. The sensitivity, specificity and accuracy are shown in Table 6.2. Thoracotomy, thoracoscopy and mediastinoscopy could be avoided in 23 patients, illustrating that EBUS, like EUS, can have a significant impact on clinical management.[37] Limitations of EBUS include inability to reach subaortic and paraesophageal lymph nodes[37] and inadequate sampling due to limited experience of the physician.[37,38] The yield of EBUS–TBNA can be significantly improved by on-site evaluation of cytology specimens and by at least 7 transbronchial needle aspirates.[39]

Peripheral pulmonary lesions can be evaluated by bronchoscopy using blind or real-time X-ray-guided transbronchial biopsies. However, two papers have addressed a novel approach to evaluating peripheral pulmonary lesions.[36,40]

In the first paper, Kurimoto et al[36] used a miniature ultrasound probe that placed a guide sheath inside the tumor, enabling easy and repetitive access to the lesion with forceps. The diagnostic yield with this technique was 81% and 69% for malignant and benign lesions, respectively. As expected, the diagnostic yield of brush cytology was inferior to that of transbronchial biopsy (TBB). Also, the size (<30 mm) and location of the lesion (left upper apical posterior segment) negatively affected the diagnostic yield of the procedure.

Shinagawa et al[40] focused on virtual bronchoscopy (VB) by CT as a tool for reaching a peripheral lesion with a ultrathin bronchoscope. They used VB to study the route to the peripheral lesion prior to the bronchoscopy and repeated the procedure in the tracheobronchial tree of the patient. Before performing the biopsy, the position of the forceps was confirmed by CT. The accuracy of this technique is shown in Table 6.2. A limitation of the procedure might be the logistical problems of a combined CT scan/bronchoscopy procedure. However, it may provide clinicians with tissue diagnosis in patients who are less suited for video-assisted thoracoscopic surgery (VATS) due to comorbidity, age or poor pulmonary function.

Prognosis

Anatomic factors

The current staging system recognizes a difference in survival between patients with tumors <3 cm (T1 tumors) and those with tumors >3 cm (T2 tumors). However, there has been a continuing debate in the literature as to whether there also exists a relationship between tumor size and outcome for tumors <3 cm. This issue has important implications for lung cancer screening as well as for future refinements of the lung cancer staging system. If survival with a subcentimeter lesion is similar to that with a 3 cm tumor, the advantage of the spiral CT scan for detecting smaller tumors will not translate into a meaningful survival benefit. In particular, the study by Patz et al[41] has stimulated this scientific debate, because, surprisingly, they did not find a correlation between tumor size and survival in 510 patients with pathologic stage IA lung cancer from a single institution after 18 years of follow-up.[41] This unexpected result could be explained by several confounding variables. The overall survival rate of 80% in this series was unusually high and, given the low number of deaths, the study might have been underpowered to detect the influence of size on survival. In addition, overall survival instead of lung cancer survival was reported, which might also have reduced the likelihood of detecting a correlation between size and survival. Furthermore, the database used by Patz et al[41] was a surgical database in which advanced cancers were not registered; because 80% of the registered cases were stage I, only 25 cases had cancers <1 cm, and approximately 90% of them were resected. Such a registry does not give a fair picture of the size–stage relationship present in a general cancer registry.[42] Since this publication, several papers have been published demonstrating that size also matters for tumors <3 cm.[43–46] Wisnivesky et al[45] found a clear size–stage relationship in the 158 794 cases available in the US National Cancer Institute (NCI) Surveillance, Epidemiology, and End Results (SEER) Registry database, even for tumors <3 cm in greatest diameter. The fact that symptomatic small cancers are more likely to be detected and entered in a general database leads to an overestimation of the rate of dissemination of small cancers. Thus, it is even probable that the rate of stage I lung cancer for tumors <15 mm in an asymptomatic screening population is even higher than the 58% in the SEER database.[45] The disease-specific cure rates for lung cancer ranged from 69% (95% CI 64–74%) for tumors 5–15 mm to 43% (95% CI

39–48%) for tumors >45 mm 160 months after diagnosis. This long follow-up period makes lead-time bias as an explanation for a better survival less likely,[46] because the survival curves become almost parallel after 12 years, suggesting that even the smallest tumors that metastasized before resection should have had time enough to progress and lead to death of the individual within this 12-year follow-up period. Wisniveusky concluded that smaller tumor size is associated with improved curability, and that subclassification by size within stage I tumors may be important – a conclusion supported by others.[43,44] On the other hand, Takeda et al[44] retrospectively evaluated the records of 603 pathologically N0 NSCLC cases after complete resection in the period 1992–1996. No significant difference was found in 5-year survival for tumors <2 cm ($n = 171$), 2–3 cm ($n = 202$) and 3–5 cm ($n = 170$), but tumors >5 cm ($n = 60$) had a worse prognosis, with 5-year survival rates of 79.6%, 72.7%, 68.1% and 46.6%, respectively.[44]

Identification of patients with the highest rate of recurrence after surgery has largely been based on the TNM staging system, but several investigators have found that the maximum standardized uptake value of FDG-PET (SUV_{max}) is also predictive of survival. In a retrospective study of 100 patients with NSCLC or carcinoid tumors stage pT1–4,N0–2,M0 treated by surgical resection, it was found that the primary tumor size and the SUV_{max} were independent prognostic factors, and, when combined together, a subgroup with an extremely poor prognosis was identified.[47] Vesselle et al[48] also investigated retrospectively the relationship between tumor stage and SUV_{max} in 178 NSCLC patients, but they normalized the SUV_{max} to tumor size in order to correct for physical partial-volume effects, which might lead to lower SUV_{max} in smaller tumors based on measurement artifacts and not on biologic differences. Indeed, they found a relationship between SUV_{max} and tumor stage, but when corrected for partial volume, this relationship disappeared, and the SUV_{max} of the primary tumor was no longer prognostic for survival.[48]

Stage IA BAC, which is defined as a non-invasive adenocarcinoma without evidence of stromal, vascular or pleural invasion, appears to have an excellent prognosis, with no lymph node involvement and a 5-year disease-free survival rate of 100%.[49] Limited resection might therefore be curative in patients with focal BAC without evidence of invasive features or lymph node involvement. A recently detected marker for invasiveness of BAC is the squamous cell carcinoma-related oncogene (SCCRO). SCCRO expression increases with progressively more invasive histologic type from pure BAC, through bronchioloalveolar carcinoma with focal invasion, towards adenocarcinoma with bronchioloalveolar features.[50]

Another anatomic prognostic factor appears to be the number of hilar or intralobar lymph node stations involved. The prognosis of single-station N1 disease was found to be significantly better than for multiple N1 disease, with a 5-year survival rate of 45% vs 32%, respectively.[44] Survival for multiple N1 disease was similar to that for single N2 disease (32% vs 31% at 5 years). Other anatomic prognostic factors found are perineural invasion and invasion of blood vessels.[51] In 72 stage I and II NSCLC patients, the overall 5-year survival rate was 62.5%: in cases of blood vessel invasion, this was only 23.5%, whereas in cases without vessel invasion, the 5-year survival rate was 74.5%. In this study, lymph vessel invasion was found to have no impact on survival. Sayar et al[52] came to the opposite conclusion, and found both lymphatic and perineural invasion to be significant prognostic factors, whereas vessel invasion was not.

Currently, metastases in lymph nodes or other tissues such as bone marrow are reported when they are >2 mm in their largest diameter with hematoxylin and eosin (H&E) staining. Smaller clusters, isolated cells or cells detected only by immunohistochemistry (IHC) or PCR fall in the categories described by the terms micrometastases, occult metastases or minimal residual disease.[53] Although a number of tumor-specific molecular characteristics have been identified in cytokeratin-positive epithelial cells in bone marrow, indicating that these cells are indeed tumor cells, the controversy about their clinical significance is continuing. In 212 bone marrow specimens from patients with NSCLC, 34.4% of specimens were cytokeratin-positive without relation to age, gender, cell type, TNM status or 5-year survival.[54] In another large series of 351 NSCLC patients, cytokeratin positivity in bone marrow aspirates was associated with poor prognosis for stage II and IIIA,[55] but for stage I disease only the detection of cytokeratin-positive cells in the regional lymph nodes was a poor prognostic sign in both univariate and multivariate analyses.[55]

Sardari et al[56] classified NSCLC into three new categories on the basis of growth patterns indicated on H&E staining: (1) destructive (angiogenetic) growth, with destruction of the lung parenchyma and formation of tumor-associated stroma at the interface with the surrounding normal tissue; (2) a papillary (intermediate) growth pattern, with preservation of the alveolar structure of the lung parenchyma with (at the interface) formation of stromal stalks containing capillary alveolar blood vessels and subsequent angiogenesis; and (3) an alveolar (non-angiogenic) growth pattern, with preservation of the alveolar structure of the lung containing septal blood vessels but without evidence of new stroma formation at the interface. Solid tumor cell nests fill the alveolar spaces, often with necrosis in the center of the nests.[56] Based on these features, 279 stage I NSCLC patients who underwent curative resection were classified as destructive (angiogenic, $n = 196$), papillary (intermediate, $n = 38$) and alveolar (non-angiogenic, $n = 45$). Alveolar growth (hazard ratio (HR) = 1.825, 95% CI 1.117–2.980, $p = 0.016$) and papillary growth (HR = 1.977, 95% CI 1.169–3.345, $p = 0.011$) turned out to be independent predictors for poor overall and disease-free survival after 140 months of follow-up.[56] Sardari et al[56] suggest that alveolar and papillary growth is associated with a poor prognosis because vascularization of alveolar growth is more efficient. Angiogenesis in destructive growth is chaotic and inefficient and leads to less efficient growth. The clinical consequences might be that alveolar growth will probably not respond to angiogenesis inhibitors and that high-risk patients with an alveolar or papillary growth pattern may be candidates for adjuvant chemotherapy. The different growth patterns may also respond differently to chemotherapy and radiotherapy.[56] Mineo et al[57] found that stage I

NSCLC patients with vascular endothelial growth factor (VEGF) overexpression, high microvessel density (MVD), CD34 and CD105 expression, and tumor vessel invasion had shorter overall survival on univariate analysis, while those with CD34 and VEGF expression had shorter survival on multivariate analysis. Tumor vessel invasion, high MVD and CD34 expression were highly predictive of poor outcome and could also help to identify patients who might benefit from adjuvant chemotherapy.[57] Recent findings suggest that the lymphatic system fulfills not only a passive role in the metastatic process. Tumors release substances that activate growth of lymphatic vessels. Several investigators have found that tumor cells home to metastatic sites as a result of constitutive chemokine expression at those sites and the expression of their receptors on tumor cells.[57a,57b] As VEGF promotes lymphatic metastases, Tamura et al[58] investigated the accuracy of VEGF-C in patients with NSCLC for predicting the presence or absence of lymph node metastases preoperatively. Although serum VEGF-C levels overlapped to a great extent in patients with and without lymph node involvement, statistically significant higher VEGF-C concentrations were found in patients with lymph node metastases ($p < 0.001$). The performance of serum VEGF-C was slightly better than standard CT criteria in detecting locally advanced disease, but when patients were classified into quartiles based on serum levels of VEGF-C, the accuracy of the CT scan in predicting the presence of lymph node metastases could be improved.[58]

Non-anatomic factors

Gender has been reported as a predictor for NSCLC survival, but most reports are limited to selected groups of patients. In a large cohort of 4618 prospectively enrolled NSCLC patients followed for a 6-year period, male gender turned out to be an unfavorable prognostic factor for survival. Men appeared to survive to the same proportion as the group of women in the next immediately advanced TNM stage and, after considering multiple known predictors of lung cancer survival, men remained at 20% increased mortality risk compared with women following the diagnosis of NSCLC.[59] Even though men develop cardiovascular disease 10 years earlier than women, the observed gender differences could not be attributed to non-lung-cancer-related causes. The fact that women are diagnosed at earlier stages might be a consequence of more frequent consultations and more routine general medical follow-ups in women, but also lower growth rates, genetic predisposition and resistance to tumor progression are possible explanations.[59] Tammemagi et al[60] evaluated the association between stage, symptoms and survival. Only 14.8% of the 1154 NSCLC patients were diagnosed while asymptomatic. They demonstrated that adverse symptoms such as hoarseness, hemoptysis, dyspnea, neurologic symptoms, weight loss and weakness/fatigue were collectively and independently associated with male gender, African-American race/ethnicity and marital status (being spouseless). Past studies have frequently attributed race/ethnic disparities in cancer survival to stage differences, but this study for the first time demonstrated that adverse symptoms explained, independently, 43% of the race/ethnic and marital disparities in lung cancer survival beyond stage.[60] Blacks accumulate more adverse symptoms than whites prior to diagnosis, and this may reflect greater delay between the onset of symptoms and diagnosis or more aggressive disease. The study findings reinforce the need for high-risk patients to seek medical attention as soon as any lung carcinoma-associated symptoms arise.[60] The majority (80%) of patients with stage III/IV NSCLC have evidence of a systemic inflammatory response, and the magnitude of the systemic response (C-reactive protein (CRP) concentrations) was associated with increased weight loss, reduced serum albumin, reduced performance status, increased fatigue and reduced survival.[61]

Several papers have addressed the role of serum carcinoembryonic antigen (CEA) level as a prognostic marker in stage I NSCLC.[62–64] In 1000 consecutive stage I NSCLC patients, CEA levels were increased in 36.8% of patients; these levels normalized in 24.2% after surgery and remained elevated in 12.6%. Multivariate analysis demonstrated that both preoperative and postoperative CEA levels were independent prognostic determinants along with age, gender and tumor size,[62,63] and that elevated CEA levels after surgery could be used as a marker for selecting patients for adjuvant chemotherapy.[62] Even subnormal CEA level was found to be an independent prognostic indicator. The 5-year survival rate of 724 patients with stage IA NSCLC was 87% with postoperative subnormal CEA levels, 75% with normal CEA levels and 53% with high levels of CEA ($p < 0.0001$).[64] The prognostic role of CEA in predicting postoperative survival was greater for adenocarcinomas than for squamous cell carcinomas, probably because of the higher proportion of smokers among patients with squamous cell carcinomas[63] (smoking inceases CEA levels).

In the past few years, the number of studies evaluating the potential use of serum or plasma tumor DNA in cancer diagnosis and prognosis has increased steadily. The presence of cell-free DNA circulating in plasma has been described in patients with malignant and inflammatory processes. Furthermore, DNA alterations can be detected in plasma matching the genetic changes of the primary tumor. For NSCLC, both quantitative and qualitative studies suggest potential applications in disease management, but translation into the clinic is currently a matter of debate because of the difficulty of comparing and normalizing the data as a result of lack of technical standardization and relatively small studies. In a rigorously validated prospectively controlled study, it was impossible to detect a difference in DNA concentrations between cancer patients and controls by a reproducible assay for quantification of plasma DNA by real-time PCR.[65] This is in contrast to a study published by Gautschi et al.[66] They established an accurate and reproducible technique to quantify circulating DNA in two independent laboratories, and compared plasma and serum for DNA quantification, correlating DNA levels with response to chemotherapy, prognostic markers and survival. They found that the real-time PCR technique is feasible, accurate and suitable for routine clinical application, and that DNA concentration in plasma correlated significantly with lactate dehydrogenase

(LDH) levels, advanced tumor stage, poor survival and disease progression under therapy. Serum DNA levels only correlated with leukocyte counts. Gautschi et al[66] concluded that plasma is better suited for quantitative studies because it is more representative for tumor status and is enriched with tumor DNA. Neither plasma nor serum are in their opinion suitable for prediction of the response to chemotherapy.[66] By using a panel of 12 polymorphic microsatellites targeting 9 different loci known to be frequently altered in NSCLC and SCLC, Beau-Faller et al[67] were able to identify and to characterize tumor DNA in plasma of 88% (30/34) of the lung cancer patients, with a similar sensitivity in NSCLC and SCLC. A reduced panel of 6 markers showed a sensitivity of 85%.[67] Other groups, however, found similar genetic alterations in patients with other respiratory diseases (42%), making this method not suitable for this patient population.[68] Circulating antibodies to p53 do not seem to correlate with clinical parameters and survival.[66] However, in vitro mutagen sensitivity of peripheral lymphocytes to bleomycin correlated with poor overall survival and poor disease-specific survival in patients with stage III NSCLC treated with radiotherapy and chemotherapy. Compromised DNA repair may increase the risk of developing cancer and lead to biologically more aggressive tumors and decreased survival, but it may also reduce the capacity to repair DNA damage after chemotherapy and/or radiotherapy. The 6-year disease-specific survival rate was 27% in patients with high bleomycin sensitivity compared with 46% in patients without such sensitivity ($p < 0.01$), even after adjustment for smoking status, age and radiation dose.[69] There was a trend toward worse local regional control and worse disease-free survival among patients with high bleomycin sensitivity, but there was no difference between the two groups in distant metastases-free survival and radiation-related complications. These results indicate that it might be possible in the future to tailor treatment based on genotype or repair phenotype.[69]

Numerous studies have focused on improving survival in early-stage lung cancer, as 30–40% of patients relapse after curative resection. Although platinum-based adjuvant chemotherapy has been found to improve survival in patients with completely resected NSCLC, lung cancer is a very heterogeneous disease, and identification of the high-risk group most suitable for adjuvant therapy is warranted. In the period 2004–5, numerous investigators have tried to relate the expression of a single or multiple individual proteins to the prognosis in NSCLC. The results are summarized in Tables 6.3–6.6, which include studies on promoter hypermethylation (Table 6.3),[70,71] degradation of the extracellular matrix (Table 6.4),[72–79] growth factors (Table 6.5)[80–87] and cell cycle control (Table 6.6).[88–97]

Although these studies help us to understand the complex process of carcinogenesis, the evaluation of individual prognostic biomarkers – often in a small number of patients – has several limitations, including the biologic and statistical interactions of these markers with other factors that could influence patient outcome. If prospectively validated, these genetic and epigenetic biomarkers may be useful markers for prognosis as well as new targets for biologic targeted

Table 6.3   Prognostic factors in patients with non-small cell lung cancer: promoter hypermethylation

Reference (first author)	Marker	N	Stage	Survival	Independent prognostic factor
Wang[70]	$p16^{INK4A}$	119	I/II (60%)	Yes, poor	No
			IIIA (40%)	No	No
Wang[70]	RASSF1A	119	I/II (60%)	No	No
			IIIA (40%)	Yes, poor	Yes
Kim[71]	$p16^{INK4A}$, RARβP2, DAPK, MGMT	61	I/II	No	No

RARβP2, retinoic acid receptor β-promoter; DAPK, death-associated protein kinase; MGMT, O^6-methylguanine-DNA-methyltransferase.

Table 6.4   Prognostic factors in patients with non-small cell lung cancer: degradation of the extracellular matrix

Reference (first author)	Marker	N	Stage	Survival	Independent prognostic factor
Ishikawa[78]	ADAM8	363	I–IV	Higher expression in advanced disease	NR
Shintani[77]	ADAM9	In vitro	NA	Overexpression correlates with brain metastases	NA
Gouyer[79]	MMP-9	116	I/II	No	No
Gouyer[79]	TIMP-1	116	I/II	Yes, poor	Yes
Aljada[75]	TIMP-1	160	I–IIIA	Yes, poor	Yes
Yamamoto[76]	p97	207	I/II	Yes, poor	Yes
Pinto[74]	MMP-9	152	I, II (58%)	Yes, for stage I	Yes, for all stages
			IV (42%)	No	
Nishiumi[72]	MUC2	79	I,II	Yes, poor	NR
Spano[73]	CXCR4	61	I	Yes, better	NR

NR, not reported; NA, not applicable; ADAM8, disintegrin and metalloproteinase domain-8; ADAM9, disintegrin and metalloproteinase domain 9; MMP, matrix metalloproteinase; TIMP, tissue inhibitor of metalloproteinases; p97, valosin-containing protein (VCP); MUC2, human mucin core protein 2, located on chromosome 11p15; CXCR4, chemokine receptor 4 (receptor for stromal cell-derived factor 1).

therapies. Of direct clinical relevance is probably the finding that overexpression of both the epidermal growth factor receptor (EGFR) and HER2 (ERBB2/Neu) proteins in patients with stage I NSCLC is an independent predictor of recurrence and poor survival compared with either one of these proteins or no expression.[81] This is the first report to demonstrate a significant relationship between

Table 6.5 Prognostic factors in patients with non-small cell lung cancer: growth factors

Reference (first author)	Marker	N	Stage	Survival	Independent prognostic factor
Shah[85]	EGFR	63	I (63%) II, III (37%)	Yes, better	Yes
Shah[85]	Syndecan-1	63	I (63%) II,III (37%)	Yes, better	Yes
Onn[81]	EGFR and synchronous HER2 (ERBB2/Neu) overexpression	111	I	Yes, poor	NR
Pelosi[86]	HER2	345	I	No	NR
Brattström[83]	HER2 without synchronous EGFR overexpression	53	I	Yes, poor	NR
Selvaggi[80]	EGFR	130	I–IIIA	Yes, poor	Yes
Ferraro[87]	EGR1 underexpression	125	I–III	Yes, poor	Yes
Marchetti[82]	HIN-1 underexpression	91	I	Yes, poor	Yes
Ren[84]	HDGF overexpression	98	I	Yes, poor	Yes

EGFR, epidermal growth factor receptor; EGR1, early growth response gene 1; HIN-1, high in normal 1; HDGF, hepatoma-derived growth factor; NR, not reported.

Table 6.6   Prognostic factors in patients with non-small cell lung cancer: cell cycle control

Reference (first author)	Marker	N	Stage	Survival	Independent prognostic factor
Dworakowska[94]	pRb and p53	195	I-IV	No	No
Yoshida[88]	Cyclin B1 and Wee1 expression	79	I-III	Yes	Yes
Iniesta[90]	3p deletions and telomase reactivation	66	I-IV	Yes, poor	NR
Vicent[92]	CL100/MKP-1	108	I-IIIA	Yes, poor	Yes
Osoegawa[93]	Skp2 overexpression	138	I-IV	Yes, poor	Yes
Bepler[89]	RRM1 overexpression	126	I-IV	Yes, better	Yes
	PTEN overexpression	126	I-IV	Yes, better	No
Vischioni[95]	Nuclear survivin expression	53	III-IV	Yes, better	Yes
Shinohara[97]	Nuclear survivin expression	144	I-II	Yes, better	Yes
Wang[96]	p14[ARF] expression with MDM2 underexpression in tumors with wild-type p53 overexpression	94	I-IV	Yes, poor	NR
Fukuoka[91]	Synchronous nuclear BRM and BRG1 expression	229	I-IV	Yes, better	NR

pRb, retinoblastoma protein; MKP-1, mitogen-activated protein kinase phosphatase 1; Skp2, S-phase kinase-associated protein 2.

synchronous coexpression of EGFR and HER2 at the level of protein and patient prognosis in a large cohort: 111 surgically treated patients with pathologic stage I NSCLC after 160 months of follow-up. This clinical observation supports earlier preclinical studies showing that EGFR–HER2 heterodimerization leads to a higher proliferative index than that of individual homodimers. It is suggested that treatment with EGFR tyrosine kinase inhibitors might be most efficient in NSCLC patients expressing both EGFR and HER2, and that adjuvant therapy for stage I NSCLC expressing both proteins might be appealing and should be investigated in a clinical trial.[81]

The role of HER2 expression was reviewed by Meert et al[98] in a meta-analysis of 30 studies, of which 24 dealt with NSCLC. They found that HER2 expression was associated with a significant detrimental effect on survival in 13 studies, whereas 16 studies showed improved survival and 16 studies were not significant.[98] For NSCLC, the HR was 1.55 (95% CI 1.29–1.86) in favor of tumors that do not express HER2, but it was concluded that there might have been some selection bias in favor of the significant studies showing HER2 overexpression.[98]

Also, RRM1 and PTEN appear to be of prognostic significance in early-stage lung cancer.[89] RRM1 controls cell proliferation through deoxynucleotide production and metastatic propensity through *PTEN* induction. Patients with high levels of both proteins had a better overall and disease-free survival.[89] High RRM1 levels have also been associated with poor outcome in patients with metastatic NSCLC who received combination chemotherapy with gemcitabine and cisplatin,[99,100] probably through decreased cytotoxicity of gemcitabine in tumors with high RRM1 expression.

Of great interest also are the reports on survivin, which is a member of the inhibitor of apoptosis protein gene family, regulating both programmed cell death and mitosis; it is undetectable in normal tissues but is highly expressed in most malignancies.[95,97]

In 144 patients with pathologic stage I and II, nuclear staining for survivin had an increased risk of disease recurrence (HR = 2.95) and death (HR = 2.74) after 5 years of follow-up, independently of other staging factors. There was also a significant correlation between nuclear staining and negative cytoplasmic staining, indicating that nuclear localization of survivin appears to lead to reduced cytoplasmic survivin levels. In the nucleus, survivin interacts with aurora B kinase and INCENP to complete mitosis. Therefore, strong nuclear staining may represent an increased number of mitotic events, and inhibition of survivin may lead to mitotic arrest. Conversely, cytoplasmic survivin inhibits apoptosis by blocking caspase-9. It has also been shown that overexpression of survivin was associated with radioresistance, and that inhibition of survivin was capable of reversing this effect.[101] Therefore, nuclear survivin might not only be a new independent prognostic factor but also – especially because of its selective expression in tumor tissue – a new therapeutic target in selected patients and a marker of response to radiation therapy. So far, however, no correlation between the expression and localization of survivin and response to chemotherapy has been found.[95]

Another new biologic marker for NSCLC is Ki-67, a nuclear protein involved in cell proliferation regulation. In a meta-analysis, Ki-67 was found to be an independent bad prognostic factor for survival in 37 studies involving 3983 patients with an HR of 1.56 (95% CI 1.30–1.87).[111a] Data from Berger et al[102] suggest that expression of the multidrug resistance protein 1 (MRP1) is associated with a better prognosis, especially in patients not pretreated with chemotherapy. MRP1 overexpression is likely to be an inherent feature of original epithelial cells that is further activated during malignant transformation, and then downregulated during disease progression. Consequently, MRP1-overexpressing tumors are less aggressive, tend to be more differentiated and especially resistant to chemotherapy.[102] Also, polymorphisms of the DNA repair genes XPD and XRCC1 independently predicted survival in platinum-treated patients with stage III and IV NSCLC.[103]

Recent technological advances in gene expression profiling (in particular with cDNA and oligonucleotide microarrays) allow the simultaneous analysis of the expression of thousands of genes and may lead to a molecular classification of NSCLC. The initial assessments of NSCLC prognosis in postsurgical patients by gene array profiling and proteomics demonstrate that these technologies can provide a broader and more complex picture than that provided by assessment of individual proteins,[104–109] as is also concluded by Petty et al[110] in their review on this topic. Although substantial work has been done in the field of gene array and proteomic profiling in lung cancer, routine clinical applications of these methods are not yet in place. What is especially needed is validation of selected candidate genes from the exploratory dataset in an independent new cohort: the importance of this is illustrated by the work of Blackhall et al.[111] After selection of 11 potential prognostic genes and evaluation of their expression using RT–PCR in the original group of patients, their clinical significance was assessed both in the original group and in an independent validation set. By this method, the original group was separated into two groups with different disease-free survival, but these findings could not be validated in the separate validation cohort.[111] In this respect also, the paper on how to design and conduct a microarray study and what the caveats are is of great practical value.

SMALL CELL LUNG CANCER

Small cell lung cancer (SCLC) accounts for approximately 20% of all cases of lung cancer. If untreated, it has a poor prognosis in the range of 5–12 weeks; even with therapy, median survival is approximately 8 months and the 2-year survival rate less than 5%. At presentation, 80–90% of the patients have already local or distant metastases. Accurate staging is critical for treatment and prognosis. The addition of FDG-PET to conventional staging might lead to an upstaging between 8% and 33%,[112,113] and complete response, as assessed by PET, was found to be an independent predictor of disease-free survival.[112]

Therefore, FDG-PET appears to be of great value for initial staging and treatment planning in patients with presumed limited-stage disease.[113]

In a review by Buttery et al,[114] the role of the extracellular matrix (ECM) in the metastatic potential of SCLC is discussed. When SCLC cells adhere less strongly to the ECM, they are more mobile and have a higher capacity to metastasize. The more mobile tumors cells are, the more susceptible to chemotherapy-induced DNA damage and apoptosis they appear to be. This is explained through the protective effect of ECM-produced β_1 integrins, preventing chemotherapy-induced DNA caspase-3 activation and apoptosis through protein tyrosine kinase activation.[114] Chemotherapy would thus selectively spare those cancer cells most adherent and most protected by the ECM, and, with subsequent genetic damage induced by the chemotherapy, drug-resistant clones are selected. β_1 integrin and p53 are considered to be part of the same signal pathway that induces apoptosis. High expressions of both β_1 integrin and p53 were found to be independent prognostic factors, more closely related to SCLC prognosis than clinical stage.[115] Novel strategies may therefore be directed at identifying and inhibiting integrin-mediated and p53-dependent cell survival signals, which may improve response to chemotherapy.

Several investigators have addressed the prognostic significance of KIT in SCLC.[116-118] Because proliferation of malignant cells in SCLC is mediated by an autocrine loop between the transmembrane KIT receptor and its ligand stem cell factor (SCF), it was expected that KIT-expressing tumors would have a poor prognosis. In a large retrospective analysis of 203 SCLC patients, the prognostic value of KIT expression was investigated. Overall survival was better for the SCLC tumors that expressed KIT (358 days) than for those with no KIT expression (151 days, $p < 0.01$), without difference for the level of KIT expression. However, an association was found between the proportion of KIT-positive cells within a tumor and survival, with patients with <25% KIT positive cells or KIT-negative tumors having the worst prognosis and KIT expression in >75% of the cells having the best prognosis. The association of KIT expression with better prognosis might be explained by the fact that if a higher proportion of the cells are in the cell cycle, they are more susceptible to chemotherapy, which is supported by the fact that 50% of the KIT-positive tumors became negative after chemotherapy. In smaller studies of 60 and 42 SCLC patients, Boldrini et al[118] and Blackhall et al[116] respectively, did not find a significant relationship between the expression of KIT and survival, TNM stage or response to chemotherapy in tumor tissue from surgically resected or biopsies from SCLC cases. So far, the role of the KIT tyrosine kinase inhibitor imatinib is unclear, and it should probably be directed only to patients with KIT-positive tumors.[119]

The current knowledge on serum biomarkers for SCLC is reviewed by Taneja et al.[120] Of interest also is the study on the prognostic significance of serum YKL-40 levels in SCLC. The biologic function of YKL-40 in cancer patients is unknown, but it is a growth factor for connective tissue cells and a potent migration factor for endothelial cells and vascular smooth muscle cells. It appears to be a prognostic factor for SCLC independent of stage, LDH levels or performance status.[121] In 200 patients with SCLC, the prognostic significance of antibodies to Hu or voltage-gated calcium channel (VGCC) was investigated, but although Hu antibodies were found in 25% of all patients and VGCC antibodies in 5%, no correlation with disease extent or survival was found.[122] There was also no relationship between the level of Hu antibodies and the appearance of the neurologic paraneoplastic syndrome.[122]

Neuroendocrine lung tumors can be classified as low-grade typical carcinoid, intermediate-grade atypical carcinoid and high-grade SCLC and large cell neuroendocrine carcinoma (LCNEC). Because of the histologic similarities and overlap in clinical behavior between SCLC and LCNEC, it has been proposed to reclassify the two groups in one single group of high-grade neuroendocrine tumors (HGNTs). Gene expression profiling of 40 000 genes in 38 surgically resected HGNT and 11 cell lines was used in order to reveal the underlying molecular characteristics of the tumor and to define new subclasses with different prognostic significance by unsupervised hierarchical clustering.[123] All samples of typical carcinoid, large-cell carcinoma and adenocarcinoma formed distinct clusters according to histologic type. However, SCLC and LCNEC were indistinguishable and formed two prognostic groups independent of histopathologic status. Many of the genes upregulated in the poor-prognosis subgroup of HGNT were found to be neuroendocrine.[123] This study illustrates that gene expression profiling could be used for the development of gene staging to guide therapy from the moment of diagnosis.

REFERENCES

1. Hetzel M, Hetzel J, Arslandemir C et al. Reliability of symptoms to determine use of bone scans to identify bone metastases in lung cancer: prospective study. BMJ 2004; 328: 1051–2.

2. Hetzel M, Arslandemir C, Konig HH et al. F-18 NaF PET for detection of bone metastases in lung cancer: accuracy, cost-effectiveness, and impact on patient management. J Bone Miner Res 2003; 18: 2206–14.

3. Schirrmeister H, Arslandemir C, Glatting G et al. Omission of bone scanning according to staging guidelines leads to futile therapy in non-small cell lung cancer. Eur J Nucl Med Mol Imaging 2004; 31: 964–8.

4. Erturan S, Yaman M, Aydin G et al. The role of whole-body bone scanning and clinical factors in detecting bone metastases in patients with non-small cell lung cancer. Chest 2005; 127: 449–54.

5. Suzuki K, Yamamoto M, Hasegawa Y et al. Magnetic resonance imaging and computed tomography in the diagnoses of brain metastases of lung cancer. Lung Cancer 2004; 46: 357–60.

6. Benamore RE, Chippington SJ, Entwisle JJ. The value of performing head CT in screening for cerebral metastases in patients with potentially resectable non-small cell lung cancer: experience from a UK cardiothoracic centre. Clin Radiol

2005; 60: 619–20; author reply 620–1.

7. Kumaran M, Benamore RE, Vaidhyanath R et al. Ultrasound guided cytological aspiration of supraclavicular lymph nodes in patients with suspected lung cancer. Thorax 2005; 60: 229–33.

8. Line BR, White CS. Positron emission tomography scanning for the diagnosis and management of lung cancer. Curr Treat Options Oncol 2004; 5: 63–73.

9. Detterbeck FC, Falen S, Rivera MP et al. Seeking a home for a PET, Part 2: Defining the appropriate place for positron emission tomography imaging in the staging of patients with suspected lung cancer. Chest 2004; 125: 2300–8.

10. Detterbeck FC, Falen S, Rivera MP et al. Seeking a home for a PET, Part 1: Defining the appropriate place for positron emission tomography imaging in the diagnosis of pulmonary nodules or masses. Chest 2004; 125: 2294–9.

11. Detterbeck FC, Vansteenkiste JF, Morris DE et al. Seeking a home for a PET, Part 3: Emerging applications of positron emission tomography imaging in the management of patients with lung cancer. Chest 2004; 126: 1656–66.

12. Vansteenkiste J, Fischer BM, Dooms C et al. Positron-emission tomography in prognostic and therapeutic assessment of lung cancer: systematic review. Lancet Oncol 2004; 5: 531–40.

13. Schrevens L, Lorent N, Dooms C et al. The role of PET scan in diagnosis, staging, and management of non-small cell lung cancer. Oncologist 2004; 9: 633–43.

14. Vansteenkiste JF, Stroobants SG. Positron emission tomography in the management of non-small cell lung cancer. Hematol Oncol Clin North Am 2004; 18: 269–88.

15. Gould MK, Kuschner WG, Rydzak

CE et al. Test performance of positron emission tomography and computed tomography for mediastinal staging in patients with non-small-cell lung cancer: a meta-analysis. Ann Intern Med 2003; 139: 879–92.

16. Gonzalez-Stawinski GV, Lemaire A, Merchant F et al. A comparative analysis of positron emission tomography and mediastinoscopy in staging non-small cell lung cancer. J Thorac Cardiovasc Surg 2003; 126: 1900–5.

17. Kelly RF, Tran T, Holmstrom A et al. Accuracy and cost-effectiveness of [18F]-2-fluoro-deoxy-D-glucose-positron emission tomography scan in potentially resectable non-small cell lung cancer. Chest 2004; 125: 1413–23.

18. Viney RC, Boyer MJ, King MT et al. Randomized controlled trial of the role of positron emission tomography in the management of stage I and II non-small-cell lung cancer. J Clin Oncol 2004; 22: 2357–62.

19. Cerfolio RJ, Ojha B, Bryant AS et al. The accuracy of integrated PET-CT compared with dedicated PET alone for the staging of patients with non-small cell lung cancer. Ann Thorac Surg 2004; 78: 1017–23.

20. Kahn D, Menda Y, Kernstine K et al. The utility of 99mTc depreotide compared with F-18 fluorodeoxyglucose positron emission tomography and surgical staging in patients with suspected non-small cell lung cancer. Chest 2004; 125: 494–501.

21. Cheran SK, Nielsen ND, Patz EF Jr. False-negative findings for primary lung tumors on FDG positron emission tomography: staging and prognostic implications. AJR Am J Roentgenol 2004; 182: 1129–32.

22. Yap CS, Schiepers C, Fishbein MC et al. FDG-PET imaging in lung cancer: how sensitive is it for bronchioloalveolar carcinoma? Eur J

Nucl Med Mol Imaging 2002; 29: 1166–73.

23. Duysinx B, Nguyen D, Louis R et al. Evaluation of pleural disease with 18-fluorodeoxyglucose positron emission tomography imaging. Chest 2004; 125: 489–93.

24. Port JL, Kent MS, Korst RJ et al. Positron emission tomography scanning poorly predicts response to preoperative chemotherapy in non-small cell lung cancer. Ann Thorac Surg 2004; 77: 254–9.

25. Hellwig D, Graeter TP, Ukena D et al. Value of F-18-fluorodeoxyglucose positron emission tomography after induction therapy of locally advanced bronchogenic carcinoma. J Thorac Cardiovasc Surg 2004; 128: 892–9.

26. Vilmann P, Larsen SS. Endoscopic ultrasound-guided biopsy in the chest: little to lose, much to gain. Eur Respir J 2005; 25: 400–1.

27. Fritscher-Ravens A, Davidson BL, Hauber HP et al. Endoscopic ultrasound, positron emission tomography, and computerized tomography for lung cancer. Am J Respir Crit Care Med 2003; 168: 1293–7.

28. Schmulewitz N, Wildi SM, Varadarajulu S et al. Accuracy of EUS criteria and primary tumor site for identification of mediastinal lymph node metastasis from non-small-cell lung cancer. Gastrointest Endosc 2004; 59: 205–12.

29. Kramer H, van Putten JW, Post WJ et al. Oesophageal endoscopic ultrasound with fine needle aspiration improves and simplifies the staging of lung cancer. Thorax 2004; 59: 596–601.

30. Schroder C, Schonhofer B, Vogel B. Transesophageal echographic determination of aortic invasion by lung cancer. Chest 2005; 127: 438–42.

31. Eloubeidi MA, Cerfolio RJ, Chen VK et al. Endoscopic ultrasound-guided fine needle aspiration of mediastinal lymph node in patients with suspected lung cancer after positron emission tomography and computed tomography scans. Ann Thorac Surg 2005; 79: 263–8.

32. LeBlanc JK, Devereaux BM, Imperiale TF et al. Endoscopic ultrasound in non-small cell lung cancer and negative mediastinum on computed tomography. Am J Respir Crit Care Med 2005; 171: 177–82.

33. Caddy G, Conron M, Wright G et al. The accuracy of EUS–FNA in assessing mediastinal lymphadenopathy and staging patients with NSCLC. Eur Respir J 2005; 25: 410–15.

34. Wallace MB, Block MI, Gillanders W et al. Accurate molecular detection of non-small cell lung cancer metastases in mediastinal lymph nodes sampled by endoscopic ultrasound-guided needle aspiration. Chest 2005; 127: 430–7.

35. Rintoul RC, Skwarski KM, Murchison JT et al. Endobronchial and endoscopic ultrasound-guided real-time fine-needle aspiration for mediastinal staging. Eur Respir J 2005; 25: 416–21.

36. Kurimoto N, Miyazawa T, Okimasa S et al. Endobronchial ultrasonography using a guide sheath increases the ability to diagnose peripheral pulmonary lesions endoscopically. Chest 2004; 126: 959–65.

37. Yasufuku K, Chiyo M, Sekine Y et al. Real-time endobronchial ultrasound-guided transbronchial needle aspiration of mediastinal and hilar lymph nodes. Chest 2004; 126: 122–8.

38. Hsu LH, Liu CC, Ko JS. Education and experience improve the performance of transbronchial needle aspiration: a learning curve at a cancer center. Chest 2004; 125: 532–40.

39. Chin R Jr, McCain TW, Lucia MA et al. Transbronchial needle aspiration in diagnosing and staging lung cancer: how many aspirates are

needed? Am J Respir Crit Care Med 2002; 166: 377–81.

40. Shinagawa N, Yamazaki K, Onodera Y et al. CT-guided transbronchial biopsy using an ultrathin broncho-scope with virtual bronchoscopic navigation. Chest 2004; 125: 1138–43.

41. Patz EF Jr, Rossi S, Harpole DH Jr et al. Correlation of tumor size and survival in patients with stage IA non-small cell lung cancer. Chest 2000; 117: 1568–71.

42. Yankelevitz D, Wisnivesky JP, Hen-schke CI. Stage of lung cancer in relation to its size: Part 1. Insights. Chest 2005; 127: 1132–5.

43. Port JL, Kent MS, Korst RJ et al. Tumor size predicts survival within stage IA non-small cell lung cancer. Chest 2003; 124: 1828–33.

44. Takeda S, Fukai S, Komatsu H et al. Impact of large tumor size on sur-vival after resection of pathologi-cally node negative (pN0) non-small cell lung cancer. Ann Thorac Surg 2005; 79: 1142–6.

45. Wisnivesky JP, Yankelevitz D, Hen-schke CI. Stage of lung cancer in relation to its size: Part 2. Evidence. Chest 2005; 127: 1136–9.

46. Wisnivesky JP, Yankelevitz D, Hen-schke CI. The effect of tumor size on curability of stage I non-small cell lung cancers. Chest 2004; 126: 761–5.

47. Downey RJ, Akhurst T, Gonen M et al. Preoperative F-18 fluoro-deoxyglucose–positron emission tomography maximal standardized uptake value predicts survival after lung cancer resection. J Clin Oncol 2004; 22: 3255–60.

48. Vesselle H, Turcotte E, Wiens L et al. Relationship between non-small cell lung cancer fluorodeoxyglucose uptake at positron emission tomog-raphy and surgical stage with relevance to patient prognosis. Clin Cancer Res 2004; 10: 4709–16.

49. Sakurai H, Dobashi Y, Mizutani E et al. Bronchioloalveolar carcinoma of the lung 3 centimeters or less in diameter: a prognostic assessment. Ann Thorac Surg 2004; 78: 1728–33.

50. Sarkaria IS, Pham D, Ghossein RA et al. *SCCRO* expression correlates with invasive progression in bron-chioloalveolar carcinoma. Ann Tho-rac Surg 2004; 78: 1734–41.

51. Gabor S, Renner H, Popper H et al. Invasion of blood vessels as signifi-cant prognostic factor in radically resected T1–3N0M0 non-small-cell lung cancer. Eur J Cardiothorac Surg 2004; 25: 439–42.

52. Sayar A, Turna A, Solak O et al. Nonanatomic prognostic factors in resected nonsmall cell lung carci-noma: the importance of perineural invasion as a new prognostic marker. Ann Thorac Surg 2004; 77: 421–5.

53. Lugo TG, Braun S, Cote RJ et al. Detection and measurement of occult disease for the prognosis of solid tumors. J Clin Oncol 2003; 21: 2609–15.

54. Hsu CP, Shai SE, Hsia JY et al. Clin-ical significance of bone marrow microinvolvement in nonsmall cell lung carcinoma. Cancer 2004; 100: 794–800.

55. Yasumoto K, Osaki T, Watanabe Y et al. Prognostic value of cytoker-atin-positive cells in the bone mar-row and lymph nodes of patients with resected nonsmall cell lung cancer: a multicenter prospective study. Ann Thorac Surg 2003; 76: 194–201.

56. Sardari Nia P, Colpaert C, Blyweert B et al. Prognostic value of nonan-giogenic and angiogenic growth patterns in non-small-cell lung can-cer. Br J Cancer 2004; 91: 1293–300.

57. Mineo TC, Ambrogi V, Baldi A et al. Prognostic impact of VEGF, CD31, CD34, and CD105 expression and

tumour vessel invasion after radical surgery for IB–IIA non-small cell lung cancer. J Clin Pathol 2004; 57: 591–7.

57a. Arenberg D. In search of the holy grail. Lung cancer biomarkers. Chest 2004; 126: 325–6.

57b. Philips RJ, Burdick MD, Lutz M. The stromal derived factor-1 CXCL12–CXC chemokine receptor 4 biological axis in non-small cell lung cancer metastases. Am J Respir Crit Care Med 2003; 167: 1676–86.

58. Tamura M, Oda M, Tsunezuka Y et al. Chest CT and serum vascular endothelial growth factor-C level to diagnose lymph node metastasis in patients with primary non-small cell lung cancer. Chest 2004; 126: 342–6.

59. Visbal AL, Williams BA, Nichols FC 3rd et al. Gender differences in non-small-cell lung cancer survival: an analysis of 4,618 patients diagnosed between 1997 and 2002. Ann Thorac Surg 2004; 78: 209–15.

60. Tammemagi CM, Neslund-Dudas C, Simoff M et al. Lung carcinoma symptoms – an independent predictor of survival and an important mediator of African-American disparity in survival. Cancer 2004; 101: 1655–63.

61. Scott HR, McMillan DC, Forrest LM et al. The systemic inflammatory response, weight loss, performance status and survival in patients with inoperable non-small cell lung cancer. Br J Cancer 2002; 87: 264–7.

62. Okada M, Nishio W, Sakamoto T et al. Prognostic significance of perioperative serum carcinoembryonic antigen in non-small cell lung cancer: analysis of 1,000 consecutive resections for clinical stage I disease. Ann Thorac Surg 2004; 78: 216–21.

63. Okada M, Nishio W, Sakamoto T et al. Effect of histologic type and smoking status on interpretation of serum carcinoembryonic antigen value in non-small cell lung carci-

noma. Ann Thorac Surg 2004; 78: 1004–9.

64. Sawabata N, Maeda H, Yokota S et al. Postoperative serum carcinoembryonic antigen levels in patients with pathologic stage IA nonsmall cell lung carcinoma: subnormal levels as an indicator of favorable prognosis. Cancer 2004; 101: 803–9.

65. Herrera LJ, Raja S, Gooding WE et al. Quantitative analysis of circulating plasma DNA as a tumor marker in thoracic malignancies. Clin Chem 2005; 51: 113–18.

66. Gautschi O, Bigosch C, Huegli B et al. Circulating deoxyribonucleic acid as prognostic marker in non-small-cell lung cancer patients undergoing chemotherapy. J Clin Oncol 2004; 22: 4157–64.

67. Beau-Faller M, Gaub MP, Schneider A et al. Plasma DNA microsatellite panel as sensitive and tumor-specific marker in lung cancer patients. Int J Cancer 2003; 105: 361–70.

68. Khan S, Coulson JM, Woll PJ. Genetic abnormalities in plasma DNA of patients with lung cancer and other respiratory diseases. Int J Cancer 2004; 110: 891–5.

69. Chang JY, Komaki R, Sasaki R et al. High mutagen sensitivity in peripheral blood lymphocytes predicts poor overall and disease-specific survival in patients with stage III non-small cell lung cancer treated with radiotherapy and chemotherapy. Clin Cancer Res 2005; 11: 2894–8.

70. Wang J, Lee JJ, Wang L et al. Value of $p16^{INK4a}$ and $RASSF1A$ promoter hypermethylation in prognosis of patients with resectable non-small cell lung cancer. Clin Cancer Res 2004; 10: 6119–25.

71. Kim YT, Lee SH, Sung SW et al. Can aberrant promoter hypermethylation of CpG islands predict the clinical outcome of non-small cell lung cancer after curative resection? Ann Thorac Surg 2005; 79: 1180–8.

72. Nishiumi N, Abe Y, Inoue Y et al. Use of 11p15 mucins as prognostic factors in small adenocarcinoma of the lung. Clin Cancer Res 2003; 9: 5616–19.

73. Spano JP, Andre F, Morat L et al. Chemokine receptor CXCR4 and early-stage non-small cell lung cancer: pattern of expression and correlation with outcome. Ann Oncol 2004; 15: 613–17.

74. Pinto CA, Carvalho PE, Antonangelo L et al. Morphometric evaluation of tumor matrix metalloproteinase 9 predicts survival after surgical resection of adenocarcinoma of the lung. Clin Cancer Res 2003; 9: 3098–104.

75. Aljada IS, Ramnath N, Donohue K et al. Upregulation of the tissue inhibitor of metalloproteinase-1 protein is associated with progression of human non-small-cell lung cancer. J Clin Oncol 2004; 22: 3218–29.

76. Yamamoto S, Tomita Y, Hoshida Y et al. Expression level of valosin-containing protein (p97) is correlated with progression and prognosis of non-small-cell lung carcinoma. Ann Surg Oncol 2004; 11: 697–704.

77. Shintani Y, Higashiyama S, Ohta M et al. Overexpression of ADAM9 in non-small cell lung cancer correlates with brain metastasis. Cancer Res 2004; 64: 4190–6.

78. Ishikawa N, Daigo Y, Yasui W et al. ADAM8 as a novel serological and histochemical marker for lung cancer. Clin Cancer Res 2004; 10: 8363–70.

79. Gouyer V, Conti M, Devos P et al. Tissue inhibitor of metalloproteinase 1 is an independent predictor of prognosis in patients with nonsmall cell lung carcinoma who undergo resection with curative intent. Cancer 2005; 103: 1676–84.

80. Selvaggi G, Novello S, Torri V et al. Epidermal growth factor receptor overexpression correlates with a poor prognosis in completely resected non-small-cell lung cancer. Ann Oncol 2004; 15: 28–32.

81. Onn A, Correa AM, Gilcrease M et al. Synchronous overexpression of epidermal growth factor receptor and HER2-neu protein is a predictor of poor outcome in patients with stage I non-small cell lung cancer. Clin Cancer Res 2004; 10: 136–43.

82. Marchetti A, Barassi F, Martella C et al. Down regulation of high in normal-1 (HIN-1) is a frequent event in stage I non-small cell lung cancer and correlates with poor clinical outcome. Clin Cancer Res 2004; 10: 1338–43.

83. Brattstrom D, Wester K, Bergqvist M et al. HER-2, EGFR, COX-2 expression status correlated to microvessel density and survival in resected non-small cell lung cancer. Acta Oncol 2004; 43: 80–6.

84. Ren H, Tang X, Lee JJ et al. Expression of hepatoma-derived growth factor is a strong prognostic predictor for patients with early-stage non-small-cell lung cancer. J Clin Oncol 2004; 22: 3230–7.

85. Shah L, Walter KL, Borczuk AC et al. Expression of syndecan-1 and expression of epidermal growth factor receptor are associated with survival in patients with nonsmall cell lung carcinoma. Cancer 2004; 101: 1632–8.

86. Pelosi G, Del Curto B, Dell'Orto P et al. Lack of prognostic implications of HER-2/neu abnormalities in 345 stage I non-small cell carcinomas (NSCLC) and 207 stage I–III neuroendocrine tumours (NET) of the lung. Int J Cancer 2005; 113: 101–8.

87. Ferraro B, Bepler G, Sharma S et al. EGR1 predicts PTEN and survival in patients with non-small-cell lung cancer. J Clin Oncol 2005; 23: 1921–6.

88. Yoshida T, Tanaka S, Mogi A et al. The clinical significance of cyclin B1 and Wee1 expression in non-small-cell lung cancer. Ann Oncol 2004; 15: 252–6.

89. Bepler G, Sharma S, Cantor A et al. RRM1 and PTEN as prognostic parameters for overall and disease-free survival in patients with non-small-cell lung cancer. J Clin Oncol 2004; 22: 1878–85.

90. Iniesta P, Gonzalez-Quevedo R, Moran A et al. Relationship between 3p deletions and telomerase activity in non-small-cell lung cancer: prognostic implications. Br J Cancer 2004; 90: 1983–8.

91. Fukuoka J, Fujii T, Shih JH et al. Chromatin remodeling factors and BRM/BRG1 expression as prognostic indicators in non-small cell lung cancer. Clin Cancer Res 2004; 10: 4314–24.

92. Vicent S, Garayoa M, Lopez-Picazo JM et al. Mitogen-activated protein kinase phosphatase-1 is overexpressed in non-small cell lung cancer and is an independent predictor of outcome in patients. Clin Cancer Res 2004; 10: 3639–49.

93. Osoegawa A, Yoshino I, Tanaka S et al. Regulation of p27 by S-phase kinase-associated protein 2 is associated with aggressiveness in non-small-cell lung cancer. J Clin Oncol 2004; 22: 4165–73.

94. Dworakowska D, Jassem E, Jassem J et al. Prognostic relevance of altered pRb and p53 protein expression in surgically treated non-small cell lung cancer patients. Oncology 2004; 67: 60–6.

95. Vischioni B, van der Valk P, Span SW et al. Nuclear localization of survivin is a positive prognostic factor for survival in advanced non-small-cell lung cancer. Ann Oncol 2004; 15: 1654–60.

96. Wang YC, Lin RK, Tan YH et al. Wild-type p53 overexpression and its correlation with MDM2 and p14^{ARF} alterations: an alternative pathway to non-small-cell lung cancer. J Clin Oncol 2005; 23: 154–64.

97. Shinohara ET, Gonzalez A, Massion PP et al. Nuclear survivin predicts recurrence and poor survival in patients with resected nonsmall cell lung carcinoma. Cancer 2005; 103: 1685–92.

98. Meert AP, Martin B, Paesmans M et al. The role of HER-2/neu expression on the survival of patients with lung cancer: a systematic review of the literature. Br J Cancer 2003; 89: 959–65.

99. Rosell R, Scagliotti G, Danenberg KD et al. Transcripts in pretreatment biopsies from a three-arm randomized trial in metastatic non-small-cell lung cancer. Oncogene 2003; 22: 3548–53.

100. Rosell R, Danenberg KD, Alberola V et al. Ribonucleotide reductase messenger RNA expression and survival in gemcitabine/cisplatin-treated advanced non-small cell lung cancer patients. Clin Cancer Res 2004; 10: 1318–25.

101. Lu B, Mu Y, Cao C et al. Survivin as a therapeutic target for radiation sensitization in lung cancer. Cancer Res 2004; 64: 2840–5.

102. Berger W, Setinek U, Hollaus P et al. Multidrug resistance markers P-glycoprotein, multidrug resistance protein 1, and lung resistance protein in non-small cell lung cancer: prognostic implications. J Cancer Res Clin Oncol 2005; 131: 355–63.

103. Gurubhagavatula S, Liu G, Park S et al. XPD and XRCC1 genetic polymorphisms are prognostic factors in advanced non-small-cell lung cancer patients treated with platinum chemotherapy. J Clin Oncol 2004; 22: 2594–601.

104. Brenton JD, Caldas C. Predictive cancer genomics – what do we need? Lancet 2003; 362: 340–1.

105. Endoh H, Tomida S, Yatabe Y et al. Prognostic model of pulmonary

adenocarcinoma by expression profiling of eight genes as determined by quantitative real-time reverse transcriptase polymerase chain reaction. J Clin Oncol 2004; 22: 811–19.

106. Hoang CD, D'Cunha J, Tawfic SH et al. Expression profiling of non-small cell lung carcinoma identifies metastatic genotypes based on lymph node tumor burden. J Thorac Cardiovasc Surg 2004; 127: 1332–41; discussion 1342.

107. Yamagata N, Shyr Y, Yanagisawa K et al. A training-testing approach to the molecular classification of resected non-small cell lung cancer. Clin Cancer Res 2003; 9: 4695–704.

108. Lu C, Soria JC, Tang X et al. Prognostic factors in resected stage I non-small-cell lung cancer: a multivariate analysis of six molecular markers. J Clin Oncol 2004; 22: 4575–83.

109. Jiang F, Yin Z, Caraway NP et al. Genomic profiles in stage I primary non small cell lung cancer using comparative genomic hybridization analysis of cDNA microarrays. Neoplasia 2004; 6: 623–35.

110. Petty RD, Nicolson MC, Kerr KM et al. Gene expression profiling in non-small cell lung cancer: from molecular mechanisms to clinical application. Clin Cancer Res 2004; 10: 3237–48.

111. Blackhall FH, Wigle DA, Jurisica I et al. Validating the prognostic value of marker genes derived from a non-small cell lung cancer microarray study. Lung Cancer 2004; 46: 197–204.

111a. Martin B, Paesmans M, Mascaux C et al. Ki-67 expression and patient survival in lung cancer: systematic review of the literature and meta-analysis. Br J Cancer 2004; 91: 2018–25.

112. Blum R, MacManus MP, Rischin D et al. Impact of positron emission tomography on the management of patients with small-cell lung cancer: preliminary experience. Am J Clin Oncol 2004; 27: 164–71.

113. Bradley JD, Dehdashti F, Mintun MA et al. Positron emission tomography in limited-stage small-cell lung cancer: a prospective study. J Clin Oncol 2004; 22: 3248–54.

114. Buttery RC, Rintoul RC, Sethi T. Small cell lung cancer: the importance of the extracellular matrix. Int J Biochem Cell Biol 2004; 36: 1154–60.

115. Oshita F, Kameda Y, Hamanaka N et al. High expression of integrin β_1 and p53 is a greater poor prognostic factor than clinical stage in small-cell lung cancer. Am J Clin Oncol 2004; 27: 215–19.

116. Blackhall FH, Pintilie M, Michael M et al. Expression and prognostic significance of kit, protein kinase B, and mitogen-activated protein kinase in patients with small cell lung cancer. Clin Cancer Res 2003; 9: 2241–7.

117. Rohr UP, Rehfeld N, Pflugfelder L et al. Expression of the tyrosine kinase c-kit is an independent prognostic factor in patients with small cell lung cancer. Int J Cancer 2004; 111: 259–63.

118. Boldrini L, Ursino S, Gisfredi S et al. Expression and mutational status of c-kit in small-cell lung cancer: prognostic relevance. Clin Cancer Res 2004; 10: 4101–8.

119. Johnson BE, Fischer T, Fischer B et al. Phase II study of STI571 (Gleevec™) for patients with small cell lung cancer. Clin Cancer Res 2003; 9: 5880–7.

120. Taneja TK, Sharma S. Markers of small cell lung cancer. World J Surg Oncol 2004; 2: 10.

121. Johansen JS, Drivsholm L, Price PA et al. High serum YKL-40 level in patients with small cell lung cancer is related to early death. Lung Cancer 2004; 46: 333–40.

122. Monstad SE, Drivsholm L, Storstein A et al. Hu and voltage-gated calcium channel (VGCC) antibodies related to the prognosis of small-cell lung cancer. J Clin Oncol 2004; 22: 795–800.

123. Jones MH, Virtanen C, Honjoh D et al. Two prognostically significant subtypes of high-grade lung neuroendocrine tumours independent of small-cell and large-cell neuroendocrine carcinomas identified by gene expression profiles. Lancet 2004; 363: 775–81.

7
Treatment of small cell lung cancer

Morten Sørensen

In recent years the focus on lung cancer generally has increased; however, attention has mainly been directed towards non-small cell lung cancer (NSCLC), illustrated by a threefold increase in American Society of Clinical Oncology (ASCO) abstracts on NSCLC since the turn of the millennium, as opposed to an unchanged number of abstracts addressing small cell lung cancer (SCLC) in the same time period. This difference may reflect the declining proportion of lung cancer patients presenting with small cell carcinoma histology, but also the many new treatment options for NSCLC that have appeared within the last 5 years. Still, the treatment of SCLC continues to represent a major challenge. Despite a high rate of initial response, most patients will eventually relapse and long-term survival remains a disappointing 10–15%. The mainstay of treatment continues to include chemotherapy/radiotherapy in limited disease (LD), whereas patients presenting with extensive disease (ED) receive chemotherapy as the sole treatment modality. Since the publication of *Lung Cancer Therapy Annual 4*, new insights have emerged with regard to various aspects of the management of SCLC, including the delivery of radiotherapy and the combination of taxanes and topoisomerase I inhibitors with radiotherapy in LD patients and with platinum-based chemotherapy in ED patients. Recently, targeted therapies have been developed, and initial data using these novel principles show encouraging results in patients responding to induction chemotherapy. Finally, randomized data suggest that second-line chemotherapy results in a survival benefit when compared with best supportive care.

RADIOTHERAPY AND CONCURRENT CHEMOTHERAPY

Timing of radiotherapy

Since the publication of two meta-analyses[1,2] over a decade ago, it has become clear that thoracic irradiation improves local control and survival in LD patients, but the optimal way to deliver chest radiotherapy remains unresolved, including the definition of target volume, dose, fractionation and timing. Although several randomized trials have been conducted to investigate the timing of radiotherapy, a general consensus has not been reached. Recently, two meta-analyses have attempted to determine whether early or late thoracic irradiation results in the longest survival in LD SCLC patients.[3,4] Neither of the analyses were able to use individual patient data; instead, survival data were abstracted from previously reported work. The analyses differed with respect to the definition of early and late radiotherapy. Six of the seven trials included were similar in the two analyses. The Cochrane meta-analysis used the delivery of radiotherapy before or after day 30 as the discrimination point for the definition of early versus late radiotherapy based on cell kinetic data. Using these criteria, a European Organization for Research and Treatment of Cancer (EORTC) study was excluded, as radiotherapy was initiated after the 30-day time point in both arms.[5] The North American meta-analysis defined early delivery as radiotherapy commencing before 9 weeks after the start of any therapy, which made the aforementioned EORTC trial eligible for inclusion. According to a consensus decision, the investigators elected to violate these predefined criteria in order to include a Yugoslavian study starting radiotherapy on week 6 in the late arm.[6] Furthermore, they opted not to include a British study,[7] as this has only been reported in abstract form. This is in contrast to the Cochrane meta-analysis, which both included published and unpublished studies. The North Central Cancer Group Treatment (NCCTG)[8] and the Eastern Cooperative Oncology Group (ECOG)/intergroup[9] trials were excluded in both analyses, because radiotherapy was commenced on the same day in neither arm. In both analyses, the included studies are quite diverse in their design and study population, which calls for caution in the interpretation of the data. In the Danish study, radiotherapy was not delivered concomitantly with chemotherapy in neither arm, and split-course radiotherapy was used in the early radiotherapy arm, whereas sequential radiotherapy was applied in the late arm.[10] In the Japanese study, radiotherapy was also administered sequentially in the late radiotherapy arm.[11] All trials used platinum-based chemotherapy, except for the Cancer and Leukemia Group B (CALGB) trial[12] and the EORTC trial.[5] Three studies included in both analyses used twice-daily radiotherapy, as opposed to the once-daily radiotherapy used in the remaining studies. Also, guidelines for offering prophylactic cranial irradiation (PCI) varied across trials.

Fried et al[4] found a significant 2-year survival benefit, which was lost at the 3-year time point. They declined from analyzing 5-year survival data because of the small numbers of patients alive at this time point. In the Cochrane meta-analysis, 2- and 5-year survivals were not significantly different when all seven trials were taken into account. However, when excluding the trial using non-platinum-based chemotherapy, the odds ratio (OR) of survival at 5 years significantly favored early chest radiotherapy, representing a 5-year survival rate of 20.2% for early versus 13.8% for late radiotherapy. As pointed out by the authors, this conclusion should be viewed with caution, as the subanalysis excluding the non-platinum trial was a post-hoc analysis. Furthermore, the 5-year survival data rely primarily on the National Cancer Institute of Canada (NCIC) data,[13] which James et al[7] failed to confirm in their replica trial of the Canadian trial. Five-year survival data on the British trial are pending, and more firm conclusions might emerge when these data are added to the meta-analysis. Fried et al[4] also reported the benefit of early radiotherapy concurrent with platinum-based chemotherapy in their subgroup analysis restricted to trials using platinum-based chemotherapy. They found survival benefit at both the 2- and 3-year time points. Further, subgroup analyses showed a significant 2- and 3-year survival benefit of early radiotherapy in trials using twice-daily radiotherapy. In the Cochrane review, a preplanned analysis stratifying for overall treatment time of irradiation identified five studies delivering radiotherapy within less than 30 days.[6,7,11,13,14] Overall 5-year survival was significantly higher (relative risk (RR) = 0.90, 95% confidence interval (CI) 0.84–0.97; $p = 0.006$) for early radiotherapy, whereas no benefit was seen at the 2-year time point. Using the same data except for the British data,[7] in a separate report, the same authors identified a parameter designated SER (Start of any therapy to the End of Radiotherapy), which is very similar to the overall treatment time of radiotherapy as an even stronger predictor of outcome.[15] They reported a higher 5-year survival rate in the shorter SER arms (OR = 0.60, 95% CI 0.45–0.80; $p = 0.0006$). However, a low SER was also associated with an increased risk of severe esophagitis (OR = 0.47, 95% CI 0.33–0.66; $p < 0.0001$), indicating that the increased survival was achieved at the expense of more toxicity. When comparing early versus late radiotherapy, no increased incidence of severe esophagitis was seen in the Cochrane meta-analysis, although a trend towards a higher risk of developing pneumonitis was observed.

In conclusion, the data available from these two meta-analyses do not provide a definitive answer on how to combine radiotherapy with chemotherapy, but the data suggest that early is superior to late delivery of radiotherapy when given concurrently with platinum-based chemotherapy. Furthermore, the studies with the shortest overall treatment time and longest median survival times also report the largest differences between early and late radiotherapy.[6,11,13,14] One interpretation of these findings is that early radiotherapy is only beneficial when effective and intensive radio-chemotherapy is delivered to fit, good-prognosis patients who are staged thoroughly.

Split-course radiotherapy

A long-term update with a median follow-up of 7.4 years on a previously published randomized NCCTG trial[8] confirms that twice-daily split-dose radiotherapy is equal to once-daily radiotherapy given concurrently with chemotherapy.[16] Median survival times and 5-year overall survival rates were 20.6 months and 22% on the twice-daily arm compared with 20.6 months and 21% on the once-daily arm. These results are contrasted by an absolute 5-year survival benefit of 10% (26% vs 16%) associated with twice-daily compared with once-daily radiotherapy reported by the ECOG/intergroup study.[9] The two trials differ with respect to the timing and duration of radiotherapy. The ECOG/intergroup elected to deliver radiotherapy continuously over a 3-week period, starting on day 1, as opposed to split-course radiotherapy, starting on day 84 with a 2.5-week treatment break introduced to avoid severe esophagitis. Toxicity data confirm that split-course radiotherapy induced less grade 3–4 esophagitis compared with the continuous twice-daily arm in the ECOG/intergroup trial (12% vs 27%).

Since the planning of the NCCTG trial, data have implied that neither split-course nor late delivery of radiotherapy influence survival positively. Split-course twice-daily radiotherapy was equal to continuous once-daily radiotherapy with respect to survival and local control in NSCLC.[17] Similarly, in head and neck cancer, split-course radiotherapy resulted in inferior local control compared to accelerated twice-daily radiotherapy.[18] Furthermore, as mentioned above, meta-analyses imply that late is inferior to early delivery in trials using twice-daily radiotherapy.[4] Thus, it is likely that the use of late split-course radiotherapy could have compromised tumor cell kill due to accelerated repopulation during the treatment break or dissemination of chemoresistant cell clones outside the radiation field. In conclusion, late split-course twice-daily radiotherapy is not superior to once-daily radiotherapy, whereas early continuous twice-daily radiotherapy results in superior survival.

Furthermore, a recent relatively small, randomized phase III trial supported the lack of benefit when radiotherapy is applied as a split course.[19] One hundred and fourteen patients were randomly allocated to receive either continuous radiotherapy concurrent with the first two cycles of chemotherapy or split-course radiotherapy concurrent with the first three cycles of chemotherapy. All patients received a total irradiation dose of 50 Gy in once-daily fractions of either 2.0 or 2.5 Gy in the continuous and split-course arms, respectively. Chemotherapy consisted of three cycles of cisplatin/etoposide and three cycles of cyclophosphamide/vincristine/doxorubicin. PCI was offered to patients with a complete response. The study confirmed that split-course radiotherapy reduced the likelihood of esophagitis. Grade 3 and 4 esophagitis were reported in 9% of patients receiving continuous radiotherapy versus 4% of patients receiving split-course therapy. No difference in response rates was observed. Overall survival rates at 5 years were 18% and 17% for the continuous and split-course arms, respectively, corroborating that split-course radiotherapy does not provide any survival advantage.

Fractionation of radiotherapy

A retrospective analysis of 324 LD patients staged with computed tomography (CT) scanning compared twice-daily ($n = 107$) with once-daily ($n = 217$) radiotherapy concurrent with cisplatin-based chemotherapy.[20] Median doses were 50 Gy over 5 weeks and 45 Gy over 3 weeks, respectively. Patients had favorable prognostic factors, although a high proportion (24%) of patients presented with pleural effusions. Fewer patients received PCI among the once-daily treated group (108/217, 50%) compared with the twice-daily treated patients (60/107, 56%). In accordance with the ECOG/intergroup trial,[9] the 5-year survival rate was 25% in the twice-daily group, which was significantly higher than the 5-year survival rate of 12% in the once-daily treated patients. The negative consequence of twice-daily radiotherapy was a higher rate of grade 3 acute esophagitis of 22% and lung fibrosis of 31% compared with 9% and 12% in the once-daily group ($p = 0.002$ and $p < 0.001$), respectively. Multivariate analysis identified PCI, fractionation of chest radiotherapy and existence of pleural effusion as factors influencing survival. These retrospective data are very similar to those reported by the ECOG/intergroup regarding both toxicity and survival data. Evidently, the study is subject to the limitations generally associated with retrospective studies, including selection of more fit patients to the schedule of more toxic twice-daily radiotherapy.

Dose of radiotherapy

The optimal total dose of radiotherapy – whether delivered in once- or twice-daily fractions – is still to be established. The RTOG determined the maximum tolerated dose (MTD) of concurrent once-daily radiotherapy administered over a fixed period of 5 weeks with a fixed dose of cisplatin.[21] Treatment was delivered in daily fractions of 1.8 Gy to the clinical target volume in 20 fractions over 4 weeks to a total of 36 Gy. During the last and 5th weeks, fields were reduced to the gross tumor volume, including twice-daily doses on the last 3 treatment days to a total of 50.4 Gy: i.e. $36 + (1.8 \times 5) + (1.8 \times 3) = 50.4$ Gy. Doses were escalated in steps of two fractions of 1.8 Gy towards the gross tumor volume added as a second daily dose. MTD was defined as one dose level beneath the dose resulting in grade 3 and 4 non-hematologic toxicity in more than 50% of patients. Three out of five patients receiving 64.8 Gy developed grade 3 esophagitis and, consequently, 61.2 Gy was declared MTD. These data indicate that it is feasible to safely deliver higher doses than those used in both the ECOG/intergroup and NCCTG trials. Interestingly, although patient numbers were small, the 18-month survival rate was 25% versus an impressive 82% in patients receiving 50.4 and 61.2 Gy, respectively.

As early twice-daily concurrent radiotherapy has resulted in an unprecedented 5-year survival rate of 26% in LD SCLC,[8] investigators have determined the MTD of twice-daily radiotherapy. In a phase I/II study, the NCCTG escalated twice-daily fractions of 1.2 Gy to a total of 48–66 Gy in four cohorts of 3–6 patients.[22] Radiotherapy was given concurrently with etoposide and cisplatin and commenced on week 6, proceeded by two cycles of a topotecan/ paclitaxel combination. Amifostine was used as a radioprotector. Three patients experienced dose-limiting toxicity. At the dose level of 66 Gy, 1 patient died due to hypoxia after completing radiotherapy and 1 patient had grade 3 esophagitis, whereas 1 patient treated with 60 Gy had grade 4 pneumonitis. The study has been extended to a phase II trial using a dose of 60 Gy, which represents a considerably higher radiotherapy dose than the 45 Gy used in the ECOG/intergroup study.

Incorporation of newer agents with radiotherapy

A number of groups have attempted to incorporate newer agents with radio-therapy in LD patients in phase II studies (Table 7.1). Extensive use of concurrent etoposide/platinum-based chemotherapy/radiotherapy has proven this combination to be safe and manageable, and therefore the combination is the most commonly used. Other drugs such as anthracyclins and alkylating agents have been shown to be less suitable.[1] Concerns have been raised that the concurrent use of taxanes and topoisomerase I inhibitors could lead to excessive toxicity.[23] Consequently, some authors have restricted the use of new agents to a short course of induction chemotherapy followed by standard concurrent etoposide/platinum-based chemotherapy/radiotherapy.[24,25]

CALGB elected to include two new drugs, topotecan and paclitaxel, in combination with etoposide as part of induction therapy.[24] To facilitate outpatient treatment, topotecan (1.5 mg/m^2) days 2–4 and etoposide (160 mg/m^2) days 5–7 were administered orally with intravenous (IV) paclitaxel (110 mg/m^2) on day 1 repeated twice every 21 days. Thereafter, once-daily radiotherapy was given to a total of 70 Gy, concurrently with three cycles of carboplatin and etoposide. A total of 65 patients were enrolled. The primary endpoint was response rate to induction therapy, which was a modest 62%, increasing to 84% following radiotherapy/chemotherapy. Three patients suffered a toxic death. As the response rate did not reach the prespecified criteria, the authors concluded that further investigation of this regimen was not justified. The same group had previously published a similar study with the modification that the two cycles of induction chemotherapy consisted of paclitaxel (175 mg/m^2 on day 1) and topotecan (1 mg/m^2 on days 1–5) with granulocyte colony-stimulating factor (G-CSF) support.[25] Radiotherapy was delivered in once-daily fractions to a total of 70 Gy, concurrent with carboplatin and etoposide. Grade 3 and 4 dysphagia was observed in 16% of 57 patients treated with radiotherapy; 92% had a response, and median survival was 22.4 months. These two CALGB trials indicate that it is feasible to deliver a higher dose of once-daily radiotherapy than the dose of 40–60 Gy used in most recent randomized studies.

Other authors have incorporated topoisomerase I inhibitors in the treatment, as two 21-day cycles of induction therapy consisting of 40 mg/m^2 irinotecan and cisplatin, both given IV on days 1 and 8. An additional two cycles of standard etoposide and cisplatin were given concurrently with twice-daily fractions of 1.5 Gy over 15 weekdays to a total of 45 Gy.[26] Magnetic resonance imaging (MRI) or CT scan of the brain was performed in all 35 LD patients included in the trial. Induction therapy resulted in a high overall response rate of 97%, although only 3 patients achieved a complete response. The response rate increased to 100%, with 43% of patients having a complete response following radiotherapy. The median overall survival time of 25 months was in the high range of what it is seen in similar patient populations (see Table 7.1). The dose intensity relative to the planned dose was approximately 80%, both for induction and concurrent chemotherapy. In 50% of the

Table 7.1   Phase II studies incorporating irinotecan, paclitaxel and topotecan with radiotherapy in limited small cell lung cancer

Reference (first author)	No. of patients	Chemotherapy	Fraction per day	Total dose (Gy)	Day starting RT	Median survival time (months)	Complete response rate[a] (%)	Response rate of CT + RT (%)	Response rate of CT only (%)	Toxic death rate (%)	≥Grade 3 esophagitis (%)	≥Grade 3 pneumonitis (%)
Han[26]	35	iIC	bid	45	43	25.0	43	100	97	2.9	29	9
Ettinger[27]	55	cPEC	bid	45	1	25.0	75	92	–	5.7	36	9
Sohn[29]	22	cIC	qd	54	29	NA	59	82	–	0	18	NA
Miller[24]	65	iPTE	qd	70	43	16.6	43	84	62	4.6	29[b]	NA
Bogart[25]	57	iPT	qd	70	43	22.4	–	92	–	1.8	16[b]	NA
Turrisi[9]	211	cEC	bid	45	1	23.0	56	87	–	2.8	27	6
	206	cEC	qd	45	1	19.0	49	87	–	2.4	11	4
Bonner[8]	130	cEC	bid[c]	48	84	20.6	45	NA	95	3	12	8
	131	cEC	qd	50.4	84	20.6	47	NA	93	0	5	5

CT, chemotherapy; RT, radiotherapy; i, induction chemotherapy; c, concurrent chemotherapy; I, irinotecan; C, cisplatin; P, paclitaxel; E, etoposide; T, topotecan.
[a] Complete response rate after completion of both chemotherapy and radiotherapy.
[b] Grade 3 + 4 dysphagia.
[c] Split-course radiotherapy with a 2.5-week break.

patients, the second induction cycle had to be postponed as a result of late bone marrow recovery. Hematologic toxicity was more pronounced during radiotherapy, with grade 3 and 4 neutropenia, anemia and thrombocytopenia in 100%, 51% and 58% of patients, respectively. Growth factor support was allowed but not routinely used. Grade 3 and 4 esophagitis and pneumonitis occurred in 29 and 9% of patients, respectively.

Some investigators have argued that radiotherapy should be delivered as early as possible, and consequently they have incorporated paclitaxel in combination with etoposide- and cisplatin-based chemotherapy with radiotherapy starting on day 1.[27] In this phase II trial, comprising 55 patients, paclitaxel was given on day 1 at a dose of 135 mg/m^2, with 60 mg/m^2 cisplatin on day 1, and etoposide given at doses of 60 mg/m^2 IV on day 1 and orally on days 2 and 3 at a dose of 80 mg/m^2/day. A total of four cycles were given every 3 weeks, with the paclitaxel dose increasing to 175 mg/m^2 for the last three chemotherapy-alone cycles. Radiotherapy consisted of twice-daily fractions of 1.5 Gy over 15 weekdays, to a total of 45 Gy. Hematologic toxicity was frequent, with 75% of patients experiencing grade 3 and 4 neutropenia. Grade 3 and 4 esophagitis was recorded more often than in the ECOG/intergroup study (36% vs 27%). Three fatal episodes related to therapy were reported (sepsis, adult respiratory distress syndrome and late lung toxicity). The overall response rate was 92%, with 75% of patients achieving a complete response. The median survival was 25 months, which is comparable to that reported in the ECOG/intergroup trial (see Table 7.1). However, the authors find it unlikely that this three-drug combination with twice-daily radiotherapy will improve survival compared with standard etoposide and cisplatin, and therefore they have cancelled further development of this strategy.

The survival benefits seen in a Japan Clinical Oncology Group (JCOG) trial in ED patients, replacing etoposide with irinotecan,[28] have inspired Korean investigators to incorporate irinotecan in the delivery of concurrent radiotherapy to 22 LD patients.[29] They used a modified version of the JCOG regimen, splitting the dose of cisplatin in two on days 1 and 8. Radiotherapy commenced on day 1 of the second cycle in once-daily fractions of 2.0 Gy, to a total of 54 Gy. Survival data are encouraging but still immature. Although no treatment-related deaths occurred, grade 3 and 4 esophagitis, anorexia and diarrhea in this once-daily radiotherapy regimen were relatively high, in the range of 18–23%, almost reaching the frequency of esophagitis seen in large studies using twice-daily radiotherapy.[8] Randomized trials incorporating irinotecan with radiotherapy in LD are warranted, as previous trials have shown that a marginal effect in ED can translate into a robust survival benefit in LD patients.[30]

CHEMOTHERAPY

Combinations with topoisomerase I inhibitors

Despite numerous randomized trials testing various different strategies in the last two decades, survival in ED patients remains essentially unchanged and poor. In a limited number of trials, modest survival benefits have been achieved at the expense of unacceptable morbidity and treatment-related death rates. Thus, the Japanese finding that irinotecan in combination with cisplatin increased median survival time by 3.4 months compared with etoposide in combination with cis-platin sparked enthusiasm for topoisomerase I inhibitors.[28] Notably, the survival benefit was reached with acceptable toxicity, although grade 3 and 4 diarrhea occurred in 16% compared with none in the etoposide arm. The study was pre-maturely stopped after the enrollment of 152 patients out of the planned 230 patients, as recommended by a preplanned interim analysis. A confirmative ran-domized study seemed justified, as the putative superiority of irinotecan relied on a single, small, prematurely stopped trial in an Asian population with phar-mocogenetics possibly different from other ethnic groups.

Accordingly, Hanna et al[31] randomized 331 patients to either irinotecan or etoposide, both in combination with cisplatin. An unequally balanced random-ization was performed, allocating one-third of patients to etoposide and two-thirds to the irinotecan arm. In both arms, four cycles every 3 weeks were delivered. Irinotecan (65 mg/m^2) and cisplatin (30 mg/m^2) were dosed on days 1 and 8. The etoposide dose was 120 mg/m^2 on days 1–3, and cisplatin was administered as a single dose of 60 mg/m^2 on day 1. After the enrollment of 30 patients, inclusion was restricted to patients in performance status 0 and 1 due to an excessive toxic death rate among performance status 2 patients. As expected, myelotoxicity and febrile neutropenia were more frequent in the etoposide arm, whereas gastrointestinal toxicity was more common in the irinotecan arm, including 21% of patients suffering from grade 3 and 4 diar-rhea. The study could not confirm the encouraging Japanese data. No signifi-cant differences were seen in overall survival, time to progression or response rates (Table 7.2). Median survival times were 9.3 versus 10.2 months in the irinotecan/cisplatin and etoposide/cisplatin arms, respectively. A number of factors could explain the conflicting results reported in the two trials. First of all, the North American study used a modified schedule. The day 15 dose of irinotecan was omitted, as approximately 50% of the day 15 dose in the Japan-ese study could not be delivered due to toxicity. Furthermore, the cisplatin dose was split in two on days 1 and 8. Both the dose intensity and total dose of etoposide in the Noda study were approximately 80% of the planned dose in the North American study. The reduced dose might have resulted in inferior performance in the etoposide arm of the Japanese study. Median survival times on etoposide arms were 9.4 versus 10.2 months in the Japanese and US stud-ies, respectively. It is conceivable that pharmacogenetics vary in the two study populations. Polymorphisms exist between Asians and Caucasians with regard

Table 7.2   Trials evaluating topoisomerase I inhibitors in combination with platinum in extensive small cell lung cancer

Reference (first author)	No. of patients	Chemotherapy		Median survival time (months)		Response rate (%)		≥Grade 3 neutropenia (%)		≥Grade 3 diarrhea (%)	
		Topol	Etoposide	Topol	Etoposide	Topol	Etoposide	Topol	Etoposide	Topol	Etoposide
Seifart[38]	42	TP 3d[a]	–	7.6	–	60	–	48[c]	–	4.8	–
Seifart[38]	42	TP 5d[b]	–	8.7	–	62	–	64[c]	–	4.8	–
Erkardt[35]	784	TP[d]	EP	9.1	9.3	63	69	58	84	6	2
Huynh[34]	44	ICb	–	NA	–	68/37[e]	–	38	–	18	–
Schmitte[33]	59	ICb	EP	12	10	71	50	27	62	12	6
Hanna[31]	331	IP	EP	9.3	10.2	48	44	36	82	21	0
Noda[28]	153	IP	EP	12.8	9.4	84	68	65	92	16	0

Topol, topoisomerase I inhibitor; T, topotecan; P, cisplatin; I, irinotecan; Cb, carboplatin; E, etoposide.
[a] 3-day topotecan schedule.
[b] 5-day topotecan schedule.
[c] Leukocytopenia.
[d] Oral topotecan.
[e] Response rates for chemonaive and relapsed patients, respectively.

to the gene responsible for the glucuronidation of SN-38, the active metabolite of irinotecan.[32] Such polymorphism is one possible factor that could contribute to the discrepancies seen in the two studies.

In a randomized phase II design, German investigators have compared irinotecan with etoposide in a similar fashion as the JCOG, although they combined with carboplatin instead of cisplatin.[33] As in the Japanese study, irinotecan was delivered on days 1, 8 and 15 every 4 weeks. The doses of irinotecan and etoposide differed from those in the JCOG trial. Irinotecan and etoposide doses were 50 mg/m^2/day and 140 mg/m^2/day, compared with 60 mg/m^2/day and 100 mg/m^2/day in the JCOG trial. Carboplatin was dosed at area under the curve (AUC) 5. Based on preliminary data on 59 evaluable patients a significant increase in progression-free survival (9 vs 6 months; $p = 0.02$) was observed. Median survival times were 12 and 10 months on the irinotecan and etoposide arms, respectively, ($p = 0.14$) (see Table 7.2). As expected, more grade 3 and 4 thrombocytopenia (18% vs 50%) and neutropenia (27% vs 62%) were recorded on the etoposide/carboplatin arm. Also, as reported earlier, irinotecan resulted in more grade 3 and 4 diarrhea (12% vs 6%). According to the protocol, the accrual will proceed as a phase III trial, which, perhaps combined with existing data, may determine whether irinotecan or etoposide is the superior drug when combined with platinum compounds in ED patients.

Other investigators have developed a 21-day irinotecan/carboplatin regimen, omitting irinotecan on days 8 and 15.[34] All 44 patients were treated with carboplatin AUC 5, whereas irinotecan was dosed depending on whether patients had received prior chemotherapy. Chemonaive ED patients received 200 mg/m^2, as opposed to relapsed patients, who were treated with a reduced dose of 150 mg/m^2. Eighteen percent of patients experienced grade 3 and 4 diarrhea. Response rates were 68% and 37% in the chemonaive and relapsed patients, respectively, which are comparable to what is commonly achieved in these patient populations (see Table 7.2).

The Noda study also prompted the investigation of the topoisomerase I inhibitor topotecan in one of the largest randomized trials ever conducted in patients with ED SCLC.[35] In order to increase patient convenience, the oral formulation of topotecan was used. The study was designed as a non-inferiority study. The two treatments were to be considered equal if the absolute difference in the lower limit of the 95% CI for the difference in 1-year survival was less than 10%. Eckardt et al[35] randomized 784 patients to either oral topotecan or IV etoposide, both in combination with cisplatin (see Table 7.2). The first 75 patients were treated with oral topotecan at a dose of 2.3 mg/m^2 on days 1–5, with cisplatin 60 mg/m^2 on day 5. However, due to an unacceptably high rate of fatal neutropenic enterocolitis, the dose of topotecan was reduced to 1.7 mg/m^2. Grade 3 and 4 neutropenia was significantly more frequent on the etoposide arm (84% vs 58%), whereas anemia and thrombocytopenia were numerically more common on the topotecan arm. As previously seen, the oral formulation of topotecan resulted in manageable grade 3 and 4 diarrhea (6% vs 2%) and anorexia (4% vs <1%) that were slightly but significantly more frequent on the topotecan arm compared with etoposide. Conversely, etoposide caused significantly more vomiting and alopecia than topotecan. Overall survival was equal (9.1 vs 9.3 months) and the prespecified criteria for non-inferiority were met. However, a small significant, but clinically irrelevant, increase in time to progression of 1 week in favor of etoposide was observed. Overall response rates also insignificantly favored etoposide (69% vs 63%). In two randomized trials, IV etoposide outperformed oral etoposide with regard to palliation and survival in an elderly poor-prognosis population.[36,37] Thus, in younger patients with good prognosis, topotecan seems to be a drug to consider when oral treatment is preferred to IV treatment and disregarding cost issues.

The standard schedule of topotecan has been a 5-day regimen, as a higher cell kill is expected when a highly S-phase-specific drug is delivered over a protracted time period. However, a 5-day schedule is inconvenient and efforts have been made to develop a shorter treatment cycle. A 5- and 3-day IV schedule in combination with cisplatin was evaluated in 84 ED patients in a phase II trial.[38] Doses of topotecan were 1.0 and 1.5 mg/m^2/day in the 5- and 3-day schedules, respectively. In both arms, cisplatin was delivered after topotecan, as this sequence has proven safer than the reverse sequence.[39,40] Response rates and overall survival were numerically better in the 5-day arm (62% vs 60% and 8.7 vs 7.6 months; $p = 0.69$). Although not reaching significance, the 5-day schedule caused more myelotoxicity than the 3-day regimen. The frequency of anemia was more than doubled in the 5-day arm (43% vs 21%; $p = 0.09$) and also leukocytopenia was more pronounced following the 5-day treatment (64%) than the 3-day treatment (48%). Three patients on the 5-day schedule died of septicemia, resulting in a relatively high rate of toxic death of 7% compared with 2% in the 3-day arm. Both regimens seem active, although a trend towards more toxicity was noted in the 5-day arm (see Table 7.2).

A relatively high treatment-related death rate was also observed in a phase II trial[41] combining topotecan 1.0 mg/m^2 on days 1–5 with cyclophosphamide 600 mg/m^2 on day 1, despite the routine use of G-CSF (filgrastim) support. Five out of 42 (12%) pretreated or chemonaive ED patients suffered an early death during the first cycle of chemotherapy. Myelotoxicity was frequent, with rates of grade 3 and 4 neutropenia, anemia and thrombocytopenia of 74%, 36% and 50%, respectively. Similar high rates of fatal adverse effects have been reported previously when topotecan was combined with another myelosuppressive drug on day 1.[42] However, the combination of cyclophosphamide and topotecan appears active, with 41% of patients achieving an objective response, including 10% of patients with a complete response. Thus, a safer way to combine the two drugs is needed, such as investigating of the reverse sequence of administration, with cyclophosphamide being delivered after topotecan. This strategy has proved to be safe when combined with cisplatin.[39,40]

Paclitaxel combinations

Addition of a novel active agent to a standard regimen has been a commonly pursued concept in the search for a more effective combination chemotherapy. Since the establishment of paclitaxel as an active agent in SCLC, achieving a response rate in the range of 29–41% in both previously treated and untreated patients,[43–45] a number of groups have investigated the addition of paclitaxel to standard etoposide- and platinum-based chemotherapy. Niell et al[46] randomized 587 ED patients to receive either a three-drug combination, adding paclitaxel to cisplatin and etoposide supported by G-CSF, or a two-drug combination with cisplatin and etoposide (Table 7.3).[46] The same doses of etoposide and cisplatin were used in the two arms. Paclitaxel was delivered on day 1 at a dose of 175 mg/m^2 as a 4-hour infusion. Due to excessive toxicity reported in another study using a similar schedule,[47] performance status 2 patients were excluded after the enrollment of the first 60 patients.

Hematologic toxicity was comparable, but more grade 3 hearing loss, renal toxicity, and motor and sensory neuropathy were seen in the paclitaxel arm. More importantly, the toxic death rate was 6.5% in the paclitaxel arm, compared with 2.4% in the reference arm. Most deaths occurred following the first cycle of chemotherapy, and were mainly caused by neutropenic sepsis. High rates of fatal adverse events had been reported previously. A Greek randomized study (Table 7.3) using a similar design and an almost identical schedule and dose, including growth factor support, was prematurely closed after 133 patients were enrolled due to a toxic death rate of 13%.[48] Similarly, 6 out of 59 patients with ED SCLC suffered a treatment-related death in a phase II study combining paclitaxel at a dose of 175 mg/m^2 with etoposide and cisplatin.[47] In the study by Niell et al,[46] the increased toxicity did not result in any improvement in efficacy. The median failure-free and overall survival were 5.9 versus 6.4 months and 9.9 versus 10.6 months on the two-drug arm compared with the paclitaxel arm, respectively (see Table 7.3) The overall response rates were insignificantly higher in the paclitaxel arm (75% vs 68%).

These data corroborate an earlier trial randomizing both LD and ED patients to either paclitaxel or vincristine in the combination with carboplatin and etoposide phosphate.[49] Although the complete response rate was nearly doubled among the 306 ED patients included in the study, this difference did not translated into any improvement in survival data. However, when survival data were analyzed for the entire population, consisting of 614 LD and ED patients, a minor but significant survival benefit of 1 month was observed. The authors have recently reported the long-term survival after a 6-year follow-up time, confirming a survival benefit in the mixed population of ED and LD patients. Median survival and 5-year survival rate increased from 11.7 to 12.5 months (see Table 7.3) and from 6% to 14% in the paclitaxel arm ($p = 0.03$).[50] Toxicity was manageable, and the addition of paclitaxel did not lead to any excessive toxic death rate (3.6% vs 2.9%), reflecting that the dose of etoposide phosphate in the paclitaxel arm was reduced to 80% of that used in the vincristine arm, as

Table 7.3   Paclitaxel added to platinum-based chemotherapy

Reference (first author)	No. of patients	Stage	Chemotherapy		Response rate (%)		Median failure-free survival (months)		Median survival (months)		Toxic death rate (%)	
			P	Non-P	P	Non-P	P	Non-P	P	Non-P	P	Non-P
Niell[46]	587	ED	PEC	EC	75	68	6.4	5.9	10.6	9.9	6.5	2.4
Mavroudis[48]	133	LD/ED	PEC	EC	50	46	NA	NA	10.5	11.5	13	0
Smit[52]	197	ED	PCb	CyDE	54	56	3.4	4.6	6.7	6.5	NA	NA
Reck[49]	614	LD/ED	PEpCb	VEpCb	72	69	8.1	7.5	12.5	11.7	3.6	2.9
Reck[49]	306	ED	PEpCb	VEpCb	67	60	–	–	9.8	10.0	–	–
Bunn[47]	59	–	PEC	–	–	–	–	–	–	–	10	–

C, cisplatin; Cb, carboplatin; Cy, cyclophosphamide; D, doxorubicin; E, etoposide; Ep, etoposide phosphate; P, paclitaxel; V, vincristine; ED, extended disease; LD, limited disease.

opposed to the study by Niell et al,[46] which used equal doses of etoposide and cisplatin in both the arms with and without the addition of paclitaxel. Furthermore, in ED patients, the dose of etoposide phosphate was additionally reduced to 80% of the dose used in LD patients for safety reasons.[49,50] In conclusion, the addition of the myelotoxic agent paclitaxel to standard etoposide- and platinum-based chemotherapy does not seem advantageous in the palliative setting of ED SCLC patients. No gains in survival have been reported in three randomized trials, and paclitaxel adds to the risk of toxic death in frail ED patients when no reduction in the dose of etoposide is performed (see Table 7.3).

In order to minimize myelotoxicity, a different strategy would be to incorporate paclitaxel as part of a two-drug regimen. Dutch investigators have reported an exceptionally high response rate of 74% (95% CI 59–88%) in patients refractory to cyclophosphamide, doxorubin and etoposide using the combination of carboplatin and paclitaxel as second-line treatment.[51] These encouraging data served as an impetus to investigate this regimen further in a randomized trial.[52] One hundred and ninety-seven ED patients were randomly allocated to paclitaxel and carboplatin or to standard cyclophosphamide, doxorubicin and etoposide (CDE). A relatively high carboplatin dose of AUC 7 was used, whereas paclitaxel was given as a standard dose of 175 mg/m^2. Twenty percent of patients had performance status 2. In both arms, more than 90% of the planned doses were delivered. More hematologic toxicity and febrile neutropenia were seen in the standard arm. Response rates were similar (54% vs 56% in the paclitaxel and standard arms, respectively). The sample size was based on an expected progression-free survival of 5.8 months observed following CDE in a previous report by the same group.[53] However, the reported progression-free survivals in both arms were considerable shorter than expected and did not differ significantly, although a numerical increase from 3.4 to 4.6 months was observed in favor of the standard arm. Also, the median survival times in both arms were rather short (6.5 vs 6.7 months; $p = 0.68$). Of note, response rates to paclitaxel and carboplatin in these chemonaive patients were lower than reported by the same group in a previous phase II study evaluating the same regimen in relapsed patients deemed refractory to second-line therapy,[51] reflecting selection bias in small phase II trials.

Combination chemotherapy including antimetabolites

In a phase II trial, Greek investigators treated 22 patients with gemcitabine 1000 mg/m^2 on days 1 and 8 and docetaxel 75 mg/m^2 on day 8, every 21 days.[54] The combination was inactive, with no objective responses observed in this heavily pretreated group of patients that included 64% patients deemed refractory to chemotherapy. The combination of gemcitabine and vinorelbine was investigated in a two-stage Simon design phase II trial including patients with progressive or recurrent SCLC.[55] The same dose of gemcitabine as in the Greek trial was used with vinorelbine 25 mg/m^2 on days 1 and 8. After the inclusion of 17 patients, further accrual was stopped, as only 1 patient had a partial response. In a non-comparative randomized phase II trial, two gemcitabine-based chemotherapy regimens were compared as part of either a doublet or a triplet.[56] One hundred and forty chemonaive patients with ED or poor-prognosis LD were randomly allocated to cisplatin, etoposide and gemcitabine or to cisplatin and gemcitabine. Both regimens were active, with median survival times of approximately 10 months, and response rates of 57% and 63% in the doublet and triplet arms, respectively. The triplet regimen resulted in a higher complete response rate (18.6% vs 4.3%) and more hematologic toxicity. In 69 patients with previously untreated ED SCLC, gemcitabine and carboplatin resulted in a response rate of 43% and a median survival of 9.2 months, which is comparable to what is commonly seen in similar patient populations.[57] Toxicity was mild and manageable. Based on these four phase II trials evaluating various gemcitabine-based combinations, the addition of platinum to gemcitabine represents an active combination in SCLC, whereas combinations with antimicrotubule agents have limited or no activity (Table 7.4). However, the two trials evaluating combinations with antimicrotubule agents were performed on a patient population with an inherently low likelihood of response, reflected by the short median survival times of 3.2–5.4 months (Table 7.4), which equally could account for the lack of demonstrable activity.

A phase II study randomly allocated 68 previously untreated ED patients with performance status 1 or 2 to either carboplatin AUC 5 or 75 mg/m^2 cisplatin, both in combination with the antifolate pemetrexed at a dose of 500 mg/m^2.[58] Vitamin B$_{12}$ and folic acid were supplied. Response rates ranged between 48% and 62%, which are higher than those reported in early single-agent platinum phase II studies. Factors predicting for response in a relapsed SCLC population such as treatment-free interval and response to first-line therapy were not reported.

Anthracycline-based combination chemotherapy

A British trial compared anthracycline-based with cisplatin-based therapy in a mixed population of LD and ED patients.[59] Two hundred and seventy-three patients were randomly allocated to standard cisplatin and etoposide or to doxorubicin, cyclophosphamide and etoposide. In both arms, etoposide doses were split into IV and oral delivery on day 1 and days 2 and 3, respectively. Myelosuppression, infections and septicemia were significantly more pronounced on the doxorubicin arm. Grade 3 and 4 neutropenia, infections and hospitalization days due to neutropenia were 97%, 79% and 1185 days on the doxorubicin arm compared with 61%, 30% and 350 days on the platinum-based arm, respectively. No data on the risk of death due to toxicity were provided. Etoposide and cisplatin induced more grade 2 and 3 nausea. Median survival and 1-year survival rates were equal (10.1 vs 10.7 months and 37% vs 38%, respectively). Subgroup analysis comparing LD and ED patients also failed to demonstrate any survival benefit. In conclusion, doxorubicin-based

Table 7.4 Phase II trials of gemcitabine-based combinations

Reference (first author)	No. of patients	Chemotherapy	Response rate (%)	Median survival (months)	Pretreatment	Stage	Patients refractory to chemotherapy (%)
Agelaki[54]	22	GD	0	3.2	All	ED/LD	64
De Marinis[56]	70	GC	57	10	None	ED/LD	0
De Marinis[56]	70	GEC	63	9.5	None	ED/LD	0
Dudek[55]	17	GV	6	5.4	All	NA	NA
Neubauer[57]	69	GCb	43	9.2	None	ED	0

G, gemcitabine; D, docetaxel; C, cisplatin; E, etoposide; V, vinorelbine; Cb, carboplatin; ED, extended disease; LD, limited disease.

chemotherapy did not provide any benefit in this trial, and the risk of severe infections was significantly increased in the doxorubin arm.

Spanish investigators compared standard etoposide (100 mg/m^2 on days 1–3) with epirubicin (100 mg/m^2 on day 1), both in combination with cisplatin.[60] The trial was fairly large, enrolling 402 patients equally distributed between LD and ED patients. Chest radiotherapy was given after the completion of chemotherapy. Compliance with the planned dose was relatively low, with only two-thirds of the patients completing all six cycles of therapy. No differences were seen in response rates or progression-free or overall survival. Slightly fewer toxicity and treatment-related deaths were recorded in the epirubicin arm. A major concern of the study is the sequential delivery of radiotherapy, which according to meta-analyses seems inferior to early concurrent radiotherapy.[3,4] At least in LD patients, the use of epirubicin does not seem feasible, as experiences with the combination of anthracyclines and radiotherapy have been poor.[1]

Japanese authors conducted a phase I/II trial determining the recommended dose of the synthetic anthracycline amrubicin in combination with cisplatin.[61] The phase II part of the study treated chemonaive ED patients with amrubicin 40 mg/m^2 on days 1–3 and cisplatin 60 mg/m^2 on day 1 The combination resulted in an impressive response rate of 88%. Median survival was a promising 13.6 months, indicating a potential future role for this combination.

Dose-dense chemotherapy

Dose-dense chemotherapy has the theoretical potential to augment tumor cell kill. However, the role of dose-dense therapy remains controversial in SCLC due to conflicting results in various randomized studies conducted over the years. To further evaluate this treatment concept, a British trial randomly assigned 318 'better-prognosis patients' to standard ICE (ifosfamide, carboplatin and etoposide) delivered at 4-week intervals or to dose-dense ICE in similar doses but given at 2-week intervals supported by G-CSF (filgrastim) and autologous blood transfusions.[62]

Chest radiotherapy was performed according to local guidelines, which for all patients consisted of sequential radiotherapy. 'Better-prognosis' patients were selected by restricting inclusion to patients with less than one negative prognostic factor, including poor performance status, ED, low serum sodium and elevated lactate dehydrogenase (LDH) or alkaline phosphatase. More patients with absence of any negative prognostic factors were allocated to the standard arm (58 vs 49%). After completion of chemotherapy, PCI was delivered to significantly more patients on the dose-dense arm compared with the standard arm (53% vs 35%). The reason for this difference is unknown, but the rate of complete response did not differ. Approximately 10% of all patients had ED. The median relative dose intensities were 99% and 182% in the standard and dose-dense arms, respectively. Of 158 patients allocated to the dose-dense arm, 18 were subsequently transferred to the standard arms mainly because of toxicity, i.e. a delay of more than 2 weeks for the recovery of the bone marrow.

Anemia and thrombocytopenia were, as expected, significantly more pronounced in the dose-dense arm, and myelotoxicity accumulated with the number of cycles received. This tendency was more marked in the dose-dense arm. The need for red cell and platelet transfusion was significantly higher in the dose-dense arm, but the increased myelotoxicity did not translate into clinically relevant toxicities. In fact, fewer fatal and serious adverse events were recorded in the dose-dense arm ($n = 5$) compared with the standard arm ($n = 9$). Furthermore, significantly fewer cycles of dose-dense chemotherapy were complicated with neutropenic sepsis (11.6% vs 15.3%). Non-hematologic toxicity did not differ between the two arms. With respect to efficacy, no significant benefit of dose-dense therapy was observed. Response rates, median survival times and 2-year survival rates were 80% vs 88%, 13.9 vs 14.4 months and 22% vs 19% in the standard and dose-dense arms, respectively. However, due to the shorter treatment time in the dose-dense schedule, patients in this arm had a correspondingly longer treatment-free survival. The authors conclude that the dose-dense strategy has reached a plateau, and further attempts to pursue this strategy do not seem justified.

SECOND-LINE CHEMOTHERAPY

Because of its high relapse rate, the management of relapsed SCLC is a very common clinical problem. Good-quality studies to guide the decision-making process are very scarce; in particular, randomized studies are lacking. As the expected lifespan of the patient is short, the main treatment goal is palliative, including maintaining or increasing the patient's quality of life. This is contrasted by the very few studies reporting quality-of-life data. However, there is a general consensus supporting the use of second-line therapy for the fit, relapsed SCLC patient. The evidence supporting this strategy is based on numerous uncontrolled phase II trials reporting clinically meaningful response rates, ranging from 10% to 70%, in selected patients.[63] The selection of patients fit to receive salvage therapy represents a complex clinical decision. Some retrospective and prospective data are available to guide this decision. Factors that predict response to second-line treatment include response to first-line treatment, performance status and time elapsed from discontinuation of first-line treatment. Until recently, it was not known whether second-line therapy influenced survival, as no randomized trials had compared chemotherapy versus best supportive care.

To answer this important question, 141 relapsed patients were randomly allocated to oral topotecan 2.3 mg/m^2 on days 1–5 every 3 weeks or to best supportive care.[64] Prognostic and predictive factors for response were equally balanced. Approximately two-thirds of patients had performance status 0 or 1. A similar proportion had ED. The median treatment-free interval was in the range of 12 weeks. Topotecan resulted in a modest response rate of 7%, and 44% of patients achieved stable disease. As expected, hematologic toxicity was higher in the topotecan arm. Grade 3 and 4 vomiting and diarrhea were a modest 3% and 6%, respectively. Grade 3 and 4 fatigue was equal, whereas dyspnea and pain were reduced in the topotecan arm compared with best supportive care (3% vs 9% and 3% vs 6%, respectively), indicating better symptom control in the topotecan arm. Patient-reported quality of life is increasingly considered an obligatory tool in assessing palliative treatment. In accordance with this trend, one of the strengths of this trial was the inclusion of a formal evaluation of quality of life. Although these data were not reported in detail, a significantly faster rate of deterioration in quality of life was seen on the best supportive care arm. Most encouragingly, topotecan led to a significant survival benefit of 12 weeks, and the overall 6-month survival rate was 49%, compared with 26% on the best supportive care arm ($p = 0.01$). Surprisingly, subset analysis showed that even in patients with a treatment-free interval <60 days, the survival difference remained significant (23 vs 13 weeks), whereas in patients with a treatment-free interval >60 days, this significance was lost (28 vs 14 weeks; $p = 0.1$) Still, the largest numerical survival benefit was seen in patients with the longest treatment-free interval. The increase in survival was accomplished without increasing the risk of early death. On the contrary, the all-cause 30-day mortality rate was increased to 13% in the best supportive care arm compared with 7%. Sepsis occurred in 4% of patients on topotecan and 3 treatment-related deaths were recorded. This study is the first trial to suggest a benefit in survival and quality of life when treating relapsed SCLC, thus adding valuable information to guide the management of SCLC.

It is still an open question which type of second-line therapy is superior. Previous randomized trials found that a three-agent combination with cyclophosphamide, doxorubicin and vincristine (CAV) resulted in equal response rates and survival compared with intravenous topotecan.[65] Furthermore, IV and oral topotecan showed similar response in a randomized trial.[66] The results of this trial will presumably serve as an inspiration to compare other treatments with oral topotecan.

In an interesting Norwegian study, patients relapsing after their participation in a previously published two-armed phase III trial[30] were systematically crossed to the comparative regimen. Out of 286 patients enrolled in the first-line study, 56 patients were crossed over to etoposide and cisplatin after first-line cyclophosphamide, epirubicin and vincristine and 52 patients were crossed over in the reverse sequence.[67] Non-randomly, 166 patients were offered best supportive care by their treating physician. The authors focused on prognostic factors and survival in the three groups of patients, leaving out data on response rates. Not surprisingly, median survival time in the crossover population was significantly longer (5.3 months) compared with the best supportive care group (2.2 months). This difference most likely reflects the fact that significantly more patients in the best supportive care group had performance status ≥ 2 and shorter treatment-free intervals than those patients receiving second-line treatment. Also, a significantly higher proportion of the best supportive care patients were classified as having refractory disease. In the cross-over population, a Cox multivariate regression analysis identified performance status at relapse as the only prognostic factor. This in contrast to other studies reporting that the length of treatment-free interval and response to first-line induction therapy predict for response to second-line therapy.[63] However, there could be several explanations for this discrepancy; the authors reported prognostic factors instead of predictive factors, as no response rate data were available. Older data from non-randomized phase II trials have implied that second-line etoposide–cisplatin following CAV results in superior response rates of 30–40% compared with response rates of 10% following the reverse sequence.[68–70] However, this notion is challenged by the present study reporting no survival benefit when comparing those patients receiving salvage etoposide–cisplatin with those treated with cyclophosphamide, epirubicin and vincristine (3.9 vs 4.5 months). It would be of interest to compare the total survival times from initial randomization to first-line therapy in the subset of patients progressing to cross-over therapy, as the original published phase III trial reported a substantial survival benefit of nearly 5 months for LD patients allocated to first-line cisplatin and etoposide.[30]

TREATMENT OF ELDERLY AND POOR-PROGNOSIS PATIENTS

Knowledge concerning the optimal treatment of the elderly is limited, as most large randomized trials tend to exclude elderly patients. This is despite the fact that more than one-third of patients with SCLC are >70 years old and the proportion of the elderly in population is continuously increasing, as the average expected lifetime increases in the general population. Thus, studies focusing on this group of patients are highly warranted.

In patients >70 years old, Ardizzoni et al[71] evaluated two regimens of cisplatin and etoposide – full dose (FD) and reduced dose (RD) – in a two-stage randomized non-comparative phase II design. Cisplatin was administered as a split dose on days 1 and 2, and etoposide was given on days 1–3. Cisplatin doses were 25 vs 40 mg/m^2/day and etoposide doses were 60 vs 100 mg/m^2/day in the RD and FD arms, respectively. The primary endpoint was the rate of treatment success (TS), defined as the proportion of patients receiving at least three courses of the planned dose of FD chemotherapy on time and achieving an objective response without grade 3 and 4 toxicity or any chemotherapy-related complications. This seems a relevant clinically endpoint; however, the recording of validated quality-of-life data would have added valuable information in this palliative setting. The criterion for proceeding to the second stage of accrual was a TS rate >50% among the first 24 patients. The RD arm was closed to further enrollment after accrual of 28 patients in the first stage due to a low TS (36%), which was mainly due to lack of objective response. The accrual of patients on the FD arm continued through the second stage to a total of 67 patients with a TS rate of 63%. Only 1 patient on the FD arm suffered a toxic death, and the frequency of grade 3 and 4 hematologic and non-hematologic toxicity amounted to approximately 10%. Median survival times and 1-year survival rates were 31 vs 41 weeks and 18% vs 39% on the RD and FD arms, respectively. RD chemotherapy seems to compromise the chance of achieving response, resulting in inferior survival time, and indicating that the two doses used are within the range of the steep part of the dose–response curve. In conclusion, RD chemotherapy offers no advantage over FD chemotherapy, which is in accordance with previously randomized trials indicating that presumable less toxic treatment regimens can compromise the goal of palliation, symptom control and survival.[36,37]

Whether the benefit of the FD arm could be achieved without the use of G-CSF in this elderly population is an open question. Certainly, it has never been established that the addition of growth factors to platinum-based chemotherapy results in improved outcome. The split cisplatin dose concept in an elderly or poor-prognosis population was also used in a randomized phase III trial comparing split-course cisplatin with carboplatin in combination with etoposide.[72] Cisplatin was split over days 1–3 at a dose of 25 mg/m²/day and the carboplatin dose was AUC 5. More than 90% of the 220 patients were >70 years old (median age 74), and 25% of patients had performance status 2 or 3. The toxic death rate was low and acceptable in both arms, and toxicity was similar except for a higher frequency of thrombocytopenia in the carboplatin arm, as expected. Of note, cisplatin did not induce a higher incidence of grade 3 and 4 nausea compared with carboplatin (28% vs 24%). Response rates and palliation score did not differ significantly. Also, progression-free and overall median survival times and 2-year survival rates were equal (5.3 vs 4.7 months, 10.6 vs 9.8 months and 11% vs 12% for carboplatin and split-course arm, respectively). These data support the general consensus that carboplatin can substitute for cisplatin in a palliative setting without compromising clinical outcome.

In a subset analysis,[73] the NCCTG compared treatment outcome in patients under and over 70 years old participating in a previously published trial randomizing LD patients to either once-daily or split-course twice-daily concurrent radiotherapy.[8] The analysis was based on a total of 263 included patients, of whom 54 patients were >70 years old at inclusion. The 2-year and 5-year survival rates were numerically lower in the elderly group (33% vs 48% and 17% vs 22%, $p = 0.14$). Although not significant, the p value is rather low, raising the question of whether significance would be reached if a higher proportion of elderly were included in the trial. However, the data emphasize that in selected elderly patients, long-term survival can be achieved. The study confirms that elderly patients are frailer, with significantly lower performance status and more weight loss than younger patients. Accordingly, the risk of severe adverse events was significantly higher: 6% and 5.6% of the elderly suffered grade 4 pneumonitis and treatment-related deaths, respectively. In the younger patients, no episodes of pneumonitis were recorded and only 0.5% died from toxicity. Caution and thorough assessment of comorbidity are advisable when considering concurrent twice-daily radiotherapy for patients >70 years old. A discussion with each individual patient should carefully balance the risk and benefits, including the risk of early treatment-related death.

SUPPORTIVE AND NON-CYTOTOXIC TREATMENTS

Epoetin (recombinant human erythropoetin) is widely used as a supportive measure during chemotherapy for various cancers in order to avoid anemia and maintain quality of life, although detrimental effects have been suggested in head and neck cancer.[74] As tumor hypoxia causes relative radio-resistance, correcting anemia could lead to better clinical outcome in LD SCLC patients treated with concurrent radiotherapy. This hypothesis was tested in a trial randomizing to either placebo or 40 000 IU epoetin alfa given every week throughout therapy until the completion of PCI in a placebo-controlled double-blind design.[75]

The target hemoglobin level was set to 14–16 g/dl (8.1–9.9 mmol/L). As expected, in the placebo group, hemoglobin dropped to a mean of 10 g/dl compared with 13 g/dl, which was corrected by a higher proportion of patients needing transfusion in the placebo arm (52% vs 15%). This translated into a greater decline in quality of life in the placebo arm, with a trend towards significance. However, due to a significantly higher rate of vascular thrombotic events in the epoetin alfa arm (34.6% vs 7.7%), the study was prematurely closed after the inclusion of 104 patients. The authors appropriately performed such a post-hoc analysis, which identified hemoglobin level of >13 g/dl (8.1 mmol/l) at baseline as a factor predicting for these events, with a trend towards significance ($p = 0.096$). Based on these findings, the use of epoetin alfa should be discouraged on a routine basis outside clinical trials. The future development of epoetin needs thorough consideration, including the complete suspension of further evaluation. However, other options should be considered, such as the reduction of target hemoglobin levels or the administration of epoetin in combination with low-molecular-weight heparin (LMWH) in future trials.

Altinbas et al[76] randomized 84 LD and ED patients to non-platinum-based chemotherapy with or without the addition of LMWH (dalteparin, 5000 U daily). Patients with LD received radiotherapy after the completion of chemotherapy and LMWH. Treatment was safe, with no treatment-related deaths and only a few manageable bleeding episodes. Overall survival increased significantly in the LMWH arm to 13 months, compared with 8 months in the chemotherapy-alone arm. The study represents a very small sample size and should be considered a non-comparative randomized phase II trial. Accordingly, no firm conclusions can be drawn regarding the benefit of LMWH. However, the data lend renewed interest to a well-known hypothesis indicating that correcting malignancy-induced coagulopathy could improve clinical outcome. This hypothesis needs to be evaluated in properly sized randomized phase III trials.

Due to poor recruitment, a randomized study evaluating the addition of heat-killed *Mycobacterium vaccae* to standard combination chemotherapy was prematurely closed after the inclusion of 80 SCLC patients.[77] A suspension of mycobacterium (SRL 172) was injected intradermally 1 day prior to the administration of platinum- or anthracycline-based chemotherapy every 4 weeks. In the comparative arm, patients were treated with chemotherapy alone, with no placebo injections being used. No significant differences in toxicity, response rates, response duration or median survival were observed. Median survival times were 41 and 40 weeks in the SRL 172 and no-SRL 172 arms, respectively. Among the 62 patients with symptom control data available, symptom response rate was significantly higher in the SRL 172 arm compared with the chemotherapy-alone arm (93% vs 63%). Similarly, an increased response rate in symptom control in NSCLC has been reported by the same group.[78] Because of the small sample size and the lack of placebo control, it is impossible to determine whether these differences in symptom control represent a genuine immunologic effect of SRL 172.

CALGB investigated the addition of tamoxifen to standard etoposide/cisplatin in a randomized study including 307 LD patients.[79] High-dose tamoxifen was administered for 5 days at a dose of 80 mg twice-daily, starting the day before each cycle of chemotherapy. Thoracic radiotherapy was delivered concurrently with cycles 5 and 6. PCI was offered to all patients with near-complete response or better. Toxicity and survival were similar, indicating no role for tamoxifen in LD SCLC.

TARGETED THERAPIES

The advent of therapies based on mechanisms that target critical molecular pathways of tumors has evoked considerable interest. Targeted therapies are not classical cytotoxics: instead, they work by disrupting pathways in processes of tumor progression, including neovascularization, dissemination, apoptosis and signal transduction. Consequently, it is expected that these drugs have the potential to convert cancer from an acute to a chronic disease by forcing tumor cells into dormancy. Maintenance therapy of patients in remission has been used as model to test this hypothesis. In a phase II study, the potential of the antiangiogenic drug thalidomide as a maintenance therapy was explored by Cooney et al[80] based on its activity in other malignancies such as multiple myeloma. Eighteen evaluable patients out of a planned 30 with complete or partial response to induction therapy were offered maintenance therapy with daily doses of 200 mg/m^2 oral thalidomide until progression. No grade 3 or 4 toxicity was reported. At the time of presentation of the study, the 1-year survival rate was 60%, which correspond to the prespecified criteria for exploring this regimen further. French authors have also performed a randomized study evaluating maintenance thalidomide given concurrently with chemotherapy in ED SCLC patients.[81] The study was stopped prematurely due to a low accrual when 119 patients out of a planned 200 were included. Patients were treated with two cycles of etoposide, cisplatin, cyclophosphamide and epirubicin. Responding patients were randomly allocated to an additional four cycles of chemotherapy in combination with either 400 mg daily thalidomide or placebo. Out of 97 responding patients, 92 patients were randomized. In the thalidomide arm, fewer patients withdrew from therapy due to disease progression (62% vs 43%; $p = 0.06$) and thalidomide-treated patients had a significantly longer median survival (11.7 months) compared with placebo-treated patients (8.7 months). However, more patients in the thalidomide arm withdrew as a result of toxicity (55% vs 35%), mainly because of severe neuropathy. The authors conclude that further use of thalidomide is prohibited by the high rate of neuropathy, and they recommend the development of novel derivatives of thalidomide with less neuropathic potential. However, the concurrent use of cisplatin undoubtedly has contributed to the high rate of neuropathy, as no severe adverse effects were reported in the aforementioned study using 200 mg/m^2 thalidomide alone.[80] As thalidomide seems to be active in SCLC based on the promising survival data, efforts to further these treatment principles should be pursued.

Temsirolimus targets the mTOR kinase, which results in a G_1 phase cell cycle block, effectively inhibiting cell proliferation. Thus, this drug has the potential to push cancer cells into dormancy, making it an ideal candidate for maintenance therapy. Based on these data, the ECOG randomized 87 ED patients in remission to treatment with two different doses of weekly IV temsirolimus (25 vs 250 mg/m^2).[82] With a difference in dose of a factor 10, the low-dose arm could be perceived as a placebo-like arm. The sample size enabled the detection of a 4-month difference in progression-free survival with a power of 85% and a significance level of 10%. Five out of 44 patients in the low-dose arm had brain metastases, compared with no patients in the high-dose arm. Toxicity was mild. Median survival from randomization numerically favoured the high-dose arm (9.0 vs 6.5 months), and progression-free survival times were 2.5 months in the high-dose arm compared with 1.8 months in the low-dose arm. The survival data seem promising and the authors recommended further study, although the prespecified criteria of an increase in progression-free survival of 4 months were not met. Although maintenance therapy using classical cytotoxics has previously failed to show any clear clinical meaningful benefit, the emergence of these new interesting data holds promise for a role for targeted therapies as maintenance therapy.

Bortezomib was evaluated as single agent in a phase II study comprising 28 sensitive and 28 refractory relapsed SCLC patients.[83] Bortezomib is a proteasome inhibitor that induces apoptosis through a decrease in Bcl-2. Reported toxicities were thrombocytopenia and fatigue. Only one partial response was observed, indicating no role for bortezomib as a single agent in SCLC. However, the population consisted of poor-prognosis patients illustrated by a very short median survival of less than 3 months.

An interesting principle targeting the cytotoxic drug DM1 to CD56$^+$ cells by conjugating the cytotoxic to a humanized antibody with affinity to CD56 was evaluated in 10 patients with relapsed pulmonary or non-pulmonary CD56⁺ small cell carcinomas.[84] The immunoconjugate BB-10901 was delivered intravenously every week for 4 weeks in a 6-week cycle: one patient had an episode of aseptic meningitis of 1-week duration; 3 non-confirmed minor responses were observed. More mature data are awaited.

G3139, an antisense oligonucleotide directed at the *BCL2* gene, was evaluated in combination with carboplatin and etoposide in 63 chemonaive ED patients. A randomized 3:1 design was used, with every 4th patient being allocated to carboplatin and etoposide without antisense therapy.[85] Grade 4 myelotoxicity was seen in 2 out of 5 patients in the chemotherapy-alone arm. In the combination treatment arm, grade 4 myelotoxicity was more common (61% of patients). Non-hematologic toxicity was rare, although 1 patient in the combined-treatment arm died of renal failure. Responses were observed in 12 out of 18 evaluable patients on the arm including antisense therapy.

Although the epidermal growth factor receptor (EGFR) is not overexpressed in SCLC, Moore et al[86] assessed the activity of the EGFR tyrosine kinase inhibitor gefitinib in relapsed SCLC or neuroendocrine tumors. Nineteen patients with either chemosensitive ($n = 12$) or chemorefractory ($n = 7$) disease were treated with 250 mg of gefitinib as a daily oral dose. None of the patients experienced grade 3 or 4 rash or diarrhea. Two patients had stable disease for more than 90 days and 17 patients had progressive disease. Thus, it seems that gefitinib has no activity in SCLC.

Based on the findings that the target of imatinib, namely the KIT receptor tyrosine kinase, is commonly expressed in SCLC, Krug et al[87] assessed the activity of imatinib in patients with recurrent SCLC in a phase II trial. Confirming the high frequency of KIT-positive SCLC tumors, they identified 28 patients with KIT-expressing tumors out of 36 patients (78%) with assessable tumor samples using immmunohistochemistry. Twenty patients were treated with an imatinib dose of 400 mg orally twice daily. However, despite expression of KIT in all patients, no objective responses were observed, suggesting that imatinib has no activity in relapsed SCLC.

The farnesyltransferase inhibitor R115777 was evaluated in patients with sensitive relapsed SCLC.[88] The drug was administered orally twice daily at a dose of 400 mg every 21 days for a consecutive period of 14 days. Toxicity was mild. However, in this population with a high a priori chance of response, no objective responses were observed after the inclusion of 20 patients. Thus, R115777 should be regarded as an inactive drug in SCLC.

CONCLUSION

Two meta-analyses indicated that early radiotherapy starting 4–9 weeks after the initiation of therapy is superior to late delivery of radiotherapy when given concurrently with platinum-based chemotherapy in LD patients. The survival benefit was estimated to an absolute 6.4% increase in 5-year survival (20.2% vs 13.8%) according to one of the meta-analyses.[4] A number of phase II trials have evaluated the introduction of newer agents such as paclitaxel and topoisomerase I inhibitors given as induction therapy or concurrently with radiotherapy (see Table 7.1). No regimen has been singled out as superior to others. Median survival times in these small trials are in the range of what can be achieved with cisplatin–etoposide given currently with twice-daily radiotherapy in a large randomized trial.[9] Topoisomerase I inhibitors in combinations with platinum have resulted in equal survival times when compared with standard etoposide–platinum combinations in ED patients in two large randomized trials with no increase in overall toxicity, although the toxicity profile varies between the two combinations. Etoposide induced more neutropenia and irinotecan caused more diarrhea (see Table 7.2). A small, prematurely stopped, Japanese randomized trial published in 2002 indicated a survival benefit for irinotecan compared with etoposide,[28] but the results have not yet been confirmed in other trials. Paclitaxel added to standard chemotherapy resulted in increased toxicity in three randomized trials without any improvement in survival (see Table 7.3). Oral topotecan in relapsed SCLC led to a survival benefit of 3 months and better quality of life when compared with best supportive care. The benefit was achieved without any increase in risk of early death or unacceptable toxicity. Finally, survival data in responding patients hold promise for a role of targeted therapies as maintenance therapy, including the antiangiogenic agent thalidomide and temsirolimus targeting mTOR kinase.

REFERENCES

1. Pignon JP Arriagada R Ihde DC et al. A meta-analysis of thoracic radiotherapy for small cell lung cancer. N Engl J Med 1992; 327: 1618–24.

2. Warde P, Payne D. Does thoracic irradiation improve survival and local control in limited stage small cell lung carcinoma of the lung? A meta-analysis. J Clin Oncol 1992; 10: 890–5.

3. Pijls-Johannesma MC, De Ruysscher D, Lambin P et al. Early versus late chest radiotherapy for limited stage small cell lung cancer. Cochrane Database Syst Rev 2005; (1): CD004700.

4. Fried DB, Morris DE, Poole C et al. Systematic review evaluating the timing of thoracic radiation therapy in combined modality therapy for limited-stage small-cell lung cancer. J Clin Oncol 2004; 22: 4837–45.

5. Gregor A, Drings P, Burghouts J et al. Randomized trial of alternating versus sequential radiotherapy/chemotherapy in limited-disease patients with small-cell lung cancer: a European Organization for Research and Treatment of Cancer Lung Cancer Cooperative Group Study. J Clin Oncol 1997; 15: 2840–9.

6. Jeremic B, Shibamoto Y, Acimovic L et al. Initial versus delayed accelerated hyperfractionated radiation therapy and concurrent chemotherapy in limited small-cell lung cancer: a randomized study. J Clin Oncol 1997; 15: 893–900.

7. James LE, Spiro S, O'Donnel KM et al. A randomised study of timing of

thoracic irradiation in small cell lung cancer (SCLC) – Study 8. Lung Cancer 2003; 41: S23 (abstract O-69).

8. Bonner JA, Sloan JA, Shanahan TG et al. Phase III comparison of twice-daily split-course irradiation versus once-daily irradiation for patients with limited stage small-cell lung carcinoma. J Clin Oncol 1999; 17: 2681–91.

9. Turrisi AT 3rd, Kim K, Blum R et al. Twice-daily compared with once-daily thoracic radiotherapy in limited small-cell lung cancer treated concurrently with cisplatin and etoposide. N Engl J Med 1999; 17: 265–71.

10. Work E, Nielsen OS, Bentzen SM et al. Randomized study of initial versus late chest irradiation combined with chemotherapy in limited-stage small-cell lung cancer. Aarhus Lung Cancer Group. J Clin Oncol 1997; 15: 3030–7.

11. Takada M, Fukuoka M, Kawahara M et al. Phase III study of concurrent versus sequential thoracic radiotherapy in combination with cisplatin and etoposide for limited-stage small-cell lung cancer: results of the Japan Clinical Oncology Group Study 9104. J Clin Oncol 2002; 20: 3054–60.

12. Perry MC, Herndon JE 3rd, Eaton WL et al. Thoracic radiation therapy added to chemotherapy for small-cell lung cancer: an update of Cancer and Leukemia Group B Study 8083. J Clin Oncol 1998; 16: 2466–7.

13. Murray N, Coy P, Pater JL et al. Importance of timing for thoracic irradiation in the combined modality treatment of limited-stage small-cell lung cancer. The National Cancer Institute of Canada Clinical Trials Group. J Clin Oncol 1993; 11: 336–44.

14. Skarlos DV, Samantas E, Briassoulis E et al. Randomized comparison of early versus late hyperfractionated thoracic irradiation concurrently with chemotherapy in limited disease small-cell lung cancer: a randomized phase II study of the Hellenic Cooperative Oncology Group (HeCOG). Ann Oncol 2001; 12: 1231–8.

15. De Ruysscher D, Pijls M, Bentzen S et al. SER, a novel time factor predictive for long-term survival in patients with limited disease small cell lung cancer after combined chest radiotherapy and chemotherapy. Lung Cancer 2005; 49: S318 (abstract O-758).

16. Schild SE, Stella PJ, Brooks BJ et al. Results of combined-modality therapy for limited-stage small cell lung carcinoma in the elderly. Cancer 2005; 103: 2349–54.

17. Schild SE, Stella PJ, Geyer SM et al. Phase III trial comparing chemotherapy plus once-daily or twice-daily radiotherapy in stage III non-small-cell lung cancer. Int J Radiat Oncol Biol Phys 2002; 54: 370–8.

18. Fu KK, Pajak TF, Trotti A et al. A Radiation Therapy Oncology Group (RTOG) phase III randomized study to compare hyperfractionation to standard fractionation radiotherapy for head and neck squamous cell carcinomas: first report of RTOG 9003. Int J Radiat Oncol Biol Phys 2000; 48: 7–16.

19. Blackstock AW, Bogart JA, Matthews et al. Split-course versus continuous thoracic radiation therapy for limited-stage small-cell lung cancer: final report of a randomized phase III trial. Clin Lung Cancer 2005; 6: 287–92.

20. Komaki R, Allen P, Glisson G et al. Hyperfractionated/accelerated thoracic radiation therapy (HFXRT) increased survival compared to daily RT (QDRT) for limited small cell lung cancer (LSCLC) with concurrent chemotherapy (ChT). Proc Am Soc Clin Oncol 2005; 24: 659 (abstract 7158).

21. Komaki R, Swann RS, Ettinger DS et al. Phase I study of thoracic radiation dose escalation with concurrent

chemotherapy for patients with limited small-cell lung cancer: Report of Radiation Therapy Oncology Group (RTOG) Protocol 97-12. Int J Radiat Oncol Biol Phys 2005; 62: 342–50.

22. Garces YI, Okuno SH, Schild SE et al. A phase I/II NCCTG trial of escalating doses of twice daily thoracic radiation therapy (TRT) in limited-stage small cell lung cancer (LSCLC). Proc Am Soc Clin Oncol 2005; 24: 661 (abstract 7163).

23. Raymond E, Burris HA, Rowinsky EK et al. Phase I study of daily times five topotecan and single injection of cisplatin in patients with previously untreated non-small-cell lung carcinoma. Ann Oncol 1997; 8: 1003–8.

24. Miller AA, Bogart JA Watson DM et al. Phase II trial of paclitaxel–topotecan–etoposide (PTE) followed by consolidation chemoradiotherapy for limited stage small cell lung cancer (LS-SCLC): CALGB 30002. Proc Am Soc Clin Oncol 2005; 24: 662 (abstract 7170).

25. Bogart JA, Herndon JE 2nd, Lyss AP et al. 70 Gy thoracic radiotherapy is feasible concurrent with chemotherapy for limited-stage small-cell lung cancer: analysis of Cancer and Leukemia Group B Study 39808. Int J Radiat Oncol Biol Phys 2004; 59: 460–8.

26. Han JY, Kwan HC, Lee DH et al. Phase II study of irinotecan plus cisplatin induction followed by concurrent twice-daily thoracic irradiation with etoposide plus cisplatin chemotherapy for limited disease small cell lung cancer. J Clin Oncol 2005; 23: 3488–94.

27. Ettinger DS, Berkey BA, Abrams RA et al. Study of paclitaxel, etoposide, and cisplatin chemotherapy combined with twice-daily thoracic radiotherapy for patients with limited stage small cell lung cancer: a Radiation Therapy Oncology Group 9609 phase II study. J Clin Oncol 2005; 23: 4991–8.

28. Noda K, Nishiwaki Y, Kawahara M et al. Irinotecan plus cisplatin compared with etoposide plus cisplatin for extensive small-cell lung cancer. N Engl J Med 2002; 346: 85–91.

29. Sohn J, Moon YW, Lee CG et al. Phase II trial of irinotecan and cisplatin with concurrent radiotherapy in limited-disease small cell lung cancer. Proc Am Soc Clin Oncol 2005; 24: 662 (abstract 7167).

30. Sundstrom S, Bremnes RM, Kaasa S et al. Cisplatin and etoposide regimen is superior to cyclophosphamide, epirubicin, and vincristine regimen in small-cell lung cancer: results from a randomized phase III trial with 5 years' follow-up. J Clin Oncol 2002; 20: 4665–72.

31. Hanna NH, Einhorn L, Sandler A et al. Randomized, phase III trial comparing irinotecan/cisplatin (IP) with etoposide/cisplatin (EP) in patients with previously untreated, extensive-stage (ES) small cell lung cancer (SCLC). Proc Am Soc Clin Oncol 2005; 24: 622 (abstract 7004).

32. Beutler E, Gelbart T, Demina A et al. Racial variability in the UDP-glucuronosyltransferase 1 (UGT1A1) promoter: a balanced polymorphism for regulation of bilirubin metabolism? Proc Natl Acad Sci USA 1998; 95: 8170–4.

33. Schmittel A, Fischer von Weikersthal L, Sebastian H et al. Irinotecan plus carboplatin versus etoposide plus carboplatin in extensive disease small cell lung cancer: a randomized phase II trial. Proc Am Soc Clin Oncol 2005; 24: 632 (abstract 7046).

34. Huynh MT, Fehrenbacher L, West H et al. A multi-institution phase II trial of irinotecan and carboplatin for extensive or relapsed small-cell lung cancer. Proc Am Soc Clin Oncol 2005; 24: 662 (abstract 7169).

35. Eckardt JR, von Pawel J, Manikhas G et al. Comparable activity with oral topotecan/cisplatin (TC) and IV etoposide/cisplatin (PE) as treatment

for chemotherapy-naïve patients (pts) with extensive disease small cell lung cancer (ED-SCLC): final results of a randomised phase III trial (389). Proc Am Soc Clin Oncol 2005; 24: 621 (abstract 7003).

36. Souhami RL, Spiro SG, Rudd RM et al. Five-day oral etoposide treatment for advanced small-cell lung cancer: randomized comparison with intravenous chemotherapy. J Natl Cancer Inst 1997; 89: 577–80.

37. Girling DJ. Comparison of oral etoposide and standard intravenous multidrug chemotherapy for small-cell lung cancer: a stopped multicentre randomised trial. Medical Research Council Lung Cancer Working Party. Lancet 1996; 348: 563–6.

38. Seifart U, Jensen K, Ukena J et al. Randomized phase II study comparing topotecan/cisplatin administration for 5 days versus 3 days in the treatment of extensive stage small cell lung cancer (SCLC). Lung Cancer 2005; 48: 415–22.

39. Sorensen M, Jensen PB, Herrstedt J et al. A dose escalating study of topotecan preceding cisplatin in previously untreated patients with small-cell lung cancer. Ann Oncol 2000; 11: 829–35.

40. Rowinsky EK, Kaufmann SH, Baker SD et al. Sequences of topotecan and cisplatin: phase I, pharmacologic, and in vitro studies to examine sequence dependence. J Clin Oncol 1996; 14: 3074–84.

41. Hobdy EM, Kraut E, Masters G et al. A phase II study of topotecan and cyclophosphamide with G-CSF in patients with advanced small cell lung cancer. Cancer Biol Ther 2004; 3: 89–93.

42. Miller AA, Lilenbaum RC, Lynch TJ. Treatment-related fatal sepsis from topotecan/cisplatin and topotecan/paclitaxel. J Clin Oncol 1996; 14: 1964–5.

43. Kirschling RJ, Jung SH, Jett JR. A phase II trial of Taxol and G-CSF in previously untreated patients with extensive small cell lung cancer (SCLC). Proc Am Soc Clin Oncol 1994; 13: 326 (abstract 1078).

44. Ettinger DS, Finkelstein DM, Sarma RP et al. Phase II study of paclitaxel in patients with extensive-disease small-cell lung cancer: an Eastern Cooperative Oncology Group study. J Clin Oncol 1995; 13: 1430–5.

45. Smit EF, Fokkema E, Biesma B et al. A phase II study of paclitaxel in heavily pretreated patients with small-cell lung cancer. Br J Cancer 1998; 77: 347–51.

46. Niell HB, Herndon JE, Miller AA et al. Randomized phase III intergroup trial of etoposide and cisplatin with or without paclitaxel and granulocyte colony-stimulating factor in patients with extensive-stage small-cell lung cancer: Cancer and Leukemia Group B Trial 9732. J Clin Oncol 2005; 23: 3752–9.

47. Bunn PA, Kelley K, Crowley J, et al. Preliminary toxicity results from Southwest Oncology Group Trial: a phase II trial of cisplatin, etoposide and paclitaxel with G-CSF in untreated patients with extensive small cell lung cancer. Proc Am Soc Clin Oncol 1999; 18: 468a (abstract 1807).

48. Mavroudis D, Papadakis E, Veslemes M et al. The Greek Lung Group Cooperative Group. A multicenter randomized phase III study comparing paclitaxel, cisplatin, etoposide versus cisplatin, etoposide as front line treatment in study of paclitaxel, etoposide and cisplatin in patients with small cell lung cancer. Proc Am Soc Clin Oncol 2000; 19: 484a (abstract 1894).

49. Reck M, von Pawel J, Macka H-N et al. Randomized phase III trial of paclitaxel, etoposide and carboplatin versus carboplatin, etoposide and vincristine in patients with small cell lung cancer. J Natl Cancer Inst 2003; 95: 1118–27.

50. Martin R, Hans-Nikolas M, Eckhard K et al. A randomized phase III trial of Taxol-based chemotherapy in previously untreated small cell lung cancer (SCLC): long term survival over six years. Lung Cancer 2005; 49: S325 (abstract P-784).

51. Groen HJ, Fokkema E, Biesma B et al. Paclitaxel and carboplatin in the treatment of small-cell lung cancer patients resistant to cyclophosphamide, doxorubicin, and etoposide: a non-cross-resistant schedule. J Clin Oncol 1999; 17: 927–32.

52. Smit EF, Groen HJM, Biesma B et al. Phase III study comparing cyclophosphamide, doxorubicin, and etoposide (CDE) to carboplatin and paclitaxel (CP) in patients (pts) with extensive disease small cell lung cancer (ED SCLC). Proc Am Soc Clin Oncol 2005; 24: 659 (abstract 7045).

53. Postmus PE, Scagliotti G, Groen HJ et al. Standard versus alternating non-cross-resistant chemotherapy in extensive small cell lung cancer: an EORTC phase III trial. Eur J Cancer 1996; 32A: 1498–503.

54. Agelaki S, Veslemes M, Syrigos K et al. A multicenter phase II study of the combination of gemcitabine and docetaxel in previously treated patients with small cell lung cancer. Lung Cancer 2004; 43: 329–33.

55. Dudek AZ, Lesniewski-Kmak K, Bliss RL et al. Pilot phase II study of gemcitabine and vinorelbine in patients with recurrent or refractory small cell lung cancer. Lung 2005; 183: 43–52.

56. De Marinis F, Nelli F, Lombardo M et al. A multicenter, randomized, Phase II study of cisplatin, etoposide, and gemcitabine or cisplatin plus gemcitabine as first-line treatment in patients with poor-prognosis small cell lung carcinoma. Cancer 2005; 103: 772–9.

57. Neubauer M, Heaven R, Olivares J et al. Results of a phase II study of carboplatin plus gemcitabine in patients with untreated extensive small cell lung cancer. Lung Cancer 2004; 46: 369–75.

58. Socinski MA, Weissman LL, Hart JT et al. A randomized phase II trial of pemetrexed (P) plus cisplatin (cis) or carboplatin (carbo) in extensive stage small cell lung cancer (ES-SCLC). Proc Am Soc Clin Oncol 2005; 24: 661 (abstract 7165).

59. Baka S, Lorigan P, Papakotoulas P et al. Phase III randomised trial of doxorubicin based chemotherapy compared with platinum based chemotherapy in both limited and extensive stage patients. Lung Cancer 2005; 49: S52 (abstract O-153).

60. Artel-Cortes A, Gomez-Codina J, Gonzalez-Larriba JL et al. Prospective randomized phase III trial of etoposide/cisplatin versus high-dose epirubicin/cisplatin in small-cell lung cancer. Clin Lung Cancer 2004; 6: 175–83.

61. Ohe Y, Negoro S, Matsui K et al. Phase I–II study of amrubicin and cisplatin in previously untreated patients with extensive-stage small-cell lung cancer. Ann Oncol 2005; 16: 430–6.

62. Lorigan P, Woll PJ, O'Brien ME et al. Randomized phase III trial of dose-dense chemotherapy supported by whole-blood hematopoietic progenitors in better-prognosis small-cell lung cancer. J Natl Cancer Inst 2005; 97: 666–74.

63. Huisman C, Postmus PE, Giaccone G et al. Second-line chemotherapy in relapsing or refractory non-small-cell lung cancer: a review. J Clin Oncol 2000; 18: 3722–30.

64. O'Brien M, Ciuleanu T, Tsekov H et al. Survival benefit of oral topotecan plus supportive care versus supportive care alone in relapsed, resistant SCLC. Lung Cancer 2005; 49: S54 (abstract O-157).

65. von Pawel J, Schiller JH, Shepherd FA et al. Topotecan versus cyclophosphamide, doxorubicin, and

vincristine for the treatment of recurrent small-cell lung cancer. J Clin Oncol 1999; 17: 658–67.

66. von Pawel J, Gatzemeier U, Pujol JL et al. Phase II comparator study of oral versus intravenous topotecan in patients with chemosensitive small-cell lung cancer. J Clin Oncol 2001; 19: 1743–9.

67. Sundstrom S, Bremnes RM, Kaasa S et al. Second-line chemotherapy in recurrent small cell lung cancer. Results from a crossover schedule after primary treatment with cisplatin and etoposide (EP-regimen) or cyclophosphamide, epirubicin, and vincristin (CEV-regimen). Lung Cancer 2005; 48: 251–61.

68. Shepherd FA, Evans WK, MacCormick R et al. Cyclophosphamide, doxorubicin, and vincristine in etoposide- and cisplatin-resistant small cell lung cancer. Cancer Treat Rep 1987; 71: 941–4.

69. Sculier JP, Klastersky J, Libert P et al. Cyclophosphamide, doxorubicin and vincristine with amphotericin B in sonicated liposomes as salvage therapy for small cell lung cancer. Eur J Cancer 1990; 26: 919–21.

70. Roth BJ, Johnson DH, Einhorn LH et al. Randomized study of cyclophosphamide, doxorubicin, and vincristine versus etoposide and cisplatin versus alternation of these two regimens in extensive small-cell lung cancer: a phase III trial of the Southeastern Cancer Study Group. J Clin Oncol 1992; 10: 282–91.

71. Ardizzoni A, Favaretto A, Boni L et al. Platinum–etoposide chemotherapy in elderly patients with small-cell lung cancer: results of a randomized multicenter phase II study assessing attenuated-dose or full-dose with lenograstim prophylaxis – a Forza Operativa Nazionale Italiana Carcinoma Polmonare and Gruppo Studio Tumori Polmonari Veneto (FONICAP–GSTPV) study. J Clin Oncol 2005; 23: 569–75.

72. Kunitoh H, Okamoto H Watanabe K et al. Randomized phase III trial of carboplatin (Cb) or cisplatin (P) in combination with etoposide (E) in elderly or poor-risk patients with extensive disease small cell lung cancer (ED-SCLC): report of a Japan Clinical Oncology Group Trial (JCOG9702). Lung Cancer 2005; 49: S53 (abstract O-155).

73. Schild SE, Stella PJ, Brooks BJ et al. Results of combined-modality therapy for limited-stage small cell lung carcinoma in the elderly. Cancer 2005; 103: 2349–54.

74. Henke M, Laszig R, Rube C et al. Erythropoietin to treat head and neck cancer patients with anaemia undergoing radiotherapy: randomised, double-blind, placebo-controlled trial. Lancet 2003; 362: 1255–60.

75. Goss G, Feld R, Bezjak A et al. Impact of maintaining Hb with epoetin alfa on time to progression (TTP), overall survival (OS), quality of life (QOL) and transfusion reduction in limited disease SCLC patients. Lung Cancer 2005; 49: S53 (abstract O-154).

76. Altinbas M, Coskun HS, Er O et al. A randomized clinical trial of combination chemotherapy with and without low-molecular-weight heparin in small cell lung cancer. J Thromb Haemost 2004; 2: 1266–71.

77. Harper-Wynne CL, Sumpter K, Ryan C et al. Addition of SRL 172 to standard chemotherapy in small cell lung cancer (SCLC) improves symptom control. Lung Cancer 2005; 47: 289–90.

78. O'Brien ME, Anderson H, Kaukel E et al. SRL172 (killed *Mycobacterium vaccae*) in addition to standard chemotherapy improves quality of life without affecting survival, in patients with advanced non-small-cell lung cancer: phase III results. Ann Oncol 2004; 15: 906–14.

79. McClay EF, Bogart J, Herndon JE

2nd et al. A phase III trial evaluating the combination of cisplatin, etoposide, and radiation therapy with or without tamoxifen in patients with limited-stage small cell lung cancer: Cancer and Leukemia Group B Study (9235). Am J Clin Oncol 2005; 28: 81–90.

80. Cooney MM, Subbiah R, Chapman A et al. Phase II trial of maintenance daily oral thalidomide in patients with extensive-stage small cell lung cancer (ES-SCLC) in remission. Proc Am Soc Clin Oncol 2005; 24: 661 (abstract 7166).

81. Pujol J, Breton J, Gervais R et al. A prospective randomized phase III, double-blind, placebo-controlled study of thalidomide in extended-disease (ED) SCLC patients after response to chemotherapy (CT). Lung Cancer 2005; 49: S54 (abstract O-159).

82. Pandya K, Levy D, Hidalgo M et al. A randomized phase II ECOG trial of two dose levels of temsirolimus (CCI-779) in patients with extensive stage small cell lung cancer in remission after induction therapy. Lung Cancer 2005; 49: S54 (abstract O-158).

83. Johl J, Chansky K, Lara PN et al. The proteasome inhibitor PS-341 (bortezomib) in platinum (plat)-treated extensive-stage small cell lung cancer (E-SCLC): a SWOG (0327) phase II trial. Proc Am Soc Clin Oncol 2005; 24: 632 (abstract 7047).

84. Fossela F, McCann J, Tolcher H et al. Phase II trial of BB-10901 (huN901-DM1) given weekly for four consecutive weeks every 6 weeks in patients with relapsed SCLC and CD56-positive small cell carcinoma. Proc Am Soc Clin Oncol 2005; 24: 660 (abstract 7159).

85. Rudin CM, Slgia R, Wang MR et al. CALGB 30103: a randomized phase II study of carboplatin and etoposide (CE) with or without G3139 in patients with extensive stage small cell lung cancer (ES-SCLC). Proc Am Soc Clin Oncol 2005; 24: 662 (abstract 7168).

86. Moore AM, Estes D, Govindan R et al. A Phase II trial of gefitinib in patients with chemosensitive and chemorefractory relapsed neuroendocrine cancer. A Hoosier Oncology Group Trial. Proc Am Soc Clin Oncol 2005; 24: 660 (abstract 7160).

87. Krug LM, Crapanzano JP, Azzoli CG et al Imatinib mesylate lacks activity in small cell lung carcinoma expressing c-kit protein: a phase II clinical trial. Cancer 2005; 103: 2128–31.

88. Heymach JV, Johnson DH, Khuri FR et al. Phase II study of the farnesyl transferase inhibitor R115777 in patients with sensitive relapse small-cell lung cancer. Ann Oncol 2004; 15: 1187–93.

8
Treatment of non-small cell lung cancer

Heine H Hansen

The treatment of non-small cell lung cancer (NSCLC) has been undergoing major changes in recent years: increasingly, a multimodality approach is being adopted, applying surgery, radiotherapy and chemotherapy, given either sequentially or concomitantly in selected groups of patients. Also, refinements of presently available treatments continue to take place and new treatment options are being developed; often based on recent knowledge of the biology of the disease, they have resulted in targeted therapy. In addition, various modes of palliative treatment are expanding, e.g. the use of endobronchial radiotherapy and the application of various types of stents.

The management of NSCLC is usually based on evidence from randomized trials, even though it should be realized that patients included in clinical trials are not representative of the patient population as a whole. This fact has been noted by Foeglé et al[1] in Europe and Potosky et al[2] in the USA. Foeglé et al[1] conducted a retrospective population-based study of a sample of 1738 patients diagnosed with primary NSCLC in a French department between 1982 and 1997. The proportion of women, metastatic cases and adenocarcinoma changed significantly over time, as did their management. The use of chemotherapy alone increased from 9.7% to 28.1% ($p < 0.0001$), while the use of radiotherapy alone decreased from 32.2% to 9.4% ($p < 0.0001$). The 5-year survival probability was 15.7% for all patients and 32.6% for those with resectable disease. Despite changes in treatment in accordance with new developments, overall survival did not improve over time. It is not unlikely that more patients with poor performance status (PS) were diagnosed during the latter part of the study period. This could at least partially explain the absence of overall improvement in survival.

Potosky et al[2] focused on receipt of specific therapies in clinical practice patterns in the USA by assessing a randomly selected cohort of nearly 900 NSCLC patients diagnosed in 1996 who were treated in diverse healthcare settings in 10 distinct geographic regions. Patterns of initial therapy focused on the investigation of differences of receipt of recommended therapies according to multiple clinical and non-clinical patient characteristics. Overall, 52% of NSCLC patients received recommended therapy. Approximately 69%, 48% and 41% of patients with stages I–II, III or IV NSCLC received recommended therapy, respectively. For all stages combined, the use of recommended therapy was significantly inversely associated with age and stage at diagnosis. Recommended therapy was also more common in white than in black patients, and in married than in single patients. Stage-specific analyses revealed a significant decline in the use of recommended surgery with increasing age at diagnosis for early-stage NSCLC only, and a significantly lower use of recommended therapy (primarily chemotherapy/radiotherapy) for stage III black and Hispanic patients compared with white patients.

A similar pattern was described by Campling et al,[3] who performed a population-based study of lung carcinoma in Pennsylvania, USA. The Pennsylvania Cancer Registry was used to identify all patients who were diagnosed with lung carcinoma in the state of Pennsylvania from 1995 to 1999. Patients who were treated within the Veterans Administration (VA) Health Care Network were identified by hospital code. A total of 48 994 patients were diagnosed with lung carcinoma in Pennsylvania during this period, including 856 patients in the VA system (6 women). The analysis was restricted to male patients ($n = 28\ 798$). There was no major difference in age of VA patients compared with non-VA patients, and the proportions of patients who had localized or regional stage disease were similar. The proportion of black patients was much higher in the VA population (23%) than in the non-VA population (9%). The median survival was 6.3 months for VA patients, compared with 7.9 months for patients in the rest of the state, and the 5-year overall survival rate was 12% for VA patients, compared with 15% for patients in the rest of the state. When survival was analyzed according to race, there was a significant difference in the age-adjusted survival of white patients in the VA system compared with patients in the rest of the state ($p = 0.0007$), but no significant difference was observed among black patients ($p = 0.92$). The overall survival of VA patients with lung carcinoma in Pennsylvania was inferior to that of patients in the remainder of the state, and this was due primarily to differences in survival among the white patients. Further investigation will be necessary to determine whether this disparity is caused by differences in socioeconomic status or comorbidities, or whether there are systematic differences in the diagnosis, staging or treatment of lung carcinoma between VA patients and civilian patients.

Noteworthy also is the publication by Langer et al,[4] who reviewed the treatment of 541 individuals diagnosed between 1998 and 1999 with lung cancer, either limited-disease small cell lung cancer (SCLC) or stages I–III NSCLC. Patients were sampled from 58 institutions in the USA and the purpose of the study was to analyze how closely current US practice with chemotherapy in the non-metastatic setting follows the literature. The authors conclude that combined-modality therapy is typically employed in the therapy of both limited-disease SCLC and limited–advanced-disease NSCLC. Even though the current practice in the USA generally matches evidence-based literature, a significant percentage of practitioners substitute carboplatin for cisplatin and use paclitaxel instead of vinca alkaloids or etoposide in NSCLC. These data were commented on by Jeremic[5] and also in a sharp editorial by Turrisi[6] entitled: 'Creeping phase II-ism and the medical pharmaceutical complex: weapons of mass distraction in the war against lung cancer.' Focusing on phase II trials, Turrisi ends his editorial as follows: 'Although the fame and fortune aspect does dance like sugarplums in investigators' and clinicians' heads, the infamy of false promises and misleading spin-doctoring of phase II trials and the potential misfortune of the consequences seem to be worth thinking about.' Both Jeremic and Turrisi strongly emphasize the need for larger prospective randomized trials with focus on both radiotherapy and chemotherapy in the large group of patients presenting with locoregional lung cancer.

MANAGEMENT OF RESECTABLE STAGE I, II AND IIIA

Surgery

Surgical therapy remains the mainstay in the treatment of stages I, II and IIIA of NSCLC. Mina et al,[7] reviewing all new cases in Western Australia in the calendar year of 1996, evaluated surgery in the management of lung cancer patients in Western Australia. A total of 668 patients with lung cancer were identified and 20% were treated with surgery. Lobectomy was the most frequently performed procedure (71%), followed by pneumonectomy (19%). The postoperative mortality rate was 6% (3% lobectomy, 12% pneumonectomy). At 5 years, the absolute survival rates for stage I, II, IIIA and IIIB, respectively, were 51%, 45%, 12% and 5%.

The influence of hospital volume on survival after resection for lung cancer and the use of dedicated specialist thoracic surgeons have been researched in both the USA and the UK. Bach et al[8] performed an analysis of 2118 patients from 76 hospitals, studying patients 65 years old or older who received a diagnosis of stage I, II or IIIA NSCLC between 1985 and 1996. The volume of procedures at the hospitals were positively associated with the survival of patients ($p < 0.001$). Five years after surgery, 44% of patients who underwent operations at the hospitals with the highest volume were alive, compared with 33% of patients who underwent operations at the hospitals with the lowest volume. Patients at the highest-volume hospitals also had lower rates of postoperative complications (20% vs 44%) and lower 30-day mortality rates (3% vs 6%) than those at the lowest-volume hospitals.

Also, Martin-Ucar et al[9] demonstrated in a group of 240 patients that lung cancer surgery provided by specialists within a multidisciplinary team resulted in increased surgical resection rates without compromising outcome, emphasizing the need for disease-specific specialists in the treatment of lung cancer.

With respect to surgical resection in the elderly, several studies have shed additional light on this topic. Among these studies are analyses of patients >70 years old in studies from Norway,[10] the USA[11] and the Netherlands,[12] and also an analysis of the outcome of pulmonary resection in octogenarians with stage I NSCLC by Brock et al[13] from the Johns Hopkins Medical Institutions in Baltimore, USA. From these studies, one can conclude that health status and tumor stage outweigh chronologic age in determining surgical candidates. The latter factor is corroborated by an analysis by Ambrogi et al[14] from Italy, who observed, among 247 consecutive patients undergoing surgery for stage I and II NSCLC, that cardiovascular disease seems to have a significant impact on survival and morbidity in patients undergoing surgery for lung cancer, especially in the presence of multifocal vascular disease and following major resections. In the study by Mery et al[11] from the USA, a total of 14 555 patients registered in the National Cancer Institute (NCI) Surveillance, Epidemiology, and End Results (SEER) database from 1992 to 1997 were analyzed. All patients had stage I and II primary NSCLC and were grouped into the following three categories: <65 years old (n = 5057; 35%): 65–74 years old (n = 6073; 42%) and ≥75 years old (n = 3425; 23%). The results indicated that age is an independent predictor of postsurgical survival in NSCLC patients, even after adjustment for significant covariates, and that curative surgery is performed less frequently in elderly patients. Among younger patients undergoing curative surgery, lobectomies are more commonly performed and confer a significant survival benefit over limited resections. This benefit, however, is not evident for patients >71 years old.

With respect to the quality of life of long-term survivors of NSCLC, Sarna et al[15] surveyed the status of 142 patients, of whom the majority (74%) had received lobectomy. The majority of the survivors experienced respiratory symptoms, and more than one-third reported dyspnea, including 1 of 5 patients with seriously diminished pulmonary function. Symptom burden, rather than ventilatory impairment, contributed to a diminished quality of life.

A similar group of patients resected for pathologic stage I NSCLC and tumor-free after 5 years still had a higher incidence of new lung cancer compared with the general population, which in turn had an excess in all-cause mortality in the following years.[16]

Surgical techniques are outside the scope of this chapter. The overall trend, however, is to expand the use of video-assisted thoracic surgery (VATS), which has replaced major pulmonary resection in clinical stage I lung cancer in view of its low perioperative mortality and morbidity.[17] The other trend is the increasing use of mediastinal lymph node dissection for NSCLC, a topic that was the subject of several articles, including an editorial, in 2005.[18–21] In the latter,[21] it is emphasized that thoracic surgeons specializing in lung cancer treatment should be encouraged to use complete lymph node dissection. A disturbing report from Little et al[22] presented at the Annual Meeting of the Society of Thoracic Surgeons in the USA in January 2005, highlights the need for change. He reviewed the pattern of surgical care in more than 11 000 patients with lung cancer. The analysis revealed that only 40% of patients had any lymph node biopsy. Whether a complete mediastinal lymphadenectomy will definitely improve long-term survival awaits the result of ongoing multicenter trials.

Results of the surgical treatment of more specific subgroups of patients, such as bronchioloalveolar lung cancer, primary adenosquamous lung cancer, Pancoast tumors and multiple primary adenocarcinomas, have also been published, based on retrospective analyses at single institutions.[23–28]

Radiotherapy

In spite of the intention to consider all patients with stage I, II and IIIa disease for surgery, there are patients who, although technically operable, either refuse surgery or are considered inoperable because of insufficient respiratory reserve, cardiovascular disease or general frailty. This group may therefore be considered 'medically inoperable'. Some respiratory physicians refer these patients for radical radiotherapy, whereas other physicians believe that radiotherapy has little to offer and adopt a watch policy, referring patients for palliative radiotherapy when they become symptomatic. Rowell and Williams[29] performed a meta-analysis in a Cochrane review, collecting two randomized and 35 non-randomized studies, including patients of any age with stage I–II NSCLC receiving radiotherapy at a dose >40 Gy in 20 fractions over 4 weeks or its radiobiologic equivalent. In the randomized trial comparing two radiotherapy schedules, the 2-year survival rate was superior following continuous hyperfractionated accelerated radiotherapy (CHART; 37%) compared with 60 Gy in 30 fractions over 6 weeks (24%). There were 26 non-randomized retrospective studies, including an estimated 2003 patients with an overall survival rate of 33–72% at 2 years, 17–55% at 3 years and 0–42% at 5 years. The proportion of deaths not due to cancer was 11–43%. The cancer-specific survival rate was 54–93% at 2 years and 13–39% at 5 years. Complete response rates were 33–61%, and local failure rates were 6–70%. Better response rates and survival were seen in patients with smaller tumors and in those receiving higher doses of radiotherapy, although the reasons for prescribing higher doses were not clearly stated. Worse outcome was seen in patients with prior weight loss or poor performance status. The reviewers conclude that radical radiotherapy appears to result in a better survival than might be expected had treatment not been given. A substantial, though variable, proportion of patients died during follow-up from causes other than cancer. The optimal radiation dose and treatment technique (particularly with respect to mediastinal irradiation) remain uncertain.

These data have since been complemented by an analysis from a population-based cancer registry in Southern Saxony-Anhalt, Germany.[30] Among 1696 patients with lung cancer, 188 in clinical stages I–IIIb (15.9%) were treated with radiotherapy alone. The results indicate that patients treated with 50–60 Gy under a potentially curative therapeutic regimen had a significantly lower survival than patients treated with ≥60 Gy. Ghosh et al[31] compared long-term results of surgery versus CHART in patients aged >70 years old with stage I NSCLC. A total of 215 patients aged >70 years old with pathologic stage I NSCLC were studied between 1991 and 2001. Of these patients, 149 had a lobectomy, 47 had a wedge resection and 19 had CHART. The survival rates at 1 and 5 years for patients undergoing wedge resection, lobectomy and CHART were 98% and 74% versus 97% and 68% versus 80% and 39%, respectively. Locoregional recurrence and survival after wedge resection and lobectomy in elderly patients with stage I NSCLC were comparable, and the data also suggest that CHART is a reasonable treatment option for those who are not suitable candidates for surgery. Similar results showing superiority for surgery are demonstrated by Okamoto et al[32] in elderly patients in clinical stage IB–II NSCLC based on the study of 112 elderly patients.

Finally, Burdett and Stewart[33] updated an individual patient data meta-analysis of postoperative radiotherapy (PORT) versus surgery alone in resected NSCLC. The results continue to show PORT to be detrimental, with an 18% relative increase in the risk of deaths. Similar detrimental effects were observed on local recurrence-free survival, distant recurrence-free survival and overall recurrence-free survival. There continues to be evidence that the effects of PORT are more harmful in patients with stage I disease than in those with stage II disease.

In the coming years, the use of 'high-tech' radiotherapy can be expected to improve results, as reviewed by Ling et al,[34] suggesting the potential of improving local control by the following methods: (1) improved target definition with combined use of positron emission tomography and computed tomography (PET/CT); (2) improved tumor coverage by reducing uncertainties from setup and respiratory motion; and (3) dose escalation.

Several pilot studies have been published recently, on dose escalation with accelerated hyperfractionated three-dimensional conformal radiotherapy, on the application of stereotactic hypofractionated high-dose irradiation and on the use of hypofractionated proton-beam radiotherapy.[35–39] Randomized trials comparing these techniques with standard radiotherapy are awaited with interest, including follow-up of early and late side effects, which were described in the earliest studies.[40,41] Another interesting new approach is the use of brachytherapy in connection with lobar and sublobar resection for small stage IA NSCLC, but firm conclusions from the study published by Fernando et al[42] cannot be reached because of the retrospective character of the analysis.

Postoperative chemotherapy

The results of several large randomized postoperative chemotherapy trials were summarized in the Lung Cancer Therapy Annual 4 and compared with a meta-analysis. The data are now updated and include two new meta-analyses (Table 8.1).

The meta-analysis by Sedrakyan et al[47] found an overall estimate of 13% relative reduction in mortality (hazard ratio (HR) = 0.87; 95% confidence interval (CI) 0.81–0.93; $p < 0.0001$) associated with adjuvant chemotherapy. Furthermore, the relative reduction associated with postoperative cisplatin was 11% versus 17% with UFT (uracil plus tegafur (ftorafur)). The topic of adjuvant therapy for resected NSCLC has also been reviewed recently by Juergens and Brahmer.[49]

The detailed data concerning the surgery setting of the Big Lung Trial from the UK[50] have been published in full detail in addition to the results of new studies. A total of 381 patients were randomized to chemotherapy or no

Table 8.1 Ongoing and completed randomized cisplatin-based adjuvant chemotherapy trials in stage I–IIIA NSCLC

Study	Therapy	No. of patients	MTP	MS (months)	5-YS (%)	Survival HR	Survival p
Meta-analysis[43]	Surgery alone	688	NR	56	49	0.87	0.08
	Surgery + CT	706	NR	60+	54	–	–
ALPI[44]	Surgery alone	540	28.9	48	47	0.96	NS
	Surgery + MVP	548	36.5	55.2	48	–	–
BLT[45]	Surgery alone	189	NR	32.6	NR	1.02	NS
	Surgery + CT	192	NR	33.9	NR	–	–
IALT[46]	Surgery alone	945	30	47	40.4	0.86	<0.03
	Surgery + CT	932	42	52	44.5	–	–
Meta-analysis[47]	Surgery alone	3572	NR	NR	NR	0.87	NR
	Surgery + CT	3628	NR	NR	NR	(0.81–0.93)	–
Meta-analysis[48]	Surgery alone	2843	–	–	–	0.872	0.001
	Surgery + CT	2873	–	–	–	(0.805–0.944)	–
Winton et al[51]	Surgery alone	240	Not reached	73	54	–	–
	Surgery + CT	242	–	94	69	0.60	0.04

ALPI, Adjuvant Lung Project of Italy; IALT, International Adjuvant Lung Cancer Trial; BLT, Big Lung Trial; MTP, median time to progression; 5-YS, 5-year survival rate; CT, chemotherapy; HR, hazard ratio (95% confidence intervals in parentheses); MVP, mitomycin–vinblastine–cisplatin; NR, not reported; NS, not significant.

chemotherapy. The chemotherapy was three 3-weekly cycles of cisplatin–vindesine, mitomycin–ifosfamide–cisplatin, mitomycin–vinblastine–cisplatin or vinorelbine–cisplatin. Chemotherapy was given before surgery in 3% of patients, whereas 97% received adjuvant chemotherapy; 93% had WHO performance status 0–1, 27% stage I, 38% stage II and 34% stage III; 48% of the patients had squamous cell carcinoma. Complete resection was achieved in approximately 95% of patients. At the time of evaluation, 52% of patients had died and there was no evidence of a benefit in overall survival for the chemotherapy group (HR = 1.02, 95% CI 0.77–1.35).

Additional data derive from the study performed by the Eastern Cooperative Oncology Group (ECOG) in the USA.[51] A total of 482 patients with completely resected stage IB or stage II NSCLC were randomized to vinorelbine plus cisplatin (242 patients) or observation (240 patients). Overall, survival was significantly prolonged in the chemotherapy group compared with the observation group (94 vs 73 months; HR for death = 0.69; p = 0.04), as was relapse-free survival (not reached vs 46.7 months; HR for recurrence = 0.60; $p < 0.001$). Five-year survival rates were 69% and 54%, respectively (p = 0.03).

The results of the postoperative UFT-based therapy have been complemented by recent studies by Nakagawa et al[52] and Imaizumi,[53] who in a study of 332 patients observed 5- and 8-year survival rates for the UFT group of 82.2% and 73.5% and for those for the control group of 75.9% and 61.2%, respectively (p = 0.105). Overall, the UFT administration did not significantly improve postoperative survival of pT1 NSCLC patients, but subset analyses suggested that UFT might be effective in pT1N0M0 patients (p = 0.0011). Imaizumi[53] reported the data from the Chubu Study Group in Japan. One hundred and fifty patients with T1N0 or T2N0 adenocarcinoma or squamous cell carcinoma were randomly assigned to either surgery alone or surgery with chemotherapy consisting of two courses of cisplatin and vindesine followed by UFT for a period of 2 years (PVU) or UFT alone for two 2 years. The 5-year survival rate of the control group was 66.3%, versus 87.9% in the PVU group and 67.7% for the UFT group. The differences in 5-year survival rates between the PVU group and the control group were statistically significant (p = 0.045). According to multivariate analysis, the only significantly positive factor on outcome was PVU chemotherapy after surgery.

The Japanese data on postoperative adjuvant chemotherapy with UFT in NSCLC have been highlighted by Hamada et al[54] in a meta-analysis. Among nine trials of postoperative adjuvant UFT-containing chemotherapy, six trials comparing surgery alone with surgery plus UFT were identified. Of six trials, two were three-arm trials, including cisplatin-based chemotherapy followed by UFT, and data from that arm were not included in the meta-analysis. Of 2003 eligible patients, most (98.8%) had squamous cell carcinoma or adenocarcinoma, and most had stage I disease; the tumor classification was T1 in 1308 (65.3%) and T2 in 674 (33.6%), and the nodal status was N0 in 1923 (96.0%). The two treatment groups did not differ significantly with respect to major prognostic factors. The median duration of follow-up was 6.44 years. The survival rates at 5 and 7 years were significantly higher in the surgery plus UFT group (81.5% and 76.5%, respectively) than in the surgery-alone group (77.2% and 69.5%, respectively; $p = 0.011$ and 0.001, respectively); overall pooled HR = 0.74 (95% CI 0.61–0.88; $p = 0.001$). Thus, the meta-analysis showed that postoperative adjuvant chemotherapy with UFT was associated with improved 5- and 7-year survival in a Japanese patient population composed primarily of stage I adenocarcinoma patients.

The results of all these studies have resulted in vigorous debate in several medical journals about whether or not adjuvant chemotherapy should become standard in all patients with resected NSCLC. The answers range from a qualified 'yes' to a 'not-yet' position.[55–59]

In the March 2005 issue of *Lancet Oncology*, Le Chevalier et al[60] concluded, based on an analysis of recent randomized clinical studies of platinum-based adjuvant chemotherapy and completely resected NSCLC, that 'the questions is thus no longer: "should adjuvant chemotherapy be given in resected NSCLC?" but, in view of the consistency of the results on the role of adjuvant chemotherapy, "how long will the medical community need to standardise, optimise, and individualise this approach".' On the other side, Scagliotti and Torri[56] concluded that: 'more detailed analyses of the results of recent positive trials are needed to reasonably conclude that adjuvant chemotherapy is recommended for every patient who undergoes radical surgery for early NSCLC and to exclude the potential of biases related to confounding factors'. This debate between Scagliotti and Le Chevalier was presented at a 'controversy session' at the 29th ESMO Conference in Vienna, Austria, October 29 to November 2, 2004.

Finally, in an editorial commenting on the ECOG trial, Pisters[61] concluded almost 1 year later, on the basis of previous trials with adjuvant chemotherapy and the data reported by Winton et al,[51] that the controversy surrounding adjuvant chemotherapy for resectable NSCLC is over: 'Adjuvant platinum-based chemotherapy should be recommended after complete resection of NSCLC in patients with a good performance status. Additional research will enable us to select those patients most likely to benefit from adjuvant therapy, to customize the therapy on the basis of the biology of the tumor, to lessen toxicity and increase compliance, to identify more effective regimens, and to further improve survival.'

Preoperative chemotherapy

At the American Society of Clinical Oncology (ASCO) 2005 meeting, Pisters et al[62] summarized the preliminary results of the South-Western Oncology Group S9900 phase III trial. This study tested the efficacy of surgery alone compared with surgery and preoperative chemotherapy in patients with early-stage NSCLC. The chemotherapy consisted of carboplatin and paclitaxel (paclitaxel 225 mg/m^2 over 3 hours, carboplatin area under the curve (AUC) = 6 on day

1), every 3 weeks × 3 or surgery alone. The study was designed for 600 patients, but was closed when 354 had been accrued; 51% of patients who received chemotherapy had either complete or partial response. Median overall survival was 47 months for patients receiving preoperative chemotherapy and 40 months for patients in the surgery-alone control arm (HR = 0.84; 95% CI 0.60–1.18; $p = 0.32$).

Another abstract from the ASCO meeting was presented by Scagliotti et al,[63] who tested the hypothesis of whether three cycles of gemcitabine–cisplatin administered before radical surgery provides better progression-free survival than surgery alone in patients with early stages of NSCLC. The original study design required 700 randomized patients. From December 2000 to December 2004, 267 patients from 44 European centers were randomized. The median follow-up time was 10 months and the 6-month progression-free survival rate was 89.1% vs 79.6%. The authors concluded that these early results suggest some advantage of the addition of preoperative chemotherapy.

REGIONAL PRIMARY UNRESECTABLE NSCLC

The optimal treatment for patients with primary unresectable regionally advanced NSCLC continues to include both chemotherapy and radiotherapy, given concurrently or sequentially – followed by surgical resection in selected patients, but the optimal treatment remains uncertain. The topic has been subjected to editorials and general reviews,[64–66] as well as reviews focusing on separate topics applied in the overall treatment, such as individual cytotoxic agents, e.g. docetaxel.[67] Also, the overall roles of surgery and radiotherapy have been analyzed in detail, including information about how to optimize the application of the three modalities with the aim of increasing the efficacy and decreasing the toxicity.

With respect to surgery, Patel et al[68] proposed a management algorithm for patients with stage III NSCLC that is based upon the currently available information on surgical therapy, chemotherapy and radiotherapy. Detailed analysis of the various subgroups, such as IIIA (T1–3N2 tumors) and the various stage IIIB tumors including T1–4N3, T4N2, and T4N0–1, were performed in light of the extent of local disease as well as patient performance status. Doddoli et al[69] performed a retrospective study including 100 patients with primary bronchogenic carcinoma in whom pneumonectomy had been performed after induction treatment. Four variables predicted 90-day mortality: age >60 years, male sex, postoperative respiratory event and postoperative cardiovascular event. Estimated overall survival rates in 90-day survivors were 35% and 25% at 3 and 5 years, respectively. The authors concluded that pneumonectomy after induction therapy is a high-risk procedure, and the survival benefit appears uncertain.

In another analysis, also from France, Perrot et al[70] reviewed 114 patients in whom different types of induction chemotherapy were used. Postoperative mortality occurred in 2 of 114 patients, all after pneumonectomy, while there were no deaths after lobectomy. The authors concluded that preoperative chemotherapy does not increase postoperative mortality and morbidity after NSCLC surgery, performed exclusively by thoracic surgeons. A similar conclusion was reached by Semik et al[71] from Germany, based on data from a national phase III trial comparing preoperative chemotherapy followed by twice-daily chemoradiation and consecutive surgery with preoperative chemotherapy alone followed by surgery and consecutive radiotherapy.

Long-term results of surgically staged IIIA-N2 NSCLC treated with the surgical combined-modality approach have been presented by Lorent et al from the Leuven Lung Cancer Group in Belgium.[72] Their study comprised a cohort of 131 mediastinoscopy-proven IIIA-N2 NSCLC patients receiving preoperative platinum-containing chemotherapy followed by surgery or radical radiotherapy. The median survival time and 5-year survival rate for the total group were 24 months and 21%, respectively. Involvement of subcarinal nodes at diagnosis was the most important prognostic factor ($p = 0.022$). Downstaging occurred in 34 of 70 resection specimens, with a pathologic complete response in 6 patients. On multivariate analysis, favorable prognostic factors were low pathologic T-stage ($p = 0.001$) and downstaging of mediastinal nodes in the resection specimen ($p = 0.008$).

Long-term results have also been reported by the Radiation Therapy Oncology Group (RTOG) in the USA.[73] A total of 88 eligible patients with stage II and IIIA NSCLC had surgical resection and received postoperative paclitaxel and carboplatin. Concurrent thoracic radiotherapy at 50.4 Gy in 28 fractions for 6 weeks was given during cycles 1 and 2. A boost of 10.8 Gy in six fractions was given for extracapsular nodal extension or T3 lesions. The median overall survival time was 56.3 months, with 1-, 2- and 3-year survival rates of 86%, 70% and 61%, respectively. The 1-, 2- and 3-year progression-free survival rates were 70%, 57% and 50%, respectively. Brain metastasis occurred as the sole site of first failure in 11%. A phase III trial comparing this treatment regimen with standard therapy seems warranted.

Whether induction chemotherapy followed by surgical resection is equivalent to concurrent chemotherapy has been analyzed by Taylor et al[74] in a review of 107 patients in a 10-year period in clinical stage IIIA NSCLC treated at the University of Texas MD Anderson Cancer Center. The type of radiotherapy varies considerably and so does the type of chemotherapy: therefore, the conclusions from this retrospective analysis are weak and inconclusive, even though the authors state that the two treatment approaches result in similar outcomes in terms of local control and median overall, 5-year overall, distant metastasis-free and disease-free survival.

As to the role of radiotherapy in connection with chemotherapy in stage III NSCLC, several articles have been published recently, discussing the need to redefine aspects of radiotherapy dose, volume, fractionation and timing.[75–77] In addition, new techniques have been developed, such as intensity-modulated radiation therapy (IMRT) guided by PET/CT imaging with respiratory gating, using which it is possible to escalate the dose using accelerated fractionation. Exploratory studies have, in this way, increased the dose of radiation to 70–80 Gy, given, for example, in 35 fractions.[78] Usually, radiotherapy is given concurrently with chemotherapy in stage III followed by surgery, but it has also been applied postoperatively in patients with stage IIIA NSCLC treated with induction chemotherapy followed by surgery. Taylor et al[79] have performed a retrospective analysis of such a group of patients and found that postoperative radiotherapy increases locoregional control based on the treatment of 98 patients, of whom 40 had stage IIB and 58 had stage IIIA disease.

As to clinical experience, DeCamp et al,[80] Jeremic et al[81] and Ishikura et al[82] have retrospectively analyzed their experience using either accelerated multimodality therapy or hyperfractionated radiotherapy with or without concurrent chemotherapy in patient groups comprising 105, 36 and 30 patients, respectively. All of these authors concluded that carefully designed randomized trials are necessary to give better insight into the issue of integrating hyperfractionated radiotherapy with concurrent chemotherapy in the management of stage III NSCLC. The same statement is valid also based on very many phase I and II studies published recently using either preoperative concurrent chemoradiotherapy and induction chemotherapy followed by thoracic radiotherapy with or without surgery.[83] The induction chemotherapy is often cisplatin or carboplatin combined with other cytostatic agents such as paclitaxel, vinorelbine, docetaxel and gemcitabine, or even three-drug combinations of gemcitabine, paclitaxel and cisplatin or carboplatin, irinotecan and paclitaxel.[84–92] Chemotherapy given concurrently with radiotherapy, usually with single agents such as gemcitabine, docetaxel, efaproxiral and celecoxib has been tested,[93–97] and also two-drug combinations of cisplatin or carboplatin combined with paclitaxel, doxetacel, UFT or vinorelbine have been part of the many phase II trials in stage III NSCLC administered with radiotherapy in various schedules, including hyperfractionated radiotherapy.[98–108]

Also the final results of the Toronto phase II trial, using induction chemotherapy with mitomycin, vindesine and cisplatin for stage IIIA unresectable NSCLC, have been reported.[109] In this study with 65 patients, the overall response rate was 67.7%, with three complete and 41 partial responders. Forty-seven patients went on to thoracotomy, with 35 complete resections. Pathologically, 4.6% of patients had no tumor remaining. There were three postoperative deaths as well as 5 chemotherapy-related deaths. Of the 35 patients completely resected, 19 have recurred, including 8 in the brain. The median survival for the entire 65 patients is 18.6 months, with 1-, 5- and 10-year survival rates of 66%, 29% and 22%, respectively.

Randomized trials

Turning to the randomized trials, these are depicted in Table 8.2. The questions studied in these trials range from attempts to improve the effect of radiotherapy to comparison of sequential chemoradiotherapy versus concurrent chemoradiotherapy to studies determining the optimal sequencing and integration of chemotherapy with standard daily thoracic radiotherapy.

With respect to radiotherapy, Belani et al[110] compared standard thoracic radiotherapy with 64 Gy (2 Gy daily) versus hyperfractionated accelerated radiotherapy 57.6 Gy (1.5 Gy tid for 2.5 weeks) in patients who received two cycles of carboplatin plus paclitaxel as induction therapy. Statistically significant differences were not observed and the study had to close early, but there was a positive statistical trend suggesting a survival advantage with the hyperfractionated radiotherapy. Further exploration of the hyperfractionated radiotherapy treatment strategy is thus warranted. Groen et al[111] tested the effect of continuously infused carboplatin as a radiosensitizer in locally unresectable NSCLC. A total of 160 patients were included and a dose of 60 Gy during 6 weeks of radiotherapy was given with or without carboplatin 840 mg/m^2 administered continuously during the radiotherapy. The median survival in the combination arm was 11.8 months, versus 11.7 months in the radiotherapy arm. Progression-free survival was similar, at 6.8 and 7.5 months, respectively ($p = 0.28$). Thus, the addition of continuously administered carboplatin as a radiosensitizer did not improve the overall survival.

In another European study,[112] 205 patients were randomly assigned to either sequential or concurrent treatment. In the sequential arm, patients received induction chemotherapy (cisplatin 120 mg/m^2 on days 1, 29 and 57 and vinorelbine 30 mg/m^2 weekly from day 1 to day 78) followed by thoracic radiotherapy at a dose of 66 Gy in 33 fractions (2 Gy per fraction and 5 fractions per week). In the concurrent arm, the same radiotherapy was given on day 1 with two concurrent cycles of cisplatin 20 mg/m^2/day and etoposide 50 mg/m^2/d (days 1–5 and days 29–33). Patients in both arms then received consolidation therapy with cisplatin 80 mg/m^2 on days 78 days and 106 and vinorelbine 30 mg/m^2/wk on days 78–127. There were 6 toxic deaths in the sequential arm and 10 in the concurrent arm. Median survival was 14.5 months in the sequential arm and 16.3 months in the concurrent arm (log-rank test $p = 0.24$). The 2-, 3- and 4-year survival rates were better in the concurrent arm (39%, 25% and 21%, respectively) than in the sequential arm (26%, 19% and 14%, respectively). Esophageal toxicity was significantly more frequent in the concurrent arm than in the sequential arm. The results from this study, although not statistically significant, support a trend in favor of concurrent chemoradiotherapy in patients with locally advanced NSCLC.

The European Lung Cancer Working Party[113] tested two different dose-intensity regimens as induction chemotherapy followed by thoracic irradiation in patients with advanced locoregional NSCLC. A total of 351 patients were eligible: 176 who received treatment with mitomycin 6 mg/m^2, ifosfamide 3 g/m^2 and cisplatin 50 mg/m^2 versus 175 who received the same drugs but in doses of 6 mg/m^2, 4.5 mg/m^2 and 60 mg/m^2, respectively, plus carboplatin 200 mg/m^2. Thereafter, all patients received chest irradiation (60 Gy, five times per week for 6 weeks). If the tumor became resectable after chemotherapy, surgery was performed, followed by mediastinal irradiation. As expected, hematologic toxicity was higher with the intensive dose and there was also a significantly higher objective response with the intensive treatment (46% vs 35%; $p = 0.03$), but in terms of survival there was no statistically significant difference between the two arms, with median survival times of 11.2 months for intensive treatment versus 12.5 months.

The last randomized trial was relatively small and included only 91, 71 and 92 patients with stage IIIA and IIIB NSCLC.[114] The patients were randomized either to induction chemotherapy with paclitaxel and carboplatin followed by thoracic radiotherapy 63 Gy (arm 1) or to induction chemotherapy with paclitaxel and carboplatin followed by weekly paclitaxel and carboplatin with concurrent thoracic irradiation (arm 2), or to weekly paclitaxel and carboplatin with thoracic irradiation followed by two cycles of paclitaxel and carboplatin (arm 3). Median overall survival was 13.0 months in the sequential arm (1), versus 12.7 in the induction concurrent arm (2) and 16.3 months for the concurrent treatment followed by consolidation (arm 3). During induction chemotherapy, grade 3/4 granulocytopenia occurred in 32% and 38% of patients on arms 1 and 2, respectively. The most common locoregional grade 3/4 toxicity during and after thoracic radiotherapy was esophagitis, which was more pronounced with the administration of concurrent chemoradiotherapy on arms 2 and 3 (19% and 28%, respectively). In addition to these studies, Stephens et al[115] reported on a randomized trial conducted in the UK comparing preoperative chemotherapy followed, if feasible, by resection with radiotherapy in patients with inoperable stage T3N1M0 or T1–3N2M0 NSCLC. The study was nationwide, but only 48 patients were randomized over a 4-year period (1995–99) and the study had to be closed because of failure to recruit patients.

With respect to toxicity, several publications have analyzed factors influencing toxicity using various radiotherapy schedules, including the use of three-dimensional conformal radiotherapy.[116–118] Other clinicians have initiated trials to test the ability of the cytoprotectant amifostine to reduce chemoradiotherapy-induced esophagitis.[119,120] Unfortunately, amifostine did not significantly reduce esophagitis in patients receiving hyperfractionated radiotherapy and chemotherapy, based on randomization of 243 patients to receive amifostine 500 mg/m^2 i.v. four times per week or no amifostine during treatment with induction chemotherapy with paclitaxel 225 mg/m^2 i.v. days 1 and 22 and carboplatin AUC days 1 and 22 followed by concurrent weekly paclitaxel 50 mg/m^2 i.v. and carboplatin AUC 2 plus hyperfractionated radiotherapy (69.6 Gy at 1.2 Gy bid). Nor were there any differences when quality of life was evaluated using EORTC QOL–C30/LC13 forms.

STAGE IIIB AND STAGE IV

The standard therapy for patients with advanced NSCLC is cytotoxic chemotherapy. Numerous trials have shown that chemotherapy can improve survival, enhance quality of life and be cost-effective. Although no combination regimen is clearly superior to another, the results of recent randomized trials have answered important questions about chemotherapy for patients with advanced disease.

Despite evidence of the benefit of chemotherapy to patients with advanced NSCLC, significant differences exist regarding the perceived role of chemotherapy in metastatic disease between the various specialist groups involved in the treatment of NSCLC. This was emphasized in the study by Jennens et al[121] from Australia, who forwarded a 16-question, multiple-choice questionnaire to all Australian general internists, pulmonary and palliative care physicians, medical and radiation oncologists, and thoracic surgeons to assess beliefs concerning the role of chemotherapy in metastatic NSCLC. Overall assessment of 'pessimism' and 'optimism' regarding the role of chemotherapy in metastatic NSCLC was made. A total of 1325 questionnaires were mailed, with 679 replies. There was a wide variation in knowledge between specialist groups – for instance, among medical oncologists, thoracic surgeons and general internists – and, in general, medical oncologists were more optimistic than palliative care physicians, radiation oncologists and pulmonary physicians. The study raises substantial issues regarding the beliefs of clinicians treating NSCLC and emphasizes the importance of multidisciplinary assessment.

The role of chemotherapy for advanced NSCLC has been editorialized both by Blackhall and Thatcher[122] and by Argiris and Schiller.[123] Reviews, a journal supplement and a US Food and Drug Administration (FDA) drug approval summary for pemetrexed have also been published concerning the role of single agents such as topotecan and pemetrexed in front-line chemotherapy[124–129] and pemetrexed, taxane–platinum combinations, antimetabolites and rexinoids in second-line treatment.[130–132] In addition, meta-analyses have been performed reviewing single-agent versus two-agent chemotherapy regimens in advanced NSCLC.[133] Sixty-five trials with 13 601 patients were eligible for the study. In the trials comparing a doublet regimen with a single-agent regimen, a significant increase was observed in tumor response and 1-year survival in favor of the doublet regimen. Adding a second drug improved tumor response and survival rate. The same investigators also observed that the addition of a third drug had a weaker effect on tumor response and no effect on survival.

A meta-analysis has also been performed to compare the activity, efficacy and toxicity of platinum-based versus non-platinum-based chemotherapy in patients with advanced NSCLC based on a review of randomized phase II and III trials comparing first-line palliative platinum-based chemotherapy versus the same regimen without platinum or with platinum replaced by a non-platinum agent.[134] The study included 37 assessable trials with 7633 patients. A 62% increase in the odds ratio (OR) for response was attributable to platinum-based therapy. The 1-year survival rate was not significantly prolonged when platinum-based therapies were compared with third-generation-based combination regimens. Toxicity was generally higher for platinum-based regimens. The publication resulted in a subsequent correspondence concerning the methodology of how to perform meta-analyses,[135] and the results are somewhat

Table 8.2 Stage III NSCLC – combined-modality therapies; randomized trials

Authors	No. of patients	Treatment	Radiation	Median survival (months)	Overall survival rate (%) 1-year	2-year	3-year
Belani et al[110]	59	2 cycles carboplatin (AUC 6) i.v. + paclitaxel 225 mg/m² i.v. q 3 wks	Arm 1: 64 Gy (2 Gy/d)	14.9	4	24	14
	60		Arm 2: 57.6 (1.5 Gy tid for 2.5 wks)	20.3	–	44	34
Groen[111]	82	Carboplatin 20 mg/m²/d during radiotherapy	60 Gy during 6 wks 5 fractions/wk	11.8	20	–	–
		vs					
	78	No chemotherapy		11.7	28	–	–
Sculier et al[113]	176	Mitomycin 6 mg/m² + ifosfamide 3 g/m² + cisplatin 50 mg/m²		11.5	51	–	17
	175	Mitomycin 6 mg/m² + ifosfamide 4.5 g/m² + cisplatin 60 mg/m² + carboplatin 200 mg/m²	60 Gy (2 Gy/d) 5 weekly × 6	11.8	46	–	11
Belani et al[114]	91	Paclitaxel 200 mg/m²/d + carboplatin (AUC 6) q 3 wks × 2	Followed by 63 Gy	13.0	30	17	–
		vs					
	74	Paclitaxel 200 mg/m²/d + carboplatin (AUC 6) q 3 wks × 2	Followed by 63 Gy + paclitaxel 45 mg/m² + carboplatin (AUC 2) weekly	12.7	25	15	
		vs					
	92	Radiotherapy 63 Gy + paclitaxel 45 mg/m² + carboplatin (AUC 2)	Followed by paclitaxel 200 mg/m² + carboplatin (AUC 6)	16.3	31	17	

Table 8.2   continued

Fournel et al[112]	103	Arm A: induction with cisplatin 120 mg/m^2 i.v. days 1, 29, 57 + vinorelbine 30 mg/m^2 i.v. weekly from day 1 to day 78	Followed by thoracic radiotherapy 66 Gy in 33 fractions of 2 Gy (5 fractions weekly) + consolidation cisplatin 80 mg/m^2 days 78 and 106 + vinorelbine 30 mg/m^2 days 78–127	14.5	26	14
	102	Arm B: thoracic radiotherapy (as arm A) + cisplatin 20 mg/m^2/d etoposide 50 mg/m^2/d (days 1–5 and days 29–33) + consolidation therapy (as arm A)	+ consolidation cisplatin 80 mg/m^2 days 78 and 106 + vinorelbine 30 mg/m^2 days 78–127	16.3	39	21

in contrast to a publication by Hotta et al.[136] The paper by Barlési and Pujol,[137] based on a systematic review of phase III trials, included combination chemotherapy without platinum compounds in the treatment of advanced NSCLC. The topic of platinum or non-platinum regimens was also touched upon by Androulakis and Georgoulias[138] in an editorial in *Lung Cancer* commenting on a randomized phase II study by Chen et al[139] of vinorelbine plus gemcitabine with or without cisplatin in patients with inoperable previously untreated NSCLC. Although the number of patients in the latter trial was insufficient to reach firm conclusions, there was a higher response rate for the platinum arm: 46.5% versus 23.3% for the combination of vinorelbine and gemcitabine. However, there was also more toxicity in the three-drug combination and there were no significant differences in the time to disease progression or overall survival between the two arms. The question of platinum or not was also the subject of an editorial by Bunn.[140]

With respect to patients who are long-term survivors of stage IV NSCLC, Okamoto et al[141] published their results of reviewing 222 NSCLC patients with stage IV disease treated in the period from 1990 to 1999. A total of 135 patients were treated with chemotherapy alone, while the remainder received a combination of chemotherapy and radiotherapy in addition to surgery, which was performed in 19 patients; 7.7% survived for more than 2 years and all but 1 patient had an adenocarcinoma. Among the 17 patients surviving for more than 2 years, 8 patients received surgery as the initial therapy and 16 (94.1%) received some type of local control therapy, including surgery or radiotherapy, during the treatment of their disease.

PHASE II TRIALS

Numerous phase II trials have emerged exploring the efficacy of either single agents or two-drug or three-drug combinations.

Single-agent chemotherapy

The various single agents tested in advanced NSCLC are shown in Table 8.3 and include both classical agents such as gemcitabine and docetaxel, and also a novel taxane (BMS-184476), a new antifolate (10-propargyl-10-deazaaminopterin), a new oral topoisomerase inhibitor (rubitecan), kareniticin, a compound isolated from the Indian Ocean sea hare (dolastatin) and green tea extract.[142–151] Based on response rate, no activity was observed for rubitecan,[148] which was given to patients who had not received chemotherapy before, or for dolastatin[149] or green tea extract.[145] Response rates of 14.3% and 10% were noted for BMS-184476[143] and the new antifolate, respectively.[144] Of the older drugs, Yasuda et al[150] applied paclitaxel in previously untreated advanced NSCLC using a weekly schedule of 80 mg/m^2 three times in a 4-week cycle. Encouraging results were observed, with 17 of 35 patients achieving

Table 8.3   Phase II trials – miscellaneous single agents

Authors	No. of patients	Treatment	Overall response rate (%)[a]	Median survival (weeks)	1-year overall survival rate (%)
Camps et al[143]	56	BMS-18447b[b] 60 mg/m^2 i.v. q 3 wks	14.3	10	–
Krug et al[144]	39	10-Propargyl-10-deazaaminopterin 135–150 mg/m^2 i.v. q 2 wks	10 (3–25)	13.5	56
Laurie et al[145]	17	Green tea extract 0.5–3.0 mg/day	–	–	–
Anderson et al[146]	24	Gemcitabine[c] 1000 mg/m^2 i.v. days 1, 8, 15	17	–	–
Nakamura Y et al[147]	27	Docetaxel 60 mg/m^2 i.v. q 3 wks	18.5 (6.3–38.0)	9.4	23.9
Baka et al[148]	17	Rubitecan[d] 1.5–2.0 mg/m^2 daily p.o. for 5 days repeated every week	0	8.3	–
Marks et al[149]	17	Dolastatin (LU 103793) 2.5 mg/m^2 i.v. for 5 consecutive days q 3 wks	0	9.5	–
Miller et al[142]	52	Kareniticin 1 mg/m^2 i.v. infusion for 5 days q 221 days	4	10.4	36
Yasuda et al[150]	35	Paclitaxel 80 mg/m^2 i.v. days 1, 8, 15 q 4 wks	49 (32–66)	10.5	–
West et al[151]	58	Paclitaxel 35 mg/m^2 24 h infusion over 96 h q 3 wks	14	12	50
Scagliotti et al[152]	19	Paclitaxel 200 mg/m^2 over 72 h q 3 wks	11.1 (1.4–34.7)	8.6	35

[a] 95% confidence intervals in parentheses.
[b] A novel taxane, analog of paclitaxel.
[c] Given as domiciliary chemotherapy.
[d] 9-Nitrocamptothecin.

a partial remission (49%; 95% CI 32–66%). The median survival time was 55 weeks. Noteworthy is also the study by Anderson et al[146] using domiciliary chemotherapy with gemcitabine in a feasibility study of 24 patients. Gemcitabine was given at 1000 mg/m^2 on days 1, 8 and 15 every 4 weeks, with the first course in hospital and the remaining courses at home. A total of 147 courses were given at home and only 14 in hospital on courses 2–6. Both the patients and carers reported positively on the use of domiciliary gemcitabine and preferred it over hospital administration. Further studies investigating this approach are obviously warranted.

An interesting study was performed by the Southwest Oncology Group in the USA,[151] who applied paclitaxel 35 mg/m^2/24 h continuously infused over 96 h every 21 days for up to six courses in patients with advanced bronchioloalveolar carcinoma (BAC). The objective response rate was 14% (all partial responses) and 40% of the patients demonstrated stable disease. The median progression-free and overall survivals were 5 and 12 months, respectively. Similar results were obtained by European investigators,[152] who observed a response rate of 11.1% among 19 patients with advanced BAC using a paclitaxel schedule of 200 mg/m^2 i.v. over 72 hours every 3 weeks.

The studies can serve as a historical control for BAC patients against which future therapeutic approaches can be compared.

RANDOMIZED TRIALS

Phase III

A number of combination regimens have recently been investigated in order to attempt to answer important questions about the use of chemotherapy for patients with advanced disease (Table 8.4). First of all, two-drug combinations have been compared with single agents. Lilenbaum et al[153] compared paclitaxel versus paclitaxel plus carboplatin, whereas Georgoulias et al[154] investigated single-dose docetaxel in comparison with docetaxel and cisplatin. In the study by Lilenbaum et al[153] 561 eligible patients were allocated by the Cancer and Leukemia Group B (CALGB) in the USA. The combination produced a higher response rate (29% vs 17%; $p < 0.001$), and also median survival favored the doublet arm with 8.8 months and 6.7 months, but this was not statistically significant. Median failure-free survival was 2.5 months in the paclitaxel arm and 4.6 months in the carboplatin–paclitaxel arm ($p = 0.0002$). No difference was observed in the 1-year survival rates (32% and 37%, respectively) or in overall survival distributions, with the HR being 0.91 (95% CI 0.77–1.17; $p = 0.25$). Hematologic toxicity and nausea were more frequent in the combination arm, but overall febrile neutropenia and toxic deaths were equally low in both arms. The results in elderly patients were similar to those in younger patients, and performance status 2 patients had a superior outcome when treated with combination chemotherapy.

Table 8.4   Advanced-stage NSCLC – phase III doublet chemotherapy trials

Authors	No. of patients	Treatment	Overall response rate (%)	Median survival (weeks)[a]	1-year overall survival rate (%)	2-year overall survival rate (%)
Lilenbaum et al[153]	277	Paclitaxel 225 mg/m^2 day 1 q 3 wks	17	6.7	32	6.7
		vs				
	284	Paclitaxel 225 mg/m^2 + carboplatin (AUC) day 1 q 3 wks	29	8.8	37	8.8
Georgoulias et al[154]	152	Docetaxel 100 mg/m^2 day 1	18	8.0	43	15
		vs				
	167	Docetaxel 100 mg/m^2 + cisplatin 80 mg/m^2 day 2 + rhG-CSF 150 µg/m^2 days 3–9 q 3 wks	35	10.5	44	19
Pujol et al[156]	155	Gemcitabine 1000 mg/m^2 days 1 and 8 + docetaxel 85 mg/m^2 day 8 q 3 wks	31	11.1	46	–
		vs				
	156	Cisplatin 100 mg/m^2 day 1 + vinorelbine 30 mg/m^2 days 1, 8, 15 and 22 q 4 wks	35.9	9.6	42	–
Kubota et al[162]	156	Docetaxel 60 mg/m^2 i.v. day 1 + cisplatin 80 mg/m^2 i.v. day 1 q 3–4 wks	37	11.3	47.7	24.4
		vs				
	155	Vindesine 3 mg/m^2 i.v. days 1, 8, 15 + cisplatin 80 mg/m^2 i.v. day 1 q 4 wks	21	9.6	21.4	12.3

continued

Table 8.4   continued

Authors	No. of patients	Treatment	Overall response rate (%)	Median survival (weeks)	1-year overall survival rate (%)	2-year overall survival rate (%)
Stathopoulos et al[158]	185	carboplatin (AUC 6) + paclitaxel 175 mg/m^2 i.v. q 3 wks vs	45.9	11	42.7	10.1
	175	Vinorelbine 25 mg/m^2 i.v. + paclitaxel 135 mg/m^2 i.v. q 2 wks	42.8	10	37.8	19
Georgoulias et al[155]	197	Gemcitabine 1000 mg/m^2 i.v. days 1 and 8 + docetaxel 100 mg/m^2 day 8 vs	30	9.0	34.3	14.1
	192	Vinorelbine 30 mg/m^2 i.v. days 1 and 8 + cisplatin 80 mg/m^2 i.v. + rhG-CSF 150 µg/m^2 days 9–15 q 3 wks	39.2	9.7	40.8	11.3
Wachters et al[160]	119	Gemcitabine 1125 mg/m^2 i.v. days 1 and 8 + cisplatin 80 mg/m^2 day 2 q 3 wks vs	46	10.7	45	–
	121	Gemcitabine 1125 mg/m^2 i.v. days 1 and 8 + epirubicin 100 mg/m^2 day 1 q 3 wks	36	9	35	–
Smit et al[161]	159	Paclitaxel 175 mg/m^2 day 1 + cisplatin 80 mg/m^2 day 1 vs	31.8	8.1	35.9	–
	160	Gemcitabine 1250 mg/m^2 days 1 and 8 + cisplatin 80 mg/m^2 day 1 vs	36.8	8.9	33.1	–
	161	Paclitaxel 175 mg/m^2 day 1 + gemcitabine 1250 mg/m^2 days 1 and 8 all q 3 wks	27.7	6.7	26.7	–

Table 8.4 continued

	N	Regimen				
Martoni et al[157]	137	Cisplatin 75 mg/m² day 1 + vinorelbine 25 mg/m² days 1 and 8	32.6	11	39.7	13.7
		vs				
	135	Cisplatin 75 mg/m² day 1 + gemcitabine 1200 mg/m² days 1 and 8 q 3 wks	25.9	11	44.4	16.6
Belani et al[163]	179	Cisplatin 75 mg/m² + etoposide 190 mg/m²	15	9	37	–
		vs				
	190	Carboplatin (AUC 6) + paclitaxel 225 mg/m² q 3 wks	23	8	32	–
Tan et al[159]	159	Vinorelbine 30 mg/m² i.v. days 1 and 8+ carboplatin (AUC 5) day 1 q 3 wks	20.8	8.6	34.4 (p = 0.01)	–
		vs				
	157	Vinorelbine 25 mg/m² i.v. + gemcitabine 1000 mg/m² i.v. both given days 1 and 8 q 3 wks	28.0	11.5	48.9	–

In the Greek study,[154] 167 patients received docetaxel 100 mg/m² plus cisplatin 80 mg/m² on day 2 plus recombinant human granulocyte colony-stimulating factor (rhG-CSF) 150 μg/m² on days 3–9, while 152 patients received docetaxel alone using the same doses and schedule as the other arm. The overall response rate was in favor of the two-drug combinations: 36.5% versus 21.7% ($p = 0.004$). Median overall survival was 10.5 months and 8.0 months, respectively ($p = 0.200$). The 1- and 2-year survival rates were essentially the same for the two drugs. The authors concluded that docetaxel could be a reasonable front-line chemotherapy for patients who cannot tolerate cisplatin.

The same investigators also used docetaxel in another large trial comparing docetaxel given on day 8 plus gemcitabine given on days 1 and 8 versus vinorelbine on the same days combined with cisplatin and including prophylactic rhG-CSF.[155] A total of 389 randomly assigned patients were analyzed for response and toxicity. As seen in the Table 8.4, no statistically significant differences were observed comparing median survival (9.0 vs 9.7 months) and 1-year survival rate (34.3% vs 40.8%). Overall, the docetaxel and gemcitabine combination had a better toxicity profile, with less hematologic toxicity and no nephrotoxicity or ototoxicity.

Two other European groups have also evaluated the use of vinorelbine combined with cisplatin. Pujol et al[156] compared this combination with gemcitabine and docetaxel, whereas Martoni et al[157] compared it with cisplatin and gemcitabine, with the cisplatin doses in both arms being 75 mg/m² given on day 1 and vinorelbine and gemcitabine being given on days 1 and 8 in each cycle of 3 weeks. Neither of the trials showed any significant differences between the two arms, and the overall median survivals were also quite similar on comparing the two studies, with median survival being in the range of 9.6–11.1 months. The Martoni study also included a pharmacoeconomic evaluation, which favored the cisplatin–vinorelbine combination.

In addition, Stathopoulos et al[158] designed a study that compared a paclitaxel–vinorelbine combination with carboplatin–paclitaxel in patients with advanced NSCLC. Again, no significant differences between the two combinations were noted based on response rate and survival, and the toxicity patterns were also similar, except for neutropenia, which was significantly greater for the paclitaxel–carboplatin treatment.

A similar study was conducted by Tan et al,[159] who randomized 316 patients with advanced NSCLC to either vinorelbine plus carboplatin or vinorelbine plus gemcitabine. A higher response rate (28.0% vs 20.8%), median survival (11.5 vs 8.6 months; $p = 0.01$) and 1-year survival rate (48.9% vs 34.4%) were observed for the vinorelbine plus gemcitabine combination.

The study by Wachters et al[160] with inclusion of 240 patients revealed no differences when combinations of gemcitabine plus cisplatin and gemcitabine and epirubicin were compared. Median progression-free survivals were 26 weeks and 23 weeks, respectively, with tumor response rates being 46% and 36% and median survivals 43 weeks and 36 weeks. The study included a quality-of-life evaluation, but again no differences were found between the two arms.

Another European trial was reported by Smit et al;[161] this was a three-arm randomized study of two cisplatin-based regimens and paclitaxel plus gemcitabine in advanced NSCLC performed by the Lung Cancer Group of the European Organization for Research and Treatment of Cancer (EORTC). Patients were randomly assigned to receive either paclitaxel 175 mg/m^2 or gemcitabine 1250 mg/m^2 on days 1 and 8, both combined with cisplatin 80 mg/m^2 (arms A and B) or paclitaxel 175 mg/m^2 combined with gemcitabine 1250 mg/m^2 days 1 and 8 (arm C). The primary endpoint was comparison of overall survival for B versus A and C versus A. A total of 480 patients were enrolled. No statistically or clinically significant differences were observed for primary or secondary endpoints, which included response rate and response duration, progression-free survival, toxicities, quality of life, and cost of treatment. Overall, the treatment was well tolerated in all three arms, but costs associated with the non-platinum arm were highest.

Also, Japanese and American investigators have shed additional light on the use of two-drug combinations in patients with advanced NSCLC. Kubota et al[162] published their final results comparing vindesine–cisplatin (VdsC) with the newer docetaxel–cisplatin combination (DC). In 311 chemotherapy-naive patients, the DC arm demonstrated significant improvements compared with the VdsC arm in terms of overall response rate (37% vs 21%, respectively; $p = 0.01$) and median survival time (11.3 vs 9.6 months, respectively; $p = 0.014$). The 2-year survival rate was 24% for DC compared with 12% for VdsC. Quality of life was also shown to be significantly better in the DC arm than in the VdsC arm ($p = 0.020$). Toxicity was predominantly hematologic and was more severe in the VdsC arm.

Finally, Belani et al[163] reported a study from the USA with enrollment of 369 patients who were randomized to receive either cisplatin 75 mg/m^2 and etoposide 100 mg/m^2 (179 patients) or carboplatin AUC = 6 mg/ml/min and paclitaxel 225 mg/m^2 (190 patients). The cycles were repeated every 3 weeks. The arms were well balanced, and again there was no statistically significant survival advantage for carboplatin–paclitaxel compared with cisplatin–etoposide, but there was an overall benefit in quality of life with the carboplatin–paclitaxel regimen. The article was accompanied by an editorial,[164] which pointed out that there is a trend for better median survival and 1-year survival rate in the cisplatin–etoposide arm compared with the carboplatin–paclitaxel arm, which might raise some concerns about the efficacy of the carboplatin–paclitaxel doublet, but it does also reflect a positive evaluation in the medical management of advanced NSCLC, giving options for use of a number of agents and combinations as second-line treatment. In addition, it should be emphasized that the relatively high median overall survival in some of the recent trials in patients with advanced NSCLC might be explained by the extensive use, and efficacy, of the second-line chemotherapy.

As summarized by Danson and Thatcher,[165] in a commentary on the study by Smit et al,[161] '. . . the choice of a patients' first line therapy with classical cytotoxics given similar survival, quality of life and toxicity data is likely to be determined by other considerations. These include cost, not only to the health provider but also the patient, in terms of time spent in hospital, transfusions, antibiotics and other symptomatic measures, which impact on the lifestyles of patients and carers.'

Triplet chemotherapy

The concept that the addition of a third agent to a doublet regimen will improve overall results has been tested in several randomized trials (Table 8.5).

Two British studies compared the combination of gemcitabine and carboplatin versus a standard arm of mitomycin, ifosfamide and cisplatin (MIC) or mitomycin, vinblastine and cisplatin (MVP). In the study by Danson et al,[166] the results failed to demonstrate any difference in efficacy between the newer regimen of gemcitabine and carboplatin and the older regimens of MIC and MVP. The overall response rate, median survival and 1-year survival rate were almost identical.

In the slightly larger study by Rudd et al,[167] with enrollment of 422 patients, there was a significant survival advantage for gemcitabine and carboplatin compared with MIC (HR = 0.76; 95% CI 0.61–0.93; p = 0.08). Median survival was 10 months with gemcitabine and carboplatin and 7.6 months with MIC. The 1-year survival rate was 40% with gemcitabine and carboplatin and 30% with MIC (difference 10%, 95% CI 3–18%). Overall response rates were similar (42% and 41%, respectively). The combination of gemcitabine and carboplatin caused less nausea, vomiting, constipation and alopecia and was associated with fewer admissions for administration and better quality of life.

In the study by Laack et al,[168] gemcitabine plus vinorelbine (GV) was compared with the same two agents in the same dose and schedule combined with cisplatin 75 mg/m^2 on day 2 i.v. every 3 weeks. Three hundred patients with advanced NSCLC were included, and, as shown in Table 8.5, the cisplatin regimen showed no survival benefit as first-line chemotherapy compared with the cisplatin-free GV regimen, which was substantially better tolerated.

Among the newer agents, two studies tested the potential value of matrix metalloproteinase (MMP) inhibitors (MMPIs).[169,170] MMPs belong to a family of enzymes that digest extracellular matrix and basement membrane components, and facilitate tumor growth, metastasis and angiogenesis. In both studies, an MMPI was added to a two-drug combination of either paclitaxel plus carboplatin or gemcitabine plus cisplatin, with the MMPI being BMS-275291 or prinomastat, respectively. In none of the studies did the addition of an MMPI to chemotherapy improve survival, but it added to the toxicity, necessitating discontinuation of the experimental arm in one of the studies.

Finally, the clinical activity and safety of killed *Mycobacterium vaccae* with chemotherapy was tested in a trial of 419 patients, with the chemotherapy consisting of mitomycin, vinblastine and cisplatin or carboplatin given every 3 weeks.[171] The study was non-placebo-controlled, and the overall efficacy with standard parameters, such as response rate, median survival and 1-year

Table 8.5	Phase III triplet chemotherapy studies in advanced-stage NSCLC					
Authors	No. of patients	Treatment	Overall response rate (%)	Median survival (weeks)	1-year overall survival rate (%)	2-year overall survival rate (%)
Danson et al[166]	186	Gemcitabine 1000 mg/m^2 days 1, 8, 15 + Carboplatin (AUC 5) q 4 wks vs	30	8	33.2	6.9
	186	Mitomycin 6 mg/m^2 i.v. + ifosfamide 3 g/m^2 i.v. + cisplatin 50 mg/m^2 i.v. q 3 wks or Mitomycin 8 mg/m^2 + vinblastine 6 mg/m^2 + cisplatin 50 mg/m^2 q 3 wks	33	8	32.5	11.8
Rudd et al[167]	212	Gemcitabine 1200 mg/m^2 i.v. days 1 and 8 + carboplatin (AUC 5) q 3 wks vs	42	10	40	12
	210	Mitomycin 6 mg/m^2 i.v. + ifosfamide 3 g/m^2 i.v. + cisplatin 50 mg/m^2 i.v. q 3 wks	41	7.6	30	6
Laack et al[168]	143	Gemcitabine 1000 mg/m^2 days 1 and 8 + vinorelbine 25 mg/m^2 days 1 and 8 vs	13	9	33.6	–
	144	Gemcitabine 1000 mg/m^2 days 1 and 8 + vinorelbine 25 mg/m^2 days 1 and 8 + cisplatin 75 mg/m^2 day 2 q 3 wks	28.3	8	27.5	–

continued

Table 8.5 continued

Authors	No. of patients	Treatment	Overall response rate (%)	Median survival (weeks)	1-year overall survival rate (%)	2-year overall survival rate (%)
Leigh et al[169]	387	Paclitaxel 200 mg/m^2 i.v + carboplatin (AUC 6) i.v. q 3 wks. vs	33.7	9.2	–	–
	387	Paclitaxel 200 mg/m^2 i.v. + carboplatin (AUC 6) i.v. q 3 wks + BMS-275291[a] 1200 mg daily p.o.	25.8	8.6	–	–
Bissett et al[170]	181	Gemcitabine 1250 mg/m^2 days 1 and 8 + cisplatin 75 mg/m^2 day 1 q 3 wks vs	26	11.5	43	–
	181	Gemcitabine 1250 mg/m^2 + cisplatin 75 mg/m^2 + prinomastat 15 mg/m^2 p.o daily	27	10.5	38	–
O'Brien et al[171]	210	Mitomycin 8–10 mg/m^2 i.v. + vinblastine 6 mg/m^2 i.v. + cisplatin 50–120 mg/m^2 or carboplatin (AUC 4–6) q 3 wks vs	33	7	25	–
	209	Mitomycin 8–10 mg/m^2 i.v. + vinblastine 6 mg/m^2 i.v. + cisplatin 50–120 mg/m^2 or carboplatin (AUC 4–6) q 3 wks + SRL172[b]	37	7	25	–

[a]A matrix metalloproteinase inhibitor.
[b]Killed *Mycobacterium vaccae*.

survival, did not reveal any difference between the standard arm and the experimental arm with killed *M. vaccae*.

Thus, none of the trials supports the use of three-drug combinations in first-line chemotherapy for patients with advanced NSCLC.

COMBINATION CHEMOTHERAPY

Phase II trials

Taxane-based phase II doublets

Several non-randomized and randomized trials have continued to explore doublet regimens. The majority of the phase II trials are taxane-based and the treatments and results are shown in Table 8.6.[172–184] It can be seen that both paclitaxel and docetaxel are included in these doublets and are often combined with the various platinum agents, such as cisplatin, carboplatin or oxaliplatin, using various dose schedules, for example with docetaxel given on days 1, 8 and 15 and cisplatin on day 1 in a 4-week schedule, as reported by Tsunoda et al[174] and Kaira et al,[177] or with docetaxel given on day 1 and cisplatin on days 1 and 2 in a 3-week schedule, as reported by Firvida et al.[176] Paclitaxel and docetaxel have also both been combined with irinotecan[179,184] and with epirubicin.[182] The majority of patients included in these trials had not received prior chemotherapy and the response rates ranged from 29% to 48%, with the median survival usually being in the range of 9–13 months. One exception is the phase II study of weekly docetaxel and cisplatin by Kaira et al.[177] Forty chemotherapy-naive patients (10 with stage IIIB and 30 with stage IV NSCLC) with an ECOG performance status of 0–2 were enrolled. Chemotherapy consisted of cisplatin (80 mg/m^2 i.v.) on day 1, and docetaxel (35 mg/m^2 i.v.) on days 1, 8 and 15, delivered in 4-week cycles consisting of three weekly treatments followed by 1 week of rest. There were 18 partial responses, with an overall response rate of 45% and an astonishing median survival period of 19.9 months and a 1-year survival rate of 69.4%. Toxicities were mild. The results are of interest, but selection criteria, small sample size and the use of second-line therapy and chest irradiation may all have had an impact on the results.

Gemcitabine-based phase II doublets (Table 8.7)

Several phase II trials have investigated combinations of gemcitabine with a platinum agent: gemcitabine–nedaplatin,[185] gemcitabine–oxaliplatin,[188,189] and the increasingly popular gemcitabine–carboplatin regimen.[187] Combinations such as gemcitabine plus vinorelbine,[190] pemetrexed,[186] irinotecan[191] or a taxane[192,193] have also been tested. Overall, the response rates are somewhat lower than for the taxane-based phase II doublets, whereas the median survival is in the same range. Overall, none of the phase II gemcitabine doublets produced meaningful benefits over current regimens. With respect to the role of gemcitabine in the treatment of advanced NSCLC, it is noteworthy that a

Table 8.6 Taxane-based phase II doublets

Authors	No. of patients	Treatment	Overall response rate (%)	Median survival (weeks)	1-year overall survival rate (%)
Aguiar et al[172]	27	Paclitaxel 100 mg/m² i.v. days 1 and 15, alternating with gemcitabine days 8 and 22 of a 36-day cycle	29	13	52
Yumuk et al[173]	51	Paclitaxel 112 mg/m² i.v. days 1 and 8 + carboplatin (AUC 5) day 1 q 3 wks	45	11	44
Tsunoda et al[174]	38	Docetaxel 25 mg/m² i.v. days 1, 8, 15 + cisplatin 80 mg/m² i.v. day 1 q 4 wks	31.6	11.8	46.5
De Castro et al[175]	50	Docetaxel 75 mg/m² i.v. day 8 + gemcitabine 1000 mg/m² i.v. days 1 and 8 q 3 wks	26	7	25
Firvida et al[176]	42	Docetaxel 85 mg/m² i.v. day 1 + cisplatin 40 mg/m² i.v. days 1 and 2 q 3 wks	48	10.5	36
Kaira et al[177]	40	Docetaxel 35 mg/m² days 1, 8, 15 + cisplatin 80 mg/m² day 1 q 4 wks	45	19.9	69.4
Winegarden et al[178]	38	Paclitaxel 175 mg/m² i.v. + oxaliplatin 130 mg/m² i.v. q 3 wks	34	9.2	37
Yamada et al[179]	24	Paclitaxel 80–180 mg/m² i.v. + irinotecan 60 mg/m² i.v. q 2 wks	58.3	12	54.2
Ramalingam et al[180]	45	Docetaxel 80 mg/m² i.v. + carboplatin (AUC 5) q 3 wks	29	11.9	47
Kallab et al[181]	29	Paclitaxel 100 mg/m² i.v. + carboplatin (AUC 2) weekly for 3 of every 4 wks	43.5	10.8	44
Yang et al[182]	38	Epirubicin 70 mg/m² i.v. day 1 + paclitaxel 175 mg/m² day 2 q 3 wks	44.7	11.9	49
Grunberg[183]	23	Paclitaxel 150 mg/m² i.v. day 1 + vinorelbine 13 mg/m² days 1–3 q 3 wks	30	7	–
Ziotopoulos et al[184]	39	Irinotecan 200 mg/m² i.v. + docetaxel 80 mg/m² i.v. q 3 wks	23	10.8	42

Table 8.7 Gemcitabine-based phase II doublets					
Authors	No. of patients	Treatment	Overall response rate (%)	Median survival (weeks)	1-year overall survival rate (%)
Kurata et al[185]	20	Gemcitabine 800–1000 mg/m^2 days 1 and 8 + nedaplatin 60–100 mg/m^2 day 1 q 3 wks	16.7	9.1	34.1
Monnerat et al[186]	58	Gemcitabine 1250 mg/m^2 days 1 and 8 + pemetrexed 500 mg/m^2 day 8 q 3 wks	15.5	10.1	42.6
Soo et al[187]	15	Carboplatin (AUC 5) day 1 + gemcitabine 10 mg/m^2/min at a dose rate of 600, 750 and 900 mg/m^2 days 1 and 8 q 3 wks	20	–	–
Bidoli et al[188]	19	Gemcitabine 1250 mg/m^2 i.v. days 1 and 8 + oxaliplatin 70–130 mg/m^2 i.v. day 1 q 3 wks–	13	6.5	–
Katakami et al[190]	50	Gemcitabine 1000 mg/m^2 i.v. + vinorelbine 25 mg/m^2 i.v. days 1 and 8 q 3 wks	18	13.9	55.4
Cappuzzo et al[189]	60	Gemcitabine 1000 mg/m^2 i.v. days 1 and 8 + oxaliplatin 130 mg/m^2 i.v. day 1 q 3 wks	25	7.3	36
Nishio et al[191]	21	Gemcitabine 1000 mg/m^2 i.v. q 2 wks + irinotecan 50–150 mg/m^2 i.v. q 2 wks	28	–	–
Neubauer et al[192]	50	Gemcitabine 900 mg/m^2 i.v. weekly + docetaxel 36 mg/m^2 i.v. weekly × 6 q 8 wks	20	6.9	32
Gillenwater et al[193]	39	Gemcitabine 800 mg/m^2 i.v. infusion over 80 minutes days 1, 8, 15 q 4 wks + paclitaxel 110 mg/m^2 i.v. infusion over 3 hours days 1, 8, 15 q 4 wks	35	10.4	35

meta-analysis of survival outcomes has been performed comparing gemcitabine plus platinum with other platinum-containing regimens in advanced NSCLC.[194] Data from a total of 4556 patients from 13 randomized trials investigating gemcitabine in combination with a platinum agent vs any other platinum-containing regimen were included in a meta-analysis. A significant reduction in overall mortality in favor of gemcitabine–platinum regimens was observed (HR = 0.90; 95% CI 0.84–0.96) with an absolute benefit at 1 year of 3.9%. Median survival was 9.0 months for the gemcitabine–platinum regimens and 8.2 months for the comparator regimens. There was a significant decrease in the risk of disease progression in favor of gemcitabine–platinum regimens. An absolute benefit of 4.2% at 1 year was estimated.

Phase II trial with miscellaneous doublets

Among the other agents known to have activity as single agents in NSCLC, oral or i.v. vinorelbine, irinotecan, pemetrexed and tegafur have been investigated, again often in combination with either cisplatin or carboplatin in phase II trials (Table 8.8).[195–199] The results based on overall response rates, median survival and 1-year survival rates are quite similar to what has been observed for combinations including the taxanes or gemcitabine. Noteworthy is the oral application of vinorelbine combined with carboplatin in the study by O'Brien et al.[198] The regimen was very well tolerated with a low level of toxicity and a low rate of serious adverse events. There were only 8 responses out of 52 enrolled patients, yielding a response rate of 18.2% (95% CI 6.8–29.6%), which is quite disappointing.

Phase II triplet combinations

Several trials have evaluated the tolerability and efficacy of three-drug combinations, as summarized in Table 8.9.[200–203] Cisplatin and carboplatin were the key elements in all of these studies. In two studies, cisplatin was combined with gemcitabine and ifosfamide,[200,201] while a third study combined carboplatin with paclitaxel and marimastat.[202] All three studies included a small number of patients. The overall response rates were 53% and 49% for the gemcitabine-containing regimens[200,201] versus 57% for the paclitaxel-containing combination.[202] In a fourth study, paclitaxel and vinorelbine were combined with cisplatin.[203] Focusing on toxicity, it appears that triplet chemotherapy regimens in general seem to cause a greater incidence of febrile neutropenia compared with doublet regimens.[203]

Randomized trials

Phase II trials

Evolution of randomized trials comparing various chemotherapy regimens for advanced NSCLC has been reviewed by Ioannidis et al.[204] The authors evaluated the evidence from randomized trials comparing various chemotherapy

Table 8.8   Phase II trials – miscellaneous doublets

Authors	No. of patients	Treatment	Overall response rate (%)	Median survival (weeks)	1-year overall survival rate (%)
Jassem et al[195]	56	Cisplatin 100 mg/m^2 day 1 + vinorelbine 25 mg/m^2 day 1 i.v. + vinorelbine 60 mg/m^2 p.o. days 8, 15, 22 q 4 wks	33	8.9	37
Fukuda et al[196]	59	Irinotecan 50 mg/m^2 i.v. days 1, 8, 15 + carboplatin (AUC 5) q 4 wks	34	10	37.6
Ichinose et al[197]	55	Cisplatin 60 mg/m^2 i.v. day 8 + tegafur 40–60 mg/m^2 twice a day days 1–21 q 5 wks	47	11	45
O'Brien et al[198]	52	Vinorelbine 25 mg/m^2 i.v. + carboplatin (AUC 5 i.v.) day 1 + vinorelbine p.o. 60 mg/m^2 on day 18 q 3 wks	18.2	9.3	–
Clarke et al[199]	33	Vinorelbine 15–30 mg/m^2 i.v. days 1–8 q 21 days + pemetrexed 300–700 mg/m^2 days 1–8 q 21 days	38	7.9	–

Table 8.9 Phase II – triplet combinations

Authors	No. of patients	Treatment	Overall response rate (%)	Median survival (weeks)	1-year overall survival rate (%)
Mohedano et al[200]	30	Gemcitabine 1000 mg/m^2 i.v. days 1 and 8 + ifosfamide 3500 mg/m^2 day 2 + cisplatin 80 mg/m^2 day 2 q 3 wks	53	15	56
Bourgeois et al[201]	33	Ifosfamide 3000 mg/m^2 i.v. (24 h infusion) day 1 + gemcitabine 1000–1750 mg/m^2 days 1 and 15 + cisplatin 80–100 mg/m^2 i.v. day 15 q 4 wks	49	–	–
Goffin et al[202]	22	Carboplatin (AUC 7) i.v. + paclitaxel 175–200 mg/m^2 i.v. q 3 wks and marimastat 10–20 mg p.o. bid	57	–	–
Cortes et al[203]	46	Paclitaxel 135 mg/m^2 i.v. day 1 + cisplatin 120 mg/m^2 i.v. day 1 + vinorelbine 30 mg/m^2 i.v. days 1 and 15 q 4 wks	39	8	33

regimens for advanced NSCLC. Across 254 eligible trials (42 661 patients) no regimens were compared in more than six studies. The search was performed up until 2002 using MEDLINE, EMBASE and the Central Registry of Controlled Trials of the Cochrane Library. Twenty-six trials (10%) found statistically significant differences in survival between the compared arms. Only five reported the randomization mode, and four reported adequate allocation concealment; nine performed unaccounted interim analyses. Statistical significance was more common in larger studies ($p = 0.003$), more recent studies ($p = 0.031$), and those from countries with only one published eligible study ($p = 0.008$). Increased reported median survival was independently associated with platinum and/or taxane and combination regimens, but also with the year of publication, smaller sample size and larger representation of non-stage IV patients and patients with a better performance status. The proportion of enrolled patients with a performance status of 2 or worse decreased significantly over time (12.9% per decade; $p < 0.001$). Randomized evidence in this field is thus fragmented and subject to considerable selection biases. From the review, one can conclude that performing hundreds of underpowered chemotherapy trials represents a poor, uncoordinated research investment. Larger, well-designed and adequately reported trials may be more definite, but their targets should be carefully selected. Smaller trials are still useful, and careful meta-analyses may yield more conclusive results.

Methodologic issues in randomized controlled trials with special focus on health-related quality of life have been reviewed by Bottomley et al.[205] A systematic review using Cochrane methodology evaluated health-related quality-of-life components in randomized controlled trials. Twenty-nine published randomized controlled trials, including 8445 patients with a health-related quality of life, were identified; common limitations included no clear hypothesis, lack of a clear approach to missing data and data analysis, and limited presentation of results. It was concluded that health-related quality of life is an important endpoint because the information helps to influence treatment recommendations, but the identified weaknesses in conducting health-related quality-of-life measurement in NSCLC randomized controlled trials and the reporting of results need to be addressed.

The results of several randomized phase II trials exploring doublet regimens are given in Table 8.10.[206–210] Douillard et al[206] presented the final results of a randomized phase II trial comparing docetaxel–cisplatin with vinorelbine–cisplatin, both as first-line therapy, followed by a cross-over at progression to single-agent vinorelbine or docetaxel in advanced NSCLC. A total of 233 patients were included and response rates were 34% and 26%, respectively ($p = 0.20$). No differences were observed in median time to progression (5 months in both arms), median survival or 3-year survival. The study suggests increased activity of first-line docetaxel–cisplatin, whereas second-line vinorelbine does not provide additional clinical benefit, even though statistical significance was not reached.

Table 8.10   Randomized phase II trials

Authors	No. of patients	Treatment	Overall response rate (%)	Median survival (weeks)	1-year overall survival rate (%)
Douillard et al[206]	233	(A1) Cisplatin 100 mg/m² + docetaxel 75 mg/m² × 6 cycles, followed by docetaxel 75 mg/m² q 3 wks	34	8	36
	205	vs (B1) Cisplatin 100 mg/m² + vinorelbine 30 mg/m² days 1 and 8 q 21 d × 6 cycles, followed by vinorelbine 30 mg/m² days 1, 8 q 3 wks	26	9	35
Lilenbaum et al[207]	82	Vinorelbine 25/mg/m² i.v. + gemcitabine 1000 mg/m² days 1 and 8 q 3 wks	14.6	7.8	38.7
	83	vs Paclitaxel 200 mg/m² i.v. + carboplatin (AUC 6) day 1 q 3 wks	16.9	8.6	31.9
Rocha Lima et al[208]	39	Gemcitabine 1000 mg/m² i.v. days 1 and 8 + irinotecan 100 mg/m² days 1 and 8 q 3 wks	12.8	7.95	23
	39	vs Gemcitabine 1000 mg/m² i.v. days 1 and 8 + docetaxel 40 mg/m² i.v. days 1 and 8	23.1	12.8	51
Scagliotti et al[209]	80	Pemetrexed 500 mg/m² day 1 + carboplatin (AUC 6) day 1	31.6	10.5	43.9
	59	vs Pemetrexed 500 mg/m² day 1 + oxaliplatin 120 mg/m² day 1 q 3 wks	26.8	10.5	49.9
Ma et al[210]	31	Pemetrexed 500 mg/m² i.v. day 1 followed by gemcitabine 1000 mg/m² days 1 and 8	31	11.4	–
	62	vs Gemcitabine 1000 mg/m² i.v. day 1 followed by pemetrexed 500 mg/m² i.v. and then gemcitabine 1000 mg/m² i.v. day 8	6.5	10.3	–
		vs Gemcitabine 1000 mg/m² i.v. days 1 and 8 + pemetrexed 500 mg/m² i.v. day 8	16.1	11.8	–

Lilenbaum et al[207] compared two different combinations: vinorelbine and gemcitabine (VG) versus carboplatin and paclitaxel (CP). Patients treated with VG experienced lower toxicity, but overall quality of life was similar in both arms. Efficacy seemed comparable between VG and CP based on overall response rates of 14.6% and 16.9%, respectively, median survival and 1-year survival. The combination of vinorelbine and gemcitabine might thus be a viable alternative to platinum-based chemotherapy in patients with advanced NSCLC.

Another phase II randomized trial including 80 patients, with 78 patients being evaluable, explored the efficacy and toxicity of gemcitabine, combined with either irinotecan or docetaxel.[208] Both combinations were well tolerated and the results of the combination with gemcitabine and docetaxel are encouraging, with an overall response rate of 23.1%, a median survival of 12.8 months, and a 1-year survival rate of 51%. Obviously, the exact role of gemcitabine and docetaxel in the management of advanced NSCLC cannot be established from this small randomized phase II trial, but it might be particularly useful for patients who have experienced toxicities with a platinum regimen or for patients who may be more susceptible to platinum-related toxicity.

Of the new agents, pemetrexed has been combined with either carboplatin or oxaliplatin in an investigation by Scagliotti et al[209] whereas another study incorporated three schedules with gemcitabine in order to evaluate the optimum administration schedule of these two agents in chemotherapy-naive patients with NSCLC.[210] The design of this latter three arm trial is given in Table 8.10. The schedule of giving gemcitabine followed by pemetrexed on day 1 and gemcitabine on day 8 was closed prematurely after interim analysis because of only 1 confirmed response in the first 19 assessable patients. A comparison between the two other schedules revealed that the schedule of pemetrexed followed by gemcitabine on day 1 and gemcitabine on day 8 was less toxic than gemcitabine on day 1 and pemetrexed followed by gemcitabine on day 8, whereas the efficacies based on median survival time and time to progression were quite similar.

Other studies in patients with advanced NSCLC have included pharmacologic studies of weekly versus twice-weekly dose-intensive cisplatin and gemcitabine.[211] Dose-limiting toxicity was as expected, with hematologic toxicity being dose-limiting on the weekly schedule and ototoxicity on the 2-weekly schedule. The highest dose intensity of cisplatin could be achieved on the 2-weekly schedule, and the further development of the weekly schedule was abandoned. The maximum tolerated dose was established at 1500 mg/m² gemcitabine in combination with cisplatin 90 mg/m², and more than half of the patients achieved an objective response on the 2-weekly schedule, versus 23% in the weekly treatment arm.

Finally, Pathak et al[212] reported on the use of multiple antioxidants in patients with advanced NSCLC receiving chemotherapy alone or chemotherapy plus high-dose multiple antioxidants. A total of 136 patients were included, and no significant differences were observed in efficacy based on response rate and survival times, and toxicity profiles were also similar in both arms.

TARGETED THERAPIES IN ADVANCED NSCLC

Although chemotherapy has resulted in some progress in the overall management of patients with lung cancer in recent years, with increasing use of neoadjuvant and adjuvant strategies and of second-line chemotherapy, treatment outcomes for NSCLC continue to be disappointing. Fortunately, the picture is changing with the introduction of targeted therapies; inhibition of the epidermal growth factor receptor (EGFR) family is at the forefront, led by the tyrosine kinase inhibitors gefitinib (Iressa) and erlotinib (OSI-774 Tarceva), but angiogenesis inhibition with bevacizumab (Avastin) has also produced interesting data from recent trials. The basis for the development of gefitinib and erlotinib is described elsewhere in this book, including an up-to-date review of the available data (see Chapter 3: pp. 20–5).

The role of targeting in NSCLC has also been subjected to numerous review articles, editorials, commentaries and supplements; this has included focusing on the individual agents, including the background on which erlotinib was approved by the FDA in the USA as a monotherapy for the treatment of patients with locally advanced or metastatic NSCLC after failure of at least one prior chemotherapy regimen.[213–231] The study by the Canadian Clinical Trials Group delivered the backbone of the data for this decision.[232] The study included a total of 731 patients randomized using a 2:1 randomization scheme: 488 patients in the erlotinib arm and 243 patients in the placebo arm. EGFR status was determined for 238 of the 731 study patients for whom tissue samples were available prior to the study. A positive EGFR expression status was defined as having at least 10% of cells staining for EGFR. Survival of erlotinib-treated patients was superior to that of placebo-treated patients and the median survival duration of erlotinib-treated patients was 6.7 months, compared with 4.7 months for placebo-treated patients. Exploratory univariate analysis showed a larger survival prolongation in two subsets of patients: those who never smoked and those with EGFR-positive tumors. Erlotinib was also superior to placebo in terms of progression-free survival, and had a response rate of 8.9%, versus 0.9% for placebo. Severe rash occurred in 8% and severe diarrhea occurred in 6% of erlotinib-treated patients.

Similar results have been obtained in several phase II trials with erlotinib. The clinical and biologic features associated with EGFR have been analyzed in studies performed in the USA, Europe, South Korea, Taiwan, China and Japan.[233–239] In addition to non-smoker females and adenocarcinoma, Asian origin has turned up as an important predictive prognostic factor associated with the response and survival benefit of both gefitinib and erlotinib.[240–247]

In addition to phase III trials with the two tyrosine kinase inhibitors, several articles have been published based on experience with a compassionate-use program in patients with advanced NSCLC who have failed prior chemotherapy or were unfit for chemotherapy. Data have been accumulated from Greece, Germany, USA, Korea, Taiwan, The Netherlands and Italy, and some of the studies have specifically analyzed the efficacy and tolerability of gefitinib in patients with poor performance status or in elderly patients.[248–257] All studies have shown that gefitinib has clinical antitumor activity and also good tolerability, with higher response rates in the Asian studies than in European or European-heritage Americans.

With respect to bevacizumab, a monoclonal antibody directed against vascular endothelial growth factor (VEGF), the results of a randomized trial in 444 patients with metastatic NSCLC were presented at the ASCO meeting in 2005.[258] Bevacizumab was added to paclitaxel and carboplatin (PCB) and compared with chemotherapy alone (PC). The response rate (27% vs 10%, $p < 0.0001$), progression-free survival (6.4 months vs 4.5 months, $p < 0.0001$), and median survival (10.2 months vs 12.5 months, $p = 0.0075$) were higher in the bevacizumab arm. Both regimens were well tolerated, but hemorrhage was more frequent in the PCB arm (4.1% vs 1.0%). There were 11 treatment-related deaths (9 in the PCB arm and 2 in the PC arm), of which 5 were due to hemoptysis, all in the PCB arm. It is noteworthy that the trial excluded patients with squamous cell carcinoma, and thus mainly included patients with adenocarcinoma. The future role of antiangiogenic therapy in NSCLC with emphasis on bevacizumab has been the subject of a detailed review by Herbst and Sandler.[259]

MAINTENANCE THERAPY

In addition to including new agents and targeted molecules in the primary treatment of patients with advanced NSCLC, other efforts to optimize delivery of existing chemotherapy agents are ongoing. One approach consists of increasing the intensity of chemotherapy, which can be achieved by delivering higher dose intensities or by employing higher total doses of chemotherapy, including the use of maintenance, which involves prolongation the duration of chemotherapy, either with the same regimen as that used for induction treatment or with other agents.

A phase II trial by De Lena et al[260] explored the effect of consolidation therapy with oral vinorelbine after induction chemotherapy with oral vinorelbine and cisplatin. The objective response rate was 26.5% among 49 evaluable patients and the overall median survival time was 10 months (95% CI 7.4–14 months) and the 1-year survival rate was 42.6%.

Westeel et al[261] conducted a randomized trial to compare maintenance therapy with vinorelbine versus observation in previously untreated patients who responded to induction treatment with MIC. Patients with stage IIIB NSCLC were treated with two monthly MIC cycles followed by radiotherapy; selected patients were treated with four monthy MIC cycles. Patients who responded to induction treatment were randomly assigned to receive intravenous vinorelbine at a dose of 25 mg/m^2 weekly for 6 months or no further treatment. A total of 573 patients were registered, of whom 227 responded to induction treatment and 181 were randomly assigned (91 to maintenance vinorelbine and 90 to observation). The 1- and 2-year survival rates were 42.2% and 20.1% in the vinorelbine arm and 50.6% and 20.2% in the observation arm, respectively. There were also no differences between the two arms in the HR of survival after adjustment for stage or in progression-free survival (log-rank $p = 0.32$). Accordingly, maintenance vinorelbine did not improve survival of patients with advanced NSCLC who responded to induction MIC treatment. The data thus confirm the conclusions of Socinski et al[262] in a review article addressing the issue of optimal duration of therapy in advanced metastatic NSCLC.

TREATMENT OF ELDERLY AND POOR PERFORMANCE STATUS PATIENTS

More than 50% of cases of advanced NSCLC are diagnosed in patients > 65 years old, and approximately 30–40% in patients >70 years old. With the aging of the population, it is to be expected that the prevalence of lung cancer among the elderly will increase. During the last decade, the incidence of lung cancer has decreased among individuals ≤ 50 years old, but has increased among those ≥ 70 years old. Accordingly, NSCLC in the older person is an increasingly common problem faced by the clinical oncologist. The problem has been described in review articles, both with respect to the general management[263,264] and especially concerning the treatment of elderly patients with advanced NSCLC receiving chemotherapy.[265,266] The topic has generated considerable interest, as evidenced by multiple review articles, which have also included description of patients with poor performance status.[267,268]

The treatment of advanced NSCLC in the elderly has also been the subject of a review by an international panel of experts that met in April 2004 with subsequent publication of their results in May 2005.[269]

Also noteworthy is an analysis by US investigators based on data from the SEER–Medicare database. Altogether, 14 875 patients with stage III (49.8%) and stage IV (50.2%) disease were analyzed at the time of diagnosis: 31% received chemotherapy, 8% received surgery and 53% received radiotherapy as either initial or adjuvant treatment. Patients ≥ 75 years old, females, African-Americans and those with more than one comorbidity were significantly less likely to receive chemotherapy ($p < 0.01$). Survival was inferior for those who did not receive a platinum-containing agent ($p < 0.01$).[270]

Among the clinical trials in elderly patients with advanced NSCLC, the phase II trials have included both single agents, such as vinorelbine given orally or gemcitabine given on either a 3- or a 4-week schedule, or two-drug cisplatin combinations, with docetaxel, vinorelbine or gemcitabine being the second compound. Oral vinorelbine with doses of 60–80 mg/m² was tolerated very well and resulted in a low response rate of 11% but a median overall survival of 8.2 months in a group of 56 chemonaive patients >70 years old.[271] Slightly higher response rates were observed on the gemcitabine studies, especially on the 3-week schedule.[272,273] In the smaller phase II trials with two-drug combinations, the response rates were considerably higher, namely 52%, 50% and 35%, with somewhat longer median survival, ranging from 7.0 to 15.8 months.[274–276] Also, the use of sequential chemotherapy has been explored in phase II trials in patients with poor performance status or elderly patients with comorbidities, yielding similar results to the other phase II trials, but possibly with less toxicity.[277,278]

Two larger randomized trials have been published.[279,280] The aim of the study by Comella et al[279] was to assess whether a combination of gemcitabine with either paclitaxel or vinorelbine could be more effective than gemcitabine and paclitaxel alone in elderly or unfit advanced NSCLC patients. A total of 264 NSCLC patients >70 years old with ECOG performance status ≤2 or younger with PS = 2 were randomly treated with gemcitabine (with either paclitaxel or vinorelbine) and compared with paclitaxel or gemcitabine alone. The median survival times and 1-year survival rates were 5.1 and 29% for gemcitabine, 6.4 and 25% for paclitaxel, 9.2 and 44% for gemcitabine and paclitaxel, and 9.7 and 32% for gemcitabine and vinorelbine. Multivariate analysis showed that performance status ≤1 and doublet treatments were significantly associated with longer survival. Doublets produced no more toxicity than single agents. The authors concluded that gemcitabine and paclitaxel should be considered a reference regimen for elderly NSCLC patients with PS ≤1.

The other randomized trial by Baka et al[280] included patients with impaired performance status (Karnofsky performance ≤70) and advanced NSCLC comparing two treatment schedules of gemcitabine. Patients were randomly assigned to receive gemcitabine 1000 mg/m^2 on days 1, 8 and 15 of each 28-day cycle or gemcitabine 1500 mg/m^2 on days 1 and 8 of each 21-day cycle, both for up to six cycles. A total of 174 patients were enrolled. Only 61.5% of the patients were alive at 2 months. There was a significant improvement in performance from baseline to precycle 3 in both treatment arms, with a trend in favor of gemcitabine given in 3 out of 4 weeks. Response rate, survival and duration were similar in both arms. The article was subsequently discussed in a Letter to the Editor by Belvedere and Grossi.[281]

SECOND-LINE CHEMOTHERAPY

An increasing number of patients with NSCLC are receiving second-line chemotherapy, with single agents, combination chemotherapy or targeted therapy, as pointed out by Herbst and Kim[282] in a review article.

Several phase II studies have evaluated various types of combination chemotherapy, some with and some without platinum compounds, including new agents such as irinotecan and capecitabine and cyclooxygenase-2 (COX-2) inhibition with celocoxib combined with docetaxel.[283–287] In addition, investigations have included randomized phase II trials, with the two main topics being the scheduling of docetaxel and comparison of single agents versus two-drug combinations (Table 8.11).

With regard to docetaxel, Gridelli et al[288] performed a randomized trial of

Table 8.11	Second-line chemotherapy – phase II trials			
Authors	Treatment	Overall response rate (%)	Median survival (weeks)	1-year overall survival rate (%)
Han et al[283]	Irinotecan 90–100 mg/m^2 i.v. days 1 + 8 + capecitabine 1000 mg/m^2 p.o. days 1–14 q 3 wks	11.4	7.4	–
Chen et al[284]	Vinorelbine 20 mg/m^2 i.v. + gemcitabine 800 mg/m^2 i.v. days 1, 8, 15 q 4 wks	31.3	8.3	34.3
Koizumi et al[285]	Gemcitabine 1000 mg/m^2 i.v. days 1 and 14 + paclitaxel 110–170 mg/m^2 i.v. days 1 and 14	22	–	–
Esteban et al[290]	Docetaxel 36 mg/m^2 i.v. weekly vs Paclitaxel 80 mg/m^2 i.v. weekly	3 15	6 3	– –
Gervais et al[289]	Docetaxel 75 mg/m^2 i.v. q 3 wks vs Docetaxel 40 mg/m^2 i.v. weekly for 6 wks, then 2 wks of rest	4.8 3.2	5.8 5.5	– –
Georgoulias et al[292]	Gemcitabine 1000 mg/m^2 i.v. days 1 and 8 + irinotecan 300 mg/m^2 i.v. day 8 q 3 wks vs Irinotecan 300 mg/m^2 i.v. q 3 wks	8.4 4.2	9 7	24.5 29

Table 8.11   continued

	N	Regimen			
Gridelli et al[288]	110	Docetaxel 75 mg/m² i.v. q 3 wks	2.7	7.1	21
	110	vs Docetaxel 33.3 mg/m² i.v. weekly	5.5	6.1	33
Quoix et al[291]	93	Docetaxel 75 mg/m² i.v. q 3 wks	8.6	4.7	–
	89	vs Doxetaxel 100 mg/m² i.v. q 3 wks	7.6	6.7	–
Pectasides et al[293]	65	Docetaxel 30 mg/m² i.v. + irinotecan 60 mg/m² days 1 and 8 q 3 wks	20	6.5	37
	65	vs Docetaxel 75 mg/m² q 3 wks	14	6.4	34
Kindwall-Keller et al[286]	36	Docetaxel 36 mg/m² i.v. days 1, 8, 15 + capecitabine 625 mg/m² twice-daily days 5–18 q 4 wks	26	9.1	37
Hanna et al[296]	264	Pemetrexed 500 mg/m² day 1 q 3 wks	9.1	8.3	29.7
	274	vs Docetaxel 75 mg/m² day 1 q 3 wks	8.8	7.9	29.2
Dancey et al[295]	104	Docetaxel 100 or 75 mg/m² i.v. q 3 wks	5.8	–	–
	100	vs Best supportive care	–	–	–

two docetaxel regimens using either a weekly or a 3-weekly schedule as second-line treatment, with the doses of docetaxel being either 75 mg/m² 3-weekly or 33.3 mg/m² weekly for 6 weeks. The study comprised 220 patients with advanced NSCLC. Quality of life was assessed by the EORTC questionnaires and Daily Diary Card. Response and survival rates were similar, but the 3-week docetaxel was more toxic for leukopenia, neutropenia, febrile neutropenia and hair loss, and, in particular, grade 3–4 hematologic toxicity was significantly more frequent in the 3-weekly arm (25% vs 6%). The study strongly favors the use of a weekly docetaxel schedule as second-line treatment. A similar observation was made by Gervais et al,[289] who again randomized weekly versus 3-weekly docetaxel in a phase II trial with 125 patients. Regarding efficacy, there was a trend towards a better disease control rate in the 3-weekly schedule compared with the weekly schedule (32.2% vs 25.4%, respectively), but the median time to progression and survival were similar in both arms.

The question of weekly use of taxanes was also explored by Esteban et al,[290] who in a small study with 71 patients (all previously treated with platinum-based chemotherapy) used either docetaxel 36 mg/m² or paclitaxel 80 mg/m² administered as a 1-hour i.v. weekly infusion for 6 weeks followed by a 2-week rest. A higher non-hematologic toxicity of docetaxel was observed, particularly pulmonary toxicity and diarrhea. Further larger studies are obviously needed in order to determine whether efficacy differences exist between paclitaxel and docetaxel.

Quoix et al[291] tested two doses of docetaxel (75 and 100 mg/m²) as second-line monotherapy for NSCLC. A total of 182 patients from 24 French centers were randomized. Based on the results, the authors concluded that 75 mg/m² is the optimal docetaxel dosage, as it has a more favorable safety profile and, on balance, a similar efficacy to the 100 mg/m² dose, even though the 100 mg/m² group tended to have a higher median overall survival of 6.7 months (95% CI 4.8–7.1) versus 4.7 months (95% CI 3.8–5.9).

Of the new combinations, the efficacy and toxicity of irinotecan were tested when given with either gemcitabine or docetaxel, and showed quite similar overall results, as observed in the studies mentioned above.

Two Greek studies have tried irinotecan as second-line treatment of patients with advanced NSCLC, pretreated with platinum combinations. Georgoulias et al[292] compared irinotecan plus gemcitabine versus irinotecan alone as second-line treatment in patients progressing after docetaxel–cisplatin-based therapy. A total of 147 evaluable patients were randomized to either combination chemotherapy (n = 76) or irinotecan alone (n = 71). No significant differences were observed between the two groups in terms of the median duration of response, time to tumor progression, overall survival and 1-year survival. The combination with gemcitabine significantly improved quality-of-life aspects such as 'general mood', 'coughing' and 'intensity of symptoms' compared with irinotecan. The other study, performed by Pectasides et al,[293] compared docetaxel as a single agent versus a combination of docetaxel and irinotecan. The administration of irinotecan with docetaxel did not significantly improve response rate, time to progression, median survival or 1-year survival.

With respect to second-line therapy, docetaxel has been considered the standard of care for patients with advanced lung cancer failing upfront therapy, with Shepherd et al[294] reporting a 7% objective response rate and a 7-month median survival when compared with 4–6 months best supportive care. This study also included a quality-of-life assessment and the results have now been published in detail.[295] A total of 204 patients were included in the trial with 104 receiving either 75 mg/m^2 or 100 mg/m^2 i.v. of docetaxel and 100 receiving best supportive care. Longitudinal analysis showed statistically significant differences in patient-rated pain scores in favor of docetaxel ($p = 0.005$) compared with best supportive care. Trends in favor of docetaxel were noted on observer-rated scales for fatigue and pain for all docetaxel patients, and for total Lung Cancer Symptom Scale score for appetite and fatigue with doxetaxel 100 mg/m^2. Overall, second-line docetaxel therapy for advanced NSCLC significantly improved survival, with a trend towards less deterioration in quality of life compared with best supportive care.

The use of docetaxel as a standard treatment in patients with NSCLC has been challenged by pemetrexed, which was compared with docetaxel in a randomized phase III trial comprising 571 patients receiving either pemetrexed 500 mg/m^2 i.v. on day 1 with vitamin B$_{12}$ and folic acid, or docetaxel 75 mg/m^2 i.v. day 1 every 3 weeks.[296] Overall response rates were 9.1% and 8.8% (analysis of variance $p = 0.105$) for pemetrexed and docetaxel, respectively. Median progression-free survival was 2.9 months for each arm, and median survival was 8.3 versus 7.9 months. The 1-year survival rate was similar for both arms. With respect to toxicity, patients receiving docetaxel were more likely to have grade 3 or 4 neutropenia, a higher degree of febrile neutropenia, and also neutropenia with infections and hospitalizations for neutropenic fever (13.4% vs 1.5%). Treatment with pemetrexed thus resulted in clinically equivalent efficacy outcomes, but with significantly fewer side effects compared with docetaxel as second-line treatment, and, based on these data, pemetrexed should be considered as a standard treatment option for second-line NSCLC when available.

SUPPORTIVE CARE

Even though much attention has been given to the use of antineoplastic agents in patients with advanced NSCLC within the last couple of years, especially after the emergence of targeted therapy, supportive care, including palliation, remains an important aspect in the management of patients with NSCLC. Supportive care has been defined as every treatment given to prevent, control or relieve complications and side effects and to improve the comfort and quality of life of people who have cancer.

With respect to advanced NSCLC, Di Maio et al[297] analyzed data of patients enrolled in three randomized trials of first-line chemotherapy, conducted between 1996 and 2001 with the specific purpose of describing supportive care in these patients. The analysis was limited to the first three cycles of treatment.

Supportive care data were available for 1185 out of 1312 enrolled patients. Gastrointestinal drugs (45.7%), corticosteroids (33.4%) and analgesics (23.8%) were the most frequently observed categories. Not surprisingly, cisplatin-based treatment required an overall higher number of supportive drugs, with higher use of antiemetics and antianemics than, for instance, vinorelbine. Patients with worse performance status were more exposed to corticosteroids, whereas elderly patients were less frequently exposed to antiemetics, but they required more drugs against concomitant diseases.

The symptoms and quality of life of patients with advanced NSCLC have also been the subjects of a supplement reviewing the various methods to assess quality of life and meaningful symptom improvement in lung cancer patients.[298]

With respect to supportive care, the role of epoetin (recombinant human erythropoietin) has been reviewed by Morère,[299] and a retrospective analysis has also been performed with data obtained from a phase III trial of darbepoetin alfa (a hyperglycosylated derivative of epoietin) versus placebo in anemic patients with lung cancer receiving chemotherapy.[300] Outcomes were compared for patients with baseline hemoglobin >10–11 g/dl and <10 g/dl. Darbepoetin alfa significantly reduced transfusions compared with placebo, irrespective of hemoglobin level at treatment initiation. Darbepoetin alfa also improved fatigue compared with placebo in both hemoglobin categories. The findings also support the use of erythropoietin therapy in lung cancer patients with mild anemia undergoing chemotherapy. The same conclusions were reached in the review by Morère.[299]

Other complications in patients with NSCLC are the occurrence of skeletal metastases, and in that regard it is noteworthy that zoledronic acid has resulted in a reduction of skeletal complications in patients with bone metastases and lung cancer. In a study of 773 patients,[301] the majority of whom had NSCLC, fewer patients treated with zoledronic acid (initially 8 mg, later reduced to 4 mg) developed at least one skeletal-related event (SRE) at 21 months compared with patients treated with placebo: 39% of those treated at a 4 mg dose ($p = 0.127$) and 36% of those treated at the 8/4 mg dose ($p = 0.023$), compared with 46% of those treated with placebo. Furthermore, zoledronic acid significantly delayed the median time to first SRE (236 days with 4 mg vs 155 days with placebo; $p = 0.009$).

Of other treatment modalities, radiotherapy remains an important part of the overall treatment in the palliative setting, and it has been used in various ways. Major topics of discussion have been which regimen of palliative radiotherapy is the most effective and least toxic and whether higher doses increase survival. A Cochrane review has been published by Macbeth et al.[302] Ten randomized trials were reviewed; there were important differences in the doses of radiotherapy investigated, the patient characteristics and the outcome measures. Because of this heterogeneity, no meta-analysis was attempted. This study found no strong evidence that any regimen gives greater palliation. There was evidence for a modest increase in survival (6% at 1 year and 3% at 2 years) in patients with better performance status given higher-dose radiotherapy. The reviewers concluded that the majority of patients should be treated with short courses of palliative radiotherapy, of 1 or 2 fractions, and that more research is needed into reducing the acute toxicity of large-fraction regimens and into the role of radical compared with high-dose palliative radiotherapy.

Subsequently, a Dutch and a British randomized trial have been published. In the Dutch study,[303] 297 patients were randomized to receive either 10×3 Gy or 2×8 Gy by external-beam irradiation. The primary endpoint was a patient-assessed score of treatment effect on seven thoracic symptoms using an adapted Rotterdam Symptom Checklist. Both treatment arms were equally effective, as the average total symptom scores over the initial 39 weeks did not differ. However, the pattern in time of the scores differed significantly ($p < 0.001$). Palliation in the 10×3 Gy arm was more prolonged, with less worsening symptoms than in 2×8 Gy arm. Survival in the 10×3 Gy arm was significantly ($p = 0.03$) better than in the 2×8 Gy arm, with a 1-year survival rate of 19.6% versus 10.9%. The results thus support the use of a 10×3 Gy radiotherapy schedule.

In the British study,[304] a 10 Gy single fraction was compared with 30 Gy in 10 fractions. A total of 149 patients were analyzed and were followed carefully with regard to performance status, hospital anxiety and depression score, and a quality-of-life index before treatment, at 1 month after treatment and every 2 months thereafter. A significantly higher proportion of patients experienced palliation and complete resolution of chest pain and dyspnea with the regimen using 30 Gy in 10 fractions; no differences were observed in toxicity or in survival (22.7 weeks for 10 Gy single fraction vs 28.3 weeks for 30 Gy in 10 fractions; $p = 0.197$). The dose of palliative radiotherapy has also been the subject of an editorial.[305]

Based on a prospective randomized study, Sundstrøm et al[306] raised the question of whether immediate or delayed radiotherapy is preferable in patients with advanced NSCLC. The design and results of the study have been published previously, and the authors concluded that the data suggest – even though the results should be interpreted cautiously – that patients with minimal or no tumor-related thoracic symptoms would not benefit from immediate palliative thoracic radiotherapy with regard to improved long-term symptom control and quality of life based on either patients' or clinicians' assessments of chest/airway symptoms. Meanwhile, chest irradiation may induce significant dysphagia in otherwise symptom-free patients. According to the authors, a wait-and-see policy, i.e. delaying thoracic irradiation until symptomatically needed, appears to be safe and acceptable.

The use of hypofractionated external-beam radiotherapy has also been evaluated as a retreatment for symptomatic NSCLC in patients who have received prior chest irradiation. Reirradiation consisted of two fractions of 8 Gy on days 1 and 8, and palliation was obtained in the majority of patients, but the number of patients in the study (28) was small.[307]

OTHER TYPES OF TREATMENT

Various types of radioactive treatments have been explored. Noteworthy is the publication by Chen et al[308] from China, who used the therapeutic radionuclide iodine-131 linked to recombinant chimeric tumor necrosis treatment (TNT) antibody (^{131}I-chTNT). A total of 107 patients received two doses of ^{131}I-chTNT administered 2–4 weeks apart. All patients had experienced treatment failure after prior radiotherapy or chemotherapy. For the 10 patients with SCLC, the overall response rate was 50%, with 1 complete and 4 partial responses. For the 97 patients with NSCLC, the overall response rate was 33%, with 3 complete remissions and 29 partial remissions. A biodistribution study demonstrated excellent localization of the radioactivity in tumors in both systemically and intratumorally injected patients. The most obvious adverse side effect was mild and reversible bone marrow suppression. Further studies are obviously needed in order to establish the exact role of this new approach to treating patients with NSCLC.

Endobronchial brachytherapy and photodynamic therapy (PDT) have also been explored in the treatment of patients with malignant lung tumors. Escobar-Sacristán et al[309] described their experience in 81 patients, 76 of whom had primary lung tumors. The technique consisted of delivering high-dose irradiation from an iridium-192 source to a target volume using one or two endobronchial catheters inserted under optical or videobronchoscopic guidance. Four sessions were scheduled at weekly intervals and 500 cGy was applied per session. In total, 85% of the symptoms analyzed (hemoptysis, cough, dyspnea, expectorate and stridor) disappeared with high-dose-rate endobronchial brachytherapy. The endoscopic response was complete in 56.9% of patients and partial or less than complete in 40.74%. One major complication occurred (bronchial fistula, 1.2%), but no lethal hemoptysis. High-dose-rate endobronchial brachytherapy is a good palliative treatment for endoluminal lung neoplasms, effectively alleviating symptoms and endoscopic evidence in many cases with an acceptable rate of complications.

With regard to PDT in NSCLC, a review has been published by Maziak et al,[310] while Freitag et al[311] described their experience with this modality of treatment using sequential PDT combined with high-dose brachytherapy for patients with limited bronchogenic carcinomas. A total of 32 patients were treated, and at a mean follow-up of 24 months, 26 patients were free of residual tumor and local recurrence. All patients included in the study were technically inoperable ($n = 15$) or had recurrent bronchogenic carcinomas ($n = 17$). The tumors were limited to the bronchial wall and other metastatic disease was not evident.

In patients with inoperable lung cancer, the use of radiofrequency thermal ablation under CT guidance has also been reported in small series of patients (31, 33 and 21), either as single-modality treatment or as an adjuvant to chemotherapy and radiotherapy.[312–316] The treatment appears to be very well tolerated and the complications are minimal. The exact role of this new treatment modality remains to be defined in the overall management of patients with lung malignancies.

BRAIN METASTASES

Within the last decade, overall survival data have demonstrated a slow but steady increase in the survival of patients with NSCLC, and, as a result of this, the occurrence of brain metastases is achieving more interest, similar to the development of the management of SCLC in the 1980s, which resulted in the use of prophylactic cranial irradiation (PCI) in patients with localized disease achieving a complete remission. The topic has been analyzed in two major retrospective analyses from the Dana Faber Cancer Center in Boston and the Southwest Oncology Group (SWOG) in the USA. Mamon et al[317] reviewed the records of 177 patients with stage IIIA NSCLC treated with surgery, chemotherapy and radiotherapy. The most common site of recurrence was the brain: 34% of patients recurred in the brain as their first site of failure and 40% of patients developed brain metastases at some point in their course. In patients with non-squamous histology and residual nodal involvement after neoadjuvant therapy, the risk of brain metastases was 53% at 3 years. In the SWOG study,[318] 422 patients were analyzed, of whom 64% had experienced disease progression. All patients had stage IIIA/B NSCLC and all were treated with concurrent cisplatin–etoposide and radiation, with a surgery arm in two of the four protocols. Fifty-four relapses (20%) were in the brain only; 17 (6.5%) were in the brain and other sites simultaneously. Again, non-squamous histology was a significant predictor, together with young patient age, for increased risk of early relapse with brain metastases. Both studies thus support the designs of ongoing trials of PCI in stage III NSCLC, as discussed in detail by Carolan et al.[319]

The treatment of isolated brain metastases in patients also undergoing surgery has been studied by Furák et al[320] and Getman et al[321] based on 65 patients and 32 patients, respectively, who were operated on for lung cancer brain metastases. The number of patients is thus relatively small, and the conclusions from the two studies differ. Furák et al[320] recommend lung surgery after brain metastasectomy in synchronous patients with N0, N1 and single-level N2 diseases, whereas Getman et al[321] question the value of lung resection in patients with isolated synchronous brain metastases. The former viewpoint is supported by data from Iwasaki et al,[322] who recommend surgical treatment for primary lung and brain metastases as long as there is stringent selection of patients.

With respect to treatment of brain metastases, radiotherapy is the preferred modality in addition to surgery, using either whole-brain irradiation or stereotactic radiosurgery.[323]

Turning to chemotherapy, single-agent gefitinib has demonstrated activity according to Hotta et al,[324] who observed 1 complete remission and 5 partial remissions in 14 patients with NSCLC and brain metastases, with the majority of patients having received prior cisplatin-based chemotherapy. Similar results have been obtained by Chiu et al[325] in a larger trial, with an objective response in 7 out of 21 patients with NSCLC and brain metastases.

Adrenal metastases

The adrenal gland is a common site of metastases from lung carcinoma, but the patients are rarely suitable for surgical resection. The experience from an Italian institute has been reported by Lucchi et al,[326] who, in an 8-year period, performed laparoscopic adrenalectomy in 14 patients who had undergone lung resection for NSCLC with suspected or confirmed solitary adrenal gland metastases. All the patients had enlarged adrenal glands on abdominal ultrasound or CT. All but 2 patients underwent at least one adrenal fine-needle aspiration. All the patients underwent careful staging to exclude other sites of metastasis. In 7 cases, a preoperative cytologic diagnosis of metastasis was established. The pathologic examination confirmed an NSCLC metastasis in 11 cases, while in 4 cases it was a cortical adenoma. Regarding the 10 patients with NSCLC metastases, 3 were still alive and well at 37–80 months from the lung resection. One patient (who underwent bilateral adrenalectomy) was still alive at 44 months with local relapse. Even though this series was small, laparoscopic adrenalectomy should be considered in patients with solitary adrenal gland metastasis operated on for NSCLC.

REFERENCES

1. Foeglé J, Hédelin G, Lebitasy MP et al. Non-small-cell lung cancer in a French department (1982–1997): management and outcome. Br J Cancer 2005; 92: 459–66.

2. Potosky AL, Saxman S, Wallace RB et al. Population variations in the initial treatment of non-small-cell lung cancer. J Clin Oncol 2004; 22: 3261–8.

3. Campling BG, Hwang W-T, Zhang J et al. A population-based study of lung carcinoma in Pennsylvania. Cancer 2005; 104: 833–40.

4. Langer CJ, Moughan J, Movsas B et al. Patterns of care survey (PCS) in lung cancer: how well does current U.S. practice with chemotherapy in the non-metastatic setting follow the literature? Lung Cancer 2005; 48: 93–102.

5. Jeremic B. Patterns of care survey (PCS) in chemotherapy (CHT) in nonmetastatic lung cancer. Lung Cancer 2005; 48: 103–5.

6. Turrisi AT. Creeping phase II-ism and the medical pharmaceutical complex: weapons of mass distraction in the war against lung cancer. J Clin Oncol 2005; 23: 4827–9.

7. Mina K, Byrne MJ, Ryan G et al. Surgical management of lung cancer in Western Australia in 1996 and its outcomes. ANZ J Surg 2004; 74: 1076–81.

8. Bach PB, Cramer LD, Schrag D et al. The influence of hospital volume on survival after resection for lung cancer. N Engl J Med 2001; 345: 181–8.

9. Martin-Ucar A, Waller DA, Atkins JL et al. The beneficial effects of

specialist thoracic surgery on the resection rate for non-small-cell lung cancer. Lung Cancer 2004; 46: 227–32.

10. Rostad H, Naalsund A, Strand T-E et al. Results of pulmonary resection for lung cancer in Norway, patients older than 70 years. Eur J Cardiothorac Surg 2005; 27: 325–8.

11. Mery CM, Pappas AN, Bueno R et al. Similar long-term survival of elderly patients with non-small cell lung cancer treated with lobectomy or wedge resection within the Surveillance, Epidemiology, and End Results database. Chest 2005; 128: 237–45.

12. Birim Ö, Zuydendorp HM, Maat APWM et al. Lung resection for non-small-cell lung cancer in patients older than 70: mortality, morbidity, and late survival compared with the general population. Ann Thorac Surg 2003; 76: 1796–801.

13. Brock MV, Kim MP, Hooker CM et al. Pulmonary resection in octogenarians with stage I nonsmall cell lung cancer: a 22-year experience. Ann Thorac Surg 2004; 77: 271–7.

14. Ambrogi V, Pompeo E, Elia S et al. The impact of cardiovascular comorbidity on the outcome of surgery for stage I and II non-small-cell lung cancer. Eur J Cardiothorac Surg 2003; 23: 811–17.

15. Sarna L, Evangelista L, Tashkin D et al. Impact of respiratory symptoms and pulmonary function on quality of life of long-term survivors of non-small cell lung cancer. Chest 2004; 125: 439–45.

16. Pasini F, Verlato G, Durante E et al. Persistent excess mortality from lung cancer in patients with stage I non-small-cell lung cancer, disease-free after 5 years. Br J Cancer 2003; 88: 1666–8.

17. Ohtsuka T, Nomori H, Horio H et al. Is major pulmonary resection by video-assisted thoracic surgery an adequate procedure in clinical stage I lung cancer? Chest 2004; 125: 1742–6.

18. Doddoli C, Aragon A, Barlesi F et al. Does the extent of lymph node dissection influence outcome in patients with stage I non-small-cell lung cancer? Eur J Cardiothorac Surg 2005; 27: 680–5.

19. Kuzdzal J, Zielinski M, Papla B et al. Transcervical extended mediastinal lymphadenectomy – the new operative technique and early results in lung cancer staging. Eur J Cardiothorac Surg 2005; 27: 384–90.

20. Yoshimasu T, Miyoshi S, Oura S et al. Limited mediastinal lymph node dissection for non-small cell lung cancer according to intraoperative histologic examinations. J Thorac Cardiovasc Surg 2005; 130: 433–7.

21. Allen MS. Mediastinal lymph node dissection for non-small cell lung cancer. J Thorac Cardiovasc Surg 2005; 130: 241–2.

22. Little AG. TS Evaluation Study Group. Patterns of surgical care of lung cancer patients. Abstract presented at Society of Thoracic Surgeons 41st Annual Meeting, Tampa, January 24–26, 2005.

23. Furák J, Troján I, Szóke T et al. Bronchioloalveolar lung cancer: occurrence, surgical treatment and survival. Eur J Cardiothorac Surg 2003; 23: 818–23.

24. Nakagawa K, Yasumitu T, Fukuhara K et al. Poor prognosis after lung resection for patients with adenosquamous carcinoma of the lung. Ann Thorac Surg 2003; 75: 1740–4.

25. Gawrychowski J, Brulinski K, Malinowski E et al. Prognosis and survival after radical resection of primary adenosquamous lung carcinoma. Eur J Cardiothorac Surg 2005; 27: 686–92.

26. Pitz CC, de la Riviére AB, van Swieten HA et al. Surgical treatment of

Pancoast tumours. Eur J Cardiothorac Surg 2004; 26: 202–8.

27. Goldberg M, Gupta D, Sasson AR et al. The surgical management of superior sulcus tumors: a retrospective review with long-term follow-up. Ann Thorac Surg 2005; 79: 1174–9.

28. Nakata M, Sawada S, Yamashita M et al. Surgical treatments for multiple primary adenocarcinoma of the lung. Ann Thorac Surg 2004; 78: 1194–9.

29. Rowell NP, Williams CJ. Radical radiotherapy for stage I/II non-small cell lung cancer in patients not sufficiently fit for or declining surgery (medically inoperable). Cochrane Database System Rev 2003; (1): CD002935.

30. Bollmann A, Blankenburg Y, Haerting J et al. Survival of patients in clinical stages I–IIIb of non-small-cell lung cancer treated with radiation therapy alone. Strahlenther Onkol 2004; 180: 488–96.

31. Ghosh S, Sujendran V, Alexiou C et al. Long term results of surgery versus continuous hyperfractionated accelerated radiotherapy (CHART) in patients aged >70 years with stage 1 non-small cell lung cancer. Eur J Cardiothorac Surg 2003; 24: 1002–7.

32. Okamoto T, Maruyama R, Shojl F et al. Clinical patterns and treatment outcome of elderly patients in clinical stage IB/II non-small cell lung cancer. J Surg Oncol 2004; 87: 134–8.

33. Burdett S, Stewart L. Postoperative radiotherapy in non-small-cell lung cancer: update of an individual patient data meta-analysis. Lung Cancer 2005; 47: 81–3.

34. Ling CC, Yorke E, Amols H et al. High-tech will improve radiotherapy of NSCLC: a hypothesis waiting to be validated. Int J Radiat Oncol Biol Phys 2004; 60: 3–7.

35. Thirion P, Holmberg O, Collins CD et al. Escalated dose for non-small-cell lung cancer with accelerated hypofractionated three-dimensional conformal radiation therapy. Radiother Oncol 2004; 71: 163–6.

36. Bradley J, Graham MV, Winter K et al. Toxicity and outcome results of RTOG 9311: a phase I–II dose-escalation study using three-dimensional conformal radiotherapy in patients with inoperable non-small-cell lung carcinoma. Int J Radiat Oncol Biol Phys 2005; 61: 318–28.

37. Onishi H, Araki T, Shirato H et al. Stereotactic hypofractionated high-dose irradiation for stage I nonsmall cell lung carcinoma. Cancer 2004; 101: 1623–31.

38. Bush DA, Slate JD, Shin BB et al. Hypofractionated proton beam radiotherapy for stage I lung cancer. Chest 2004; 126: 1198–203.

39. Zimmermann FB, Geinitz H, Schill S et al. Stereotactic hypofractionated radiation therapy for stage I non-small cell lung cancer. Lung Cancer 2005; 48: 107–14.

40. Takeda T, Takeda A, Kunieda E et al. Radiation injury after hypofractionated stereotactic radiotherapy for peripheral small lung tumors: serial changes on CT. AJR Am J Roentgenol 2004; 182: 1123–8.

41. Miller KL, Shafman TD, Anscher MS et al. Bronchial stenosis: an underreported complication of high-dose external beam radiotherapy for lung cancer? Int J Radiat Oncol Biol Phys 2005; 61: 64–9.

42. Fernando HC, Santos RS, Benfiled JR et al. Lobar and sublobar resection with and without brachytherapy for small stage IA non-small cell lung cancer. J Thorac Cardiovasc Surg 2005; 129: 261–7.

43. Non-Small Cell Lung Cancer Collaborative Group. Chemotherapy in non-small cell lung cancer: a meta-analysis using updated data on individual patients from 52 randomized

clinical trials. BMJ 1995; 311; 899–909.

44. Scagliotti G, Fossati R, Torri V et al. Randomized study of adjuvant chemotherapy for completely resected stage I, II, or IIIA non-small cell lung cancer. J Natl Cancer Inst 2003; 95: 1453–61.

45. Waller D, Stephens RJ, Spiro SG et al. The Big Lung Trial (BLT); determining the value of cisplatin-based chemotherapy for all patients with non-small cell lung cancer (NSCLC). Preliminary results in the surgical setting. Proc Am Soc Clin Oncol 2003; 22: 632.

46. The International Adjuvant Lung Cancer Trial Collaborative Group. Cisplatin-based adjuvant chemotherapy in patients with completely resected non-small cell lung cancer. N Engl J Med 2004; 350: 351–60.

47. Sedrakyan A, van Der Meulen J, Prendiville J et al. Postoperative chemotherapy for non-small cell lung cancer: a systematic review and meta-analysis. J Thorac Cardiovasc Surg 2004; 128: 414–19.

48. Hotta K, Matsuo K, Kiura K et al. Role of adjuvant chemotherapy in patients with resected non-small-cell lung cancer. J Clin Oncol 2004; 22: 3860–7.

49. Juergens RA, Brahmer JR. Adjuvant therapy for resected non-small-cell lung cancer: past, present, and future. Curr Oncol Rep 2005; 7: 248–54.

50. Waller D, Peake MD, Stephens RJ et al. Chemotherapy for patients with non-small cell lung cancer: the surgical setting of the Big Lung Trial. Eur J Cardiothoracic Surg 2004; 26: 173–82.

51. Winton T, Livingston R, Johnson D et al. Vinorelbine plus cisplatin vs. observation in resected non-small-cell lung cancer. N Engl J Med 2005; 352: 2589–97.

52. Nakagawa M, Tanaka F, Tsubota N et al. A randomized phase III trial of adjuvant chemotherapy with UFT for completely resected pathological stage I non-small-cell lung cancer: The West Japan Study Group for Lung Cancer Surgery (WJSG) – the 4th study. Ann Oncol 2005; 16: 75–80.

53. Imaizumi M. Postoperative adjuvant cisplatin, vindesine, plus uracil–tegafur chemotherapy increased survival of patients with completely resected p-stage I non-small cell lung cancer. Lung Cancer 2005; 49: 85–94.

54. Hamada C, Tanaka F, Ohta M et al. Meta-analysis of postoperative adjuvant chemotherapy with tegafur–uracil in non-small cell lung cancer. J Clin Oncol 2005; 23: 4999–5006.

55. Bunn PA. Role of adjuvant chemotherapy in stage IB–IIIA non-small cell lung cancer? Qualified, Yes! J Clin Oncol 2004; 488–96.

56. Scagliotti GV, Torri V. Should we be using adjuvant chemotherapy for non-small cell lung cancer? Not yet. J Clin Oncol 2004; 501–10.

57. Lin T, Brahner J. Adjuvant therapy for resected non-small-cell lung cancer: recent advances, emerging agents and lingering questions. Curr Oncol Rep 2004; 6: 251–8.

58. Ikhlaque N, Baumann M. Adjuvant chemotherapy for lung cancer. N Engl J Med 2004; 350: 1681–3.

59. Johnson DH. Postoperative adjuvant chemotherapy in resected non-small cell lung cancer. J Clin Oncol 2004; 497–500.

60. Le Chevalier T, Arriagada R, Pignon J-P et al. Should adjuvant chemotherapy become standard treatment in all patients with resected non-small-cell lung cancer? Lancet Oncol 2005; 6: 182–4.

61. Pisters KMW. Adjuvant chemotherapy for non-small-cell lung cancer – the smoke clears. N Engl J Med 2005; 352: 2640–2.

62. Pisters K, Vallieres E, Bunn P et al.

S9900: a phase III trial of surgery alone or surgery plus preoperative (preop) paclitaxel/carboplatin (PC) chemotherapy in early stage non-small cell lung cancer (NSCLC): preliminary results. Proc Am Soc Clin Oncol 2005; 24: 1095a (abstract 7012).

63. Scagliotti GV, Ch.E.S.T. Investigators. Preliminary results of Ch.E.S.T.: a phase III study of surgery alone or surgery plus preoperative gemcitabine–cisplatin in clinical early stages non-small cell lung cancer (NSCLC). J Clin Oncol 2005: 23(Suppl 16S): LBA7023 (abstract).

64. Vokes EE. Optimal therapy for unresectable stage III non-small-cell lung cancer. J Clin Oncol 2005; 23: 5853–5.

65. Eberhardt W, Gauler T, Hepp R et al. The role of chemotherapy in the treatment of stage III non-small-cell lung cancer. Ann Oncol 2004; 15: 71–80.

66. Eberhardt W, Stuschke M, Stamatis G. Preoperative chemoradiation approaches to locally advanced non-small-cell lung cancer: one man's pride, another man's burden? Ann Oncol 2004; 15: 365–7.

67. Scagliotti GV, Turrisi III AT. Docetaxel-based combined-modality chemoradiotherapy for locally advanced non-small cell lung cancer. Oncologist 2003; 8: 361–74.

68. Patel V, Shrager JB. Which patients with stage III non-small cell lung cancer should undergo surgical resection? Oncologist 2005; 10: 335–44.

69. Doddoli C, Barlesi F, Trousse D et al. One hundred consecutive pneumonectomies after induction therapy for non-small cell lung cancer: an uncertain balance between risks and benefits. J Thorac Cardiovasc Surg 2005; 130: 417–25.

70. Perrot E, Guibert B, Mulsant P et al. Preoperative chemotherapy does not increase complications after nonsmall cell lung cancer resection. Ann Thorac Surg 2005; 80: 423–7.

71. Semik M, Riesenbeck D, Linder A et al. Preoperative chemotherapy with or without additional radiotherapy: benefit and risk for surgery of stage III non-small cell lung cancer. Eur J Cardiothorac Surg 2004; 26: 1205–10.

72. Lorent N, De Leyn P, Verbeken E et al. Long-term survival of surgically staged IIIA-N2 non-small-cell lung cancer treated with surgical combined modality approach: analysis of a 7 year prospective experience. Ann Oncol 2004; 15: 1645–53.

73. Bradley JD, Paulus R, Graham MV et al. Phase II trial of postoperative adjuvant paclitaxel/carboplatin and thoracic radiotherapy in resected stage II and IIIA non-small-cell lung cancer: promising long-term results of the Radiation Therapy Oncology Group – RTOG 9705. J Clin Oncol 2005; 23: 3480–7.

74. Taylor NA, Liao ZX, Cox JD et al. Equivalent outcome of patients with clinical stage IIIA non-small-cell lung cancer treated with concurrent chemoradiation compared with induction chemotherapy followed by surgical resection. Int J Radiat Oncol Biol Phys 2004; 58: 204–12.

75. Gandara D, West H, Albain K et al. Defining the role of radiation therapy in combination with preoperative chemotherapy in stage III non-small cell lung cancer: rationale and design of a new intergroup study. J Clin Oncol 2004; 458–63.

76. Rengan R, Rosenzweig KE, Venkatraman E et al. Improved local control with higher doses of radiation in large-volume stage III non-small-cell lung cancer. Int J Radiat Oncol Biol Phys 2004; 60: 741–7.

77. Gaspar L. Controversies in stage IIIA N2 non-small cell lung cancer after Intergroup Trial 0139: the

radiation oncology perspective. J Clin Oncol 2004; 463–9.

78. Holloway CL, Robinson D, Murray B et al. Results of a phase I study to dose escalate using intensity modulated radiotherapy guided by combined PET/CT imaging with induction chemotherapy for patients with non-small cell lung cancer. Radiother Oncol 2004; 73: 285–7.

79. Taylor NA, Liao ZX, Stevens C et al. Postoperative radiotherapy increases locoregional control of patients with stage IIIA non-small-cell lung cancer treated with induction chemotherapy followed by surgery. Int J Radiat Oncol Biol Phys 2003; 56: 616–25.

80. DeCamp MM, Rice TW, Adelstein DJ et al. Value of accelerated multimodality therapy in stage IIIA and IIIB non-small cell lung cancer. J Thorac Cardiovasc Surg 2003; 126: 17–25.

81. Jeremic B, Milicic B, Dagovic A et al. Interfraction interval in patients with stage III non-small-cell lung cancer treated with hyperfractionated radiation therapy with or without concurrent chemotherapy. Am J Clin Oncol 2004; 27: 616–25.

82. Ishikura S, Ohe Y, Nihei K et al. A phase II study of hyperfractionated accelerated radiotherapy (HART) after induction cisplatin (CDDP) and vinorelbine (VNR) for stage III non-small-cell lung cancer (NSCLC). Int J Radiat Oncol Biol Phys 2005;44p9.5 61: 1117–22.

83. Ichinose Y, Fukuyama Y, Asoh H et al. Induction chemoradiotherapy and surgical resection for selected stage IIIB non-small-cell lung cancer. Ann Thorac Surg 2003; 76: 1810–14.

84. Marks LB, Garst J, Socinski MA et al. Carboplatin/paclitaxel or carboplatin/vinorelbine followed by accelerated hyperfractionated conformal radiation therapy: report of a prospective phase I dose escalation trial from the Caroline Conformal Therapy Consortium. J Clin Oncol 2004; 22: 4329–40.

85. Catalano G, Jereczek-Fossa BA, De Pas T et al. Three-times daily radiotherapy with induction chemotherapy in locally advanced non-small cell lung cancer. Strahlenther Onkol 2005; 6: 363–71.

86. Machtay M, Lee JH, Stevenson JP et al. Two commonly used neoadjuvant chemotherapy regimens for locally advanced stage III non-small cell lung carcinoma: long-term results and associations with pathologic response. J Thorac Cardiovasc Surg 2004; 127: 108–13.

87. Katayama H, Ueoka H, Kiura T et al. Preoperative concurrent chemotherapy with cisplatin and docetaxel in patients with locally advanced non-small-cell lung cancer. Br J Cancer 2004; 90: 979–84.

88. Beslija S, Dizdarevic Z, Lomigoric J et al. Randomized phase II study of induction chemotherapy with gemcitabine plus cisplatin followed by sequential radiotherapy versus radiotherapy alone in patients with stage III non-small cell lung cancer. J BUON 2005; 10: 347–55.

89. Byrne MJ, Phillips M, Powell A et al. Cisplatin and gemcitabine induction chemotherapy followed by concurrent chemoradiotherapy or surgery for locally advanced non-small cell lung cancer. Int Med J 2005; 35: 336–42.

90. Ardizzoni A, Scolaro T, Mereu C et al. Induction chemotherapy with carboplatin–paclitaxel followed by standard radiotherapy with concurrent daily low-dose cisplatin plus weekly paclitaxel for inoperable non-small-cell lung cancer. Am J Clin Oncol 2005; 28: 58–64.

91. De Marinis F, Nelli F, Migliorino MR et al. Gemcitabine, paclitaxel, and cisplatin as induction chemotherapy for patients with

biopsy-proven stage IIIA (N2) non-small cell lung carcinoma. Cancer 2003; 98: 1707–17.

92. Vergnenègre A, Daniel C, Lèna H et al. Doxetaxel and concurrent radiotherapy after two cycles of induction chemotherapy with cisplatin and vinorelbine in patients with locally advanced non-small-cell lung cancer. Lung Cancer 2005; 47: 395–404.

93. Brunsvig PF, Hatlevoll R, Berg R et al. Weekly docetaxel with concurrent radiotherapy in locally advanced non-small cell lung cancer; a phase I/II study with 5 years' follow-up. Lung Cancer 2005; 50: 97–105.

94. Burmeister BH, Fielding DI, Ramsay JR et al. A phase I study of moderate-dose radiation therapy and weekly gemcitabine in patients with locally advanced non-small cell lung cancer not suitable for radical chemoradiation therapy. Clin Oncol (R Coll Radiol) 2005; 17: 332–6.

95. Liao Z, Komaki R, Milas L et al. A phase I clinical trial of thoracic radiotherapy and concurrent celecoxib for patients with unfavorable performance status inoperable/unresectable non-small cell lung cancer. Clin Cancer Res 2005; 11: 3342–8.

96. Choy H, Nabid A, Stea B et al. Phase II multicenter study of induction chemotherapy followed by concurrent efaproxiral (RSR13) and thoracic radiotherapy for patients with locally advanced non-small-cell lung cancer. J Clin Oncol 2005; 23: 5918–28.

97. Schwarzenberger P, Theodossiou C, Barron S et al. Dose escalation of docetaxel concomitant with hypotractionated, once weekly chest radiotherapy for non-small-cell lung cancer. Am J Clin Oncol 2004; 27: 395–9.

98. Socinski MA, Morris DE, Halle JS et al. Induction and concurrent chemotherapy with high-dose thoracic conformal radiation therapy in unresectable stage IIIA and IIIB non-small-cell lung cancer: a dose-escalation phase I trial. J Clin Oncol 2004; 22: 4341–50.

99. Saynak M, Aksu G, Fayda M et al. The results of concomitant and sequential chemoradiotherapy with cisplatin and etoposide in patients with locally advanced non-small cell lung cancer. J BUON 2005; 10: 213–18.

100. Keene KS, Harman EM, Knauf DG et al. Five-year results of a phase II trial of hyperfractionated radiotherapy and concurrent daily cisplatin chemotherapy for stage III non-small-cell lung cancer. Am J Clin Oncol 2005; 28: 217–22.

101. Kim YS, Yoon SM, Choi EK et al. Phase II study of radiotherapy with three-dimensional conformal boost concurrent with paclitaxel and cisplatin for stage IIIB non-small-cell lung cancer. Int J Radiat Oncol Biol Phys 2005; 62: 76–81.

102. Jeremic B, Milicic B, Acimovic L et al. Concurrent hyperfractionated radiotherapy and low-dose daily carboplatin and paclitaxel in patients with stage III non-small-cell lung cancer: long-term results of a phase II study. J Clin Oncol 2005; 23: 1144–51.

103. Kiura K, Ueoka H, Tabata M et al. Phase I/II study of docetaxel and cisplatin with concurrent thoracic radiation therapy for locally advanced non-small-cell lung cancer. Br J Cancer 2003; 89: 795–802.

104. Ichinose Y, Nakai Y, Kudoh S et al. Uracil/tegafur plus cisplatin with concurrent radiotherapy for locally advanced non-small-cell lung cancer: a multi-institutional phase II trial. Clin Cancer Res 2004; 10: 4369–73.

105. Yoshizawa H, Tanaka J, Kagamu H et al. Phase I/II study of daily carboplatin, 5-fluorouracil and concurrent radiation therapy for locally

advanced non-small-cell lung cancer. Br J Cancer 2003; 89: 803–7.

106. Dediu M, Tarlea A, Iorga P et al. Split course radiation with concurrent vinorelbine and cisplatin in locally advanced non-small cell lung cancer. A phase II study. J BUON 2004; 9: 167–72.

107. Winterhalder RC, Deschler-Marini S, Landmann C et al. Vinorelbine plus low-dose cisplatin with concomitant radiotherapy for the treatment of locally advanced or inoperable non-metastasized non-small-cell lung cancer (stage I–IIIB): a phase II study. Radiother Oncol 2004; 73: 321–4.

108. Kaplan B, Altynbas M, Eroglu C et al. Preliminary results of a phase II study of weekly paclitaxel (PTX) and carboplatin (CBDCA) administered concurrently with thoracic radiation therapy (TRT) followed by consolidation chemotherapy with PTX/CBDCA for stage III unresectable non-small-cell lung cancer (NSCLC). Am J Clin Oncol 2004; 27: 603–10.

109. Burkes RL, Shepherd FA, Blackstein ME et al. Induction chemotherapy with mitomycin, vindesine, and cisplatin for stage IIIA (T1–3, N2) unresectable non-small-cell lung cancer: final results of the Toronto phase II trial. Lung Cancer 2005; 47: 103–9.

110. Belani C, Wang W, Johnson DH et al. Phase III study of the Eastern Cooperative Oncology Group (ECOG 2597): induction chemotherapy followed by either standard thoracic radiotherapy or hyperfractionated accelerated radiotherapy for patients with unresectable stage IIIA and B non-small-cell lung cancer. J Clin Oncol 2005; 23: 3760–7.

111. Groen HJM, van der Leest AHW, Fokkema E et al. Continuously infused carboplatin used as radiosensitizer in locally unresectable non-small-cell lung cancer:

a multicenter phase III study. Ann Oncol 2004; 15: 427–32.

112. Fournel P, Robinet G, Thomas P et al. Randomized phase III trial of sequential chemoradiotherapy compared with concurrent chemoradiotherapy in locally advanced non-small-cell lung cancer: Groupe Lyon–Saint-Etienne d'Oncologie Thoracique–Groupe Francais de Pneumo-Cancérologie NPC 95-01 Study. J Clin Oncol 2005; 23: 5910–17.

113. Sculier JP, Lafitte J-J, Berghmans T et al. A phase III randomised study comparing two different dose-intensity regimens as induction chemotherapy followed by thoracic irradiation in patients with advanced locoregional non-small-cell lung cancer. Ann Oncol 2004; 15: 399–409.

114. Belani C, Choy H, Bonomi P et al. Combined chemoradiotherapy regimes of paclitaxel and carboplatin for locally advanced non-small-cell lung cancer: a randomized phase II locally advanced multi-modality protocol. J Clin Oncol 2005; 23: 5883–91.

115. Stephens RJ, Girling DJ, Hopwood P et al. A randomised controlled trial of pre-operative chemotherapy followed, if feasible, by resection versus radiotherapy in patients with inoperable stage T3, N1, M0 or T1–3, N2, M0 non-small cell lung cancer. Lung Cancer 2005; 49: 395–400.

116. Socinski MA, Zhang C, Herndon J 2nd et al. Combined modality trials of the Cancer and Leukemia Group B in stage III non-small-cell lung cancer: analysis of factors influencing survival and toxicity. Ann Oncol 2004; 15: 1033–41.

117. Semrau S, Bier A, Thierbach U et al. Concurrent radiochemotherapy with vinorelbine plus cisplatin or carboplatin in patients with locally advanced non-small-cell lung cancer (NSCLC) and increased risk of

treatment complications. Strahlenther Onkol 2003; 12: 823–31.

118. Rakovitch E, Tsao M, Ung Y et al. Comparison of the efficacy and acute toxicity of weekly versus daily chemoradiotherapy for non-small-cell lung cancer: a meta-analysis. Int J Radiat Oncol Biol Phys 2004; 58: 196–203.

119. Movsas B, Scott C, Langer C et al. Randomized trial of amifostine in locally advanced non-small-cell lung cancer patients receiving chemotherapy and hyperfractionated radiation: Radiation Therapy Oncology Group Trial 98-01. J Clin Oncol 2005; 23: 2145–54.

120. Antonadou D, Petridis A, Synidinou M et al. Amifostine reduces radiochemotherapy-induced toxicities in patients with locally advanced non-small cell lung cancer. Semin Oncol 2003; 30: 2–9.

121. Jennens RR, de Boer R, Irving L et al. A survey of knowledge and bias among clinicians regarding the role of chemotherapy in metastatic non-small cell lung cancer. Chest 2004; 126: 1985–93.

122. Blackhall F, Thatcher N. Chemotherapy for advanced lung cancer. Eur J Cancer 2004; 40: 2345–8.

123. Argiris A, Schiller JH. Can current treatment for advanced non-small cell lung cancer be improved? JAMA 2004; 292: 499–500.

124. Stewart DJ. Update on the role of topotecan in the treatment of non-small cell lung cancer. Oncologist 2004; 9: 43–52.

125. Scagliotti GV, Novello S. Pemetrexed in front-line chemotherapy for advanced non-small-cell lung cancer. Oncology 2004; 18: 32–7.

126. Budde LS, Hanna NH. Antimetabolites in the management of non-small cell lung cancer. Curr Treat Options Oncol 2005; 6: 83–93.

127. Belani C, Carney D, Lee JS et al (eds). Gemcitabine and pemetrexed: progress and new perspectives in treatment of thoracic cancers. Lung Cancer 2005; 50(Suppl 1).

128. Cohen MH, Johnson JR, Wang Y-C et al. FDA drug approval summary: pemetrexed for injection (Alimta®) for the treatment for non-small cell lung cancer. Oncologist 2005; 10: 363–8.

129. Dubey S, Schiller JH. Three emerging new drugs for NSCLC: pemetrexed, bortezomib, and cetuximab. Oncologist 2005; 10: 282–91.

130. De Marinis F, De Petris L. Pemetrexed in second-line treatment of non-small-cell lung cancer. Oncology 2004; 18: 38–42.

131. Rigas JR. Taxane–platinum combinations in advanced non-small cell lung cancer: a review. Oncologist 2004; 9: 16–23.

132. Rigas JR, Dragnev KH. Emerging role of rexinoids in non-small cell lung cancer: focus on bexarotene. Oncologist 2005; 10: 22–33.

133. Delbaldo C, Michiels S, Syz N et al. Benefits of adding a drug to a single-agent or a 2-agent chemotherapy regimen in advanced non-small-cell lung cancer. A meta analysis. JAMA 2004; 292: 470–84.

134. D'Addario G, Pintilie M, Leighl NB et al. Platinum-based versus non-platinum-based chemotherapy in advanced non-small-cell lung cancer: a meta-analysis of the published literature. J Clin Oncol 2005; 23: 2926–36.

135. Tiseo M, Boni L, Ardizzoni A. Platinum-based versus non-platinum-based chemotherapy in advanced non-small-cell lung cancer: does cisplatin versus carboplatin make a difference? J Clin Oncol 2005; 23: 6276–7.

136. Hotta K, Matsuo K, Ueoka H et al. Meta-analysis of randomized clinical trials comparing cisplatin to carboplatin in patients with advanced non-small-cell lung cancer. J Clin Oncol 2004; 22: 3852–9.

137. Barlési F, Pujol J-L. Combination of chemotherapy without platinum compounds in the treatment of advanced non-small cell lung cancer: a systematic review of phase III trials. Lung Cancer 2005; 49: 289–98.

138. Androulakis N, Georgoulias V. NSCLC – platinum or not. Lung Cancer 2005; 47: 381–3.

139. Chen Y-M, Perng R-P, Shih J-F et al. A randomized phase II study of vinorelbine plus gemcitabine with/without cisplatin against inoperable non-small-cell lung cancer previously untreated. Lung Cancer 2005; 47: 373–80.

140. Bunn PA. Platinums in lung cancer: sufficient or necessary? J Clin Oncol 2005; 23: 2882–3.

141. Okamoto T, Maruyana R, Shoji F et al. Long-term survivors in stage IV non-small cell lung cancer. Lung Cancer 2005; 47: 85–91.

142. Miller AA, Herndon JE II, Gu L et al. Phase II trial of karenitecin in patients with relapsed or refractory non-small cell lung (CALGB 30004). Lung Cancer 2005; 48: 399–407.

143. Camps C, Felip E, Sanchez JM et al. Phase II trial of the novel taxane BMS-184476 as second-line in non-small-cell lung cancer. Ann Oncol 2005; 16: 597–601.

144. Krug LM, Azzoli G, Kris MG et al. 10-Propargyl-10-deazaaminopterin: an antifolate with activity in patients with previously treated non-small cell lung cancer. Clin Cancer Res 2003; 9: 2072–8.

145. Laurie SA, Miller VA, Grant SC et al. Phase I study of green tea extract in patients with advanced lung cancer. Cancer Chemother Pharmacol 2005; 55: 33–8.

146. Anderson H, Addington-Hall JM, Peake MD et al. Domiciliary chemotherapy with gemcitabine is safe and acceptable to advanced non-small-cell lung cancer patients:

results of a feasibility study. Br J Cancer 2003; 89: 2190–6.

147. Nakamura Y, Kunitoh H, Kubota K et al. Retrospective analysis of safety and efficacy of low-dose doxetaxel 60 mg/m^2 in advanced non-small cell lung cancer patients previously treated with platinum-based chemotherapy. J Clin Oncol 2003; 26: 459–64.

148. Baka S, Ranson M, Lorigan P et al. A phase II trial with RFS2000 (rubitecan) in patients with advanced non-small cell lung cancer. Eur J Cancer 2005; 41: 1547–50.

149. Marks RS, Graham DL, Sloan JA et al. A phase II study of the dolastatin 15 analogue LU 103793 in the treatment of advanced non-small-cell lung cancer. Am J Clin Oncol 2003; 26: 336–7.

150. Yasuda K, Igishi T, Kawasaki Y et al. Phase II trial of weekly paclitaxel in previously untreated advanced non-small-cell lung cancer. Oncology 2003; 65: 224–8.

151. West HL, Crowley JJ, Vance RB et al. Advanced bronchioloalveolar carcinoma: a phase II trial of paclitaxel by 96-hour infusion (SWOG 9714): a Southwest Oncology Group Study. Ann Oncol 2005; 16: 1076–80.

152. Scagliotti GV, Smit E, Bosquee L et al. A phase II study of paclitaxel in advanced bronchioloalveolar carcinoma (EORTC trial 08956). Lung Cancer 2005; 50: 91–6.

153. Lilenbaum RC, Herndon JE II, List MA et al. Single-agent versus combination chemotherapy in advanced non-small-cell lung cancer: the Cancer and Leukemia Group B (Study 9730). J Clin Oncol 2005; 23: 190–6.

154. Georgoulias V, Ardavanis A, Agelidou A et al. Docetaxel versus docetaxel plus cisplatin as front-line treatment of patients with advanced non-small-cell lung cancer: a randomized, multicenter phase III trial. J Clin Oncol 2004; 22: 2602–9.

155. Georgoulias V, Ardavanis A, Tsiafaki X et al. Vinorelbine plus cisplatin versus doxetaxel plus gemcitabine in advanced non-small-cell lung cancer: a phase III randomized trial. J Clin Oncol 2005; 23: 2937–45.

156. Pujol J-L, Breton J-L, Gervais R et al. Gemcitabine–doxetaxel versus cisplatin–vinorelbine in advanced or metastatic non-small-cell lung cancer: a phase III study addressing the case for cisplatin. Ann Oncol 2005; 16: 602–10.

157. Martoni A, Marino A, Sperandi F et al. Multicentre randomised phase III study comparing the same dose and schedule of cisplatin plus the same schedule of vinorelbine or gemcitabine in advanced non-small cell lung cancer. Eur J Cancer 2005; 41: 81–92.

158. Stathopoulos GP, Veslemes M, Georgatou N et al. Front-line paclitaxel–vinorelbine versus paclitaxel–carboplatin in patients with advanced non-small-cell lung cancer: a randomized phase III trial. Ann Oncol 2004; 15: 1048–55.

159. Tan EH, Szczesna A, Krzakowski M et al. Randomized study of vinorelbine–gemcitabine versus vinorelbine–carboplatin in patients with advanced non-small cell lung cancer. Lung Cancer 2005; 49: 233–40.

160. Wachters FM, van Putten JW, Kramer H et al. First-line gemcitabine with cisplatin or epirubicin in advanced non-small-cell lung cancer: a phase III trial. Br J Cancer 2003; 89: 1192–9.

161. Smit EF, van Meerbeeck JPAM, Lianes P et al. Three-arm randomized study of two cisplatin-based regimens and paclitaxel plus gemcitabine in advanced non-small-cell lung cancer: a phase III trial of the European Organization for Research and Treatment of Cancer Lung Cancer Group – EORTC 08975. J Clin Oncol 2003; 21: 3909–17.

162. Kubota K, Watanabe K, Kunitoh H et al. Phase III randomized trial of docetaxel plus cisplatin versus vindesine plus cisplatin in patients with stage IV non-small-cell lung cancer: the Japanese Taxotere Lung Cancer Study Group. J Clin Oncol 2004; 22: 254–61.

163. Belani CP, Lee JS, Socinski MA et al. Randomized phase III trial comparing cisplatin–etoposide to carboplatin–paclitaxel in advanced or metastatic non-small cell lung cancer. Ann Oncol 2005; 16: 1069–75.

164. Besse B, Soria JC, Le Chevalier T. Front-line doublets in advanced non-small cell lung cancer. The golden age for second line chemotherapy. Ann Oncol 2005; 16: 977–8.

165. Danson S, Thatcher N. The context of the problem. Commentary to Smith EF, van Meerbeeck JP, Lianes P et al (in J Clin Oncol 2003; 21: 3909–17). Cancer Treat Rev 2004; 30: 309–14.

166. Danson S, Middleton MR, O'Byrne KJ et al. Phase III trial of gemcitabine and carboplatin versus mitomycin, ifosfamide, and cisplatin or mitomycin, vinblastine, and cisplatin in patients with advanced nonsmall cell lung carcinoma. Cancer 2003; 98: 542–53.

167. Rudd RM, Gower NH, Spiro SG et al. Gemcitabine plus carboplatin versus mitomycin, ifosfamide, and cisplatin in patients with stage IIIB or IV non-small-cell lung cancer: a phase III randomized study of the London Lung Cancer Group. J Clin Oncol 2005; 23: 142–53.

168. Laack E, Dickgreber N, Müller T et al. Randomized phase III study of gemcitabine and vinorelbine, and cisplatin in the treatment of advanced non-small-cell lung cancer: from the German and Swiss Lung Cancer Study Group. J Clin Oncol 2004; 22: 2348–56.

169. Leighl NB, Paz-Ares L, Douillard J-Y et al. Randomized phase III study of

matrix metalloproteinase inhibitor BMS-275291 in combination with paclitaxel and carboplatin in advanced non-small-cell lung cancer: National Cancer Institute of Canada – Clinical Trials Group Study BR. 18. J Clin Oncol 2005; 23: 2831–9.

170. Bissett D, O'Byrne KJ, von Pawel J et al. Phase III study of matrix metalloproteinase inhibitor prinomastat in non-small-cell lung cancer. J Clin Oncol 2005; 23: 842–9.

171. O'Brien MER, Anderson H, Kaukel E et al. SRL172 (killed *Mycobacterium vaccae*) in addition to standard chemotherapy improves quality of life without affecting survival, in patients with advanced non-small-cell lung cancer: phase III results. Ann Oncol 2004; 15: 906–14.

172. Aquiar D, Aguiar J, Bohn U. Alternating weekly administration of paclitaxel and gemcitabine: a phase II study in patients with advanced non-small-cell lung cancer. Cancer Chemother Pharmacol 2005; 55: 152–8.

173. Yumuk PF, Turhal NS, Gumus M et al. Results of paclitaxel (day 1 and 8) and carboplatin given on every three weeks in advanced (stage III–IV) non-small cell lung cancer. BMC Cancer 2005; 5: 10.

174. Tsunoda T, Koizumi T, Hayasaka M et al. Phase II study of weekly docetaxel combined with cisplatin in patients with advanced non-small-cell lung cancer. Cancer Chemother Pharmacol 2004; 54: 173–7.

175. De Castro J, Lorenzo A, Morales S et al. Phase II study of a fixed dose-rate infusion of gemcitabine associated with docetaxel in advanced non-small-cell lung carcinoma. Cancer Chemother Pharmacol 2005; 55: 197–202.

176. Firvida JL, Amenedo M, Rodríguez R et al. Docetaxel plus fractionated cisplatin is a safe and active schedule as first-line treatment of patients with advanced non-small cell lung cancer: results of a phase II study. Invest New Drugs 2004; 22: 481–7.

177. Kaira K, Takise A, Minato K et al. Phase II study of weekly docetaxel and cisplatin in patients with non-small cell lung cancer. Anticancer Drugs 2005; 16: 455–60.

178. Winegarden JD, Mauer AM, Otterson GA et al. A phase II study of oxaliplatin and paclitaxel in patients with advanced non-small-cell lung cancer. Ann Oncol 2004; 15: 915–20.

179. Yamada K, Ikehara M, Tanaka G et al. Dose escalation study of paclitaxel in combination with fixed-dose irinotecan in patients with advanced non-small cell lung cancer (JCOG 9807). Oncology 2004; 66: 94–100.

180. Ramalingam S, Dobbs TW, Einzig AI et al. Carboplatin and docetaxel in advanced non-small-cell lung cancer: results of a multicenter phase II study. Cancer Chemother Pharmacol 2004; 53: 439–44.

181. Kallab AM, Nalamolu Y, Dainer PM et al. A phase II study of weekly paclitaxel and carboplatin in previously untreated patients with advanced non-small-cell lung cancer. Med Oncol 2005; 22: 145–51.

182. Yang C-H, Chen M-C, Cheng A-L et al. Survival outcome of inoperable non-small cell lung cancer patients receiving conventional dose epirubicin and paclitaxel as first-line treatment. Oncology 2005; 68: 350–5.

183. Grunberg SM, Dugan MC, Greenblatt MC. Phase I/II trial of paclitaxel and vinorelbine in advanced non-small cell lung cancer. Cancer Invest 2005; 23: 392–8.

184. Ziotopoulos P, Androulakis N, Mylonaki E et al. Front-line treatment of advanced non-small cell lung cancer with irinotecan and doxetacel: a multicentre phase II

study. Lung Cancer 2005; 50: 115–22.

185. Kurata T, Tamura K, Yamamoto N et al. Combination phase I study of nedaplatin and gemcitabine for advanced non-small-cell lung cancer. Br J Cancer 2004: 90: 2092–6.

186. Monnerat C, Le Chevalier T, Kelly K et al. Phase II study of pemetrexed–gemcitabine combination in patients with advanced-stage non-small cell lung cancer. Clin Cancer Res 2004; 10: 5439–46.

187. Soo RA, Lim HL, Wang LZ et al. Phase I trial of fixed dose-rate gemcitabin in combination with carboplatin in chemonaive advanced non-small cell lung cancer: a Cancer Therapeutics Research Group study. Cancer Chemother Pharmacol 2003; 52: 153–8.

188. Bidoli P, Stani SC, Mariani L et al. Phase I study of escalating doses of oxaliplatin in combination with fixed dose gemcitabine in patients with non-small cell lung cancer. Lung Cancer 2004; 43: 203–8.

189. Cappuzzo F, Novello S, De Marinis F et al. Phase II study of gemcitabine plus oxaliplatin as first-line chemotherapy for advanced non-small-cell lung cancer. Br J Cancer 2005; 93: 29–34.

190. Katakami N, Sugiura T, Nogami T et al. Combination chemotherapy of gemcitabine and vinorelbine for patients in stage IIIB–IV non-small cell lung cancer: a phase II study of the West Japan Thoracic Oncology Group (WJTOG) 9908. Lung Cancer 2004; 43: 93–100.

191. Nishio M, Ohyanagi F, Taguch F et al. Phase I study of combination chemotherapy with gemcitabine and irinotecan for non-small cell lung cancer. Lung Cancer 2005; 48: 115–19.

192. Neubauer MA, Garfield, DH, Kuerfler PR et al. Results of a phase II multicenter trial of weekly docetaxel and gemcitabine as first-line

therapy for patients with advanced non-small cell lung cancer. Lung Cancer 2005; 47: 121–7.

193. Gillenwater HH, Stinchcombe TE, Qaqish BF et al. A phase II trial of weekly paclitaxel and gemcitabine infused at a constant rate in patients with advanced non-small cell lung cancer. Lung Cancer 2005; 47: 413–19.

194. Le Chevalier T, Scagliotti G, Natale R et al. Efficacy of gemcitabine plus platinum chemotherapy compared with other platinum containing regimens in advanced non-small-cell lung cancer: a meta-analysis of survival outcomes. Lung Cancer 2005; 47: 69–80.

195. Jasssem J, Kosmidis P, Ramlau R et al. Oral vinorelbine in combination with cisplatin: a novel active regimen in advanced non-small-cell lung cancer. Ann Oncol 2003; 14: 1634–9.

196. Fukuda M, Oka M, Soda H et al. Phase II study of irinotecan combined with carboplatin in previously untreated non-small-cell lung cancer. Cancer Chemother Pharmacol 2004; 54: 573–7.

197. Ichinose Y, Yoshimori K, Sakai H et al. S-1 plus cisplatin combination chemotherapy in patients with advanced non-small cell lung cancer: a multi-institutional phase II trial. Clin Cancer Res 2004; 10: 7860–4.

198. O'Brien ME, Szczesna A, Karnicka H et al. Vinorelbine alternating oral and intravenous plus carboplatin in advanced non-small-cell lung cancer: results of a multicentre phase II study. Ann Oncol 2004; 15: 921–7.

199. Clarke, SJ, Boyer, MJ, Millward M et al. A phase I/II study of pemetrexed and vinorelbine in patients with non-small cell lung cancer. Lung Cancer 2005; 49: 401–12.

200. Mohedano NM, Rovira PS, Barriuso AL et al. Triplet chemotherapy combination with gemcitabine, cis-

platin and ifosfamide in patients with advanced non-small-cell lung cancer. Am J Clin Oncol 2003; 26: 363–5.

201. Bourgeois H, Billiart I, Chabrun V et al. Phase I study with dose escalation of gemcitabine and cisplatin in combination with ifosfamide (GIP) in patients with non-small-cell lung carcinoma. Am J Clin Oncol 2004; 27: 89–95.

202. Goffin JR, Anderson IC, Supko JG et al. Phase I trial of the matrix metalloproteinase inhibitor marimastat combined with carboplatin and paclitaxel in patients with advanced non-small cell lung cancer. Clin Cancer Res 2005; 11: 3417–24.

203. Cortes J, Rodriguez J, Calvo E et al. Paclitaxel, cisplatin, and vinorelbine combination chemotherapy in metastatic non-small-cell lung cancer. Am J Clin Oncol 2004; 27: 299–303.

204. Ioannidis JP, Polycarpou A, Ntais C et al. Randomised trials comparing chemotherapy regimens for advanced non-small cell lung cancer: biases and evaluation over time. Eur J Cancer 2003; 39: 2278–87.

205. Bottomley A, Efficace F, Thomas R et al. Health-related quality of life in non-small-cell lung cancer: methodologic issues in randomized controlled trials. J Clin Oncol 2003; 21: 2982–92.

206. Douillard J-Y, Gervais R, Dabouis G et al. Sequential two-line strategy for stage IV non-small-cell lung cancer: docetaxel–cisplatin versus vinorelbine–cisplatin followed by cross-over to single-agent docetaxel or vinorelbine at progression: final results of a randomised phase II study. Ann Oncol 2005; 16: 81–9.

207. Lilenbaum RC, Chen C-S, Chidiac T et al. Phase II randomized trial of vinorelbine and gemcitabine versus carboplatin and paclitaxel in advanced non-small-cell lung cancer. Ann Oncol 2005; 16: 97–101.

208. Rocha Lima CM, Rizvi NA, Zhang C et al. Randomized phase II trial of gemcitabine plus irinotecan or docetaxel in stage IIIB or stage IV NSCLC. Ann Oncol 2004; 15: 410–18.

209. Scagliotti G, Kortsik C, Dark GG et al. Pemetrexed combined with oxaliplatin or carboplatin as first-line treatment in advanced non-small cell lung cancer: a multicenter, randomized, phase II trial. Clin Cancer Res 2005; 11: 690–6.

210. Ma CX, Nair S, Thomas S et al. Randomized phase II trial of three schedules of pemetrexed and gemcitabine as front-line therapy for advanced non-small-cell lung cancer. J Clin Oncol 2005; 23: 5929–37.

211. Crul M, Schoemaker NE, Pluim D et al. Randomized phase I clinical and pharmacologic study of weekly versus twice-weekly dose-intensive cisplatin and gemcitabine in patients with advanced non-small cell lung cancer. Clin Cancer Res 2003; 9: 3526–33.

212. Pathak AK, Bhutani M, Guleria R et al. Chemotherapy alone vs. chemotherapy plus high dose multiple antioxidants in patients with advanced non small cell lung cancer. J Am Coll Nutr 2005; 24: 16–21.

213. Rosell R, Felip E, Garcia-Campelo R et al. The biology of non-small-cell lung cancer: identifying new targets for rational therapy. Lung Cancer 2004; 46: 135–48.

214. Maione P, Rossi A, Airoma G et al. The role of targeted therapy in non-small cell lung cancer. Crit Rev Oncol Hematol 2004; 51: 29–44.

215. Gridelli C. Targeted therapies in the treatment of non small cell lung cancer: reality and hopes. Curr Opin Oncol 2004; 16: 126–9.

216. Gridelli C, Rossi A, Maione P. Treatment of non-small cell lung

cancer and targeted therapies: where are we? Curr Opin Oncol 2005; 17: 114–17.

217. Perrone F, Di Maio M, Budillon A et al. Targeted therapies and non-small cell lung cancer: methodological and conceptual challenge for clinical trials. Curr Opin Oncol 2005; 17: 123–9.

218. Ciardiello F, De Vita F, Orditura M et al. The role of EGFR inhibitors in nonsmall cell lung cancer. Curr Opin Oncol 2004; 16: 130–5.

219. Pao W, Miller VA. Epidermal growth factor receptor mutations, small-molecule kinase inhibitors, and non-small-cell lung cancer: current knowledge and future directions. J Clin Oncol 2005; 23: 2556–68.

220. Doroshow JH. Targeting EGFR in non-small-cell lung cancer. N Engl J Med 2005; 353: 200–2.

221. Kim DW, Choy H. Potential role for epidermal growth factor receptor inhibitors in combined-modality therapy for non-small-cell lung cancer. Int J Radiat Oncol Biol Phys 2004; 59: 11–20.

222. Sridhar SS, Seymour L, Shepherd FA. Inhibitors of epidermal-growth-factor receptors: a review of clinical research with a focus on non-small-cell lung cancer. Lancet Oncol 2003; 4: 397–406.

223. Ciardiello F, De Vita F, Orditura M et al. The role of EGFR inhibitors in nonsmall cell lung cancer. Curr Opin Oncol 2004; 16: 130–5.

224. Sharma R, Boyer M, Clarke S et al. Gefitinib in advanced non-small cell lung cancer. Int Med J 2005; 35: 77–82.

225. Ranson M, Wardell S. Gefitinib, a novel, orally administered agent for the treatment of cancer. J Clin Pharm Ther 2004; 29: 95–103.

226. Birnbaum A, Ready N. Gefitinib therapy for non-small cell lung cancer. Curr Treat Option Oncol 2005; 6: 75–81.

227. Goss G (ed). New hope for patients with non-small-cell lung cancer: gefitinib and other innovative therapies. EJC Suppl 2003; 1(8): 1–33.

228. Thatcher N (ed). Gefitinib (Iressa) in NSCLC: a real alternative to chemotherapy. Eur Resp Rev 2004; 13: 119–41.

229. Cohen MH, Johnson JR, Chen Y-F et al. FDA drug approval summary: erlotinib (Tarceva®) tablets. Oncologist 2005; 10: 461–6.

230. Comis RL. The current situation: erlotinib (Tarceva®) and gefitinib (Iressa®) in non-small-cell lung cancer. Oncologist 2005; 10: 467–70.

231. Shah NT, Kris MG, Pao W et al. Practical management of patients with non-small-cell lung cancer treated with gefitinib. J Clin Oncol 2005; 23: 165–74.

232. Shepherd FA, Rodrigues Pereira J et al. Erlotinib in previously treated non-small cell lung cancer. N Eng J Med 2005; 353: 123–32.

233. Tsao M-S, Sakurada A, Cutz J-C et al. Erlotinib in lung cancer – molecular and clinical predictors of outcome. N Engl J Med 2005; 353: 133–44.

234. Pérez-Soler R, Chachoua A, Hammon LA et al. Determinants of tumor response and survival with erlotinib in patients with non-small-cell lung cancer. J Clin Oncol 2004; 22: 3238–47.

235. Han S-W, Kim T-Y, Hwang PG et al. Predictive and prognostic impact of epidermal growth factor receptor mutation in non-small-cell lung cancer patients treated with gefitinib. J Clin Oncol 2005; 23: 2493–501.

236. Shigematsu H, Lin L, Takahashi T et al. Clinical and biological features associated with epidermal growth factor receptor gene mutations in lung cancer. J Natl Cancer Inst 2005; 97: 339–46.

237. Parra HS, Cavina R, Latteri F et al. Analysis of epidermal growth factor receptor expression as a predictive factor for response to gefitinib (Iressa, ZD1839) in non-small-cell lung cancer. Br J Cancer 2004; 91: 208–12.

238. Berghmans T, Meert AP et al. Prognostic role of epidermal growth factor receptor in stage III nonsmall cell lung cancer. Eur Respir J 2005; 25: 329–35.

239. Swinson DEB, Cox G, O'Byrne KJ. Coexpression of epidermal growth factor receptor with related factors is associated with a poor prognosis in non-small-cell lung cancer. Br J Cancer 2004; 91: 1301–7.

240. Miller VA, Kris MG, Shah N. Bronchioloalveolar pathologic subtype and smoking history predict sensitivity to gefitinib in advanced non-small-cell lung cancer. J Clin Oncol 2004; 22: 1103–9.

241. Hsieh R-K, Lim K-H, Kuo HT et al. Female sex and bronchioloalveolar pathologic subtype predict EGFR mutations in non-small cell lung cancer. Chest 2005; 128: 317–21.

242. Mohamed MK, Ramalingam S, Lin Y et al. Skin rash and good performance status predict improved survival with gefitinib in patients with advanced non-small cell lung cancer. Ann Oncol 2005; 16: 780–5.

243. Kim K-S, Jeong J-Y, Kim Y-C et al. Predictors of the response to gefitinib in refractory non-small cell lung cancer. Clin Cancer Res 2005; 11: 2244–51.

244. Kaneda H, Tamura K, Kurata T et al. Retrospective analysis of the predictive factors associated with the response and survival benefit of gefitinib in patients with advanced non-small-cell lung cancer. Lung Cancer 2004; 46: 247–54.

245. Zhang X-T, Li L-Y, Mu X-L et al. The EGFR mutation and its correlation with response of gefitinib in previously treated Chinese patients with advanced non-small-cell lung cancer. Ann Oncol 2005; 16: 1334–42.

246. Huang S-F, Liu H-P, Li L-H et al. High frequency of epidermal growth factor receptor mutations with complex patterns in non-small cell lung cancers related to gefitinib responsiveness in Taiwan. Clin Cancer Res 204; 10: 8195–203.

247. Lim S-T, Wong E-H, Chuah K-L et al. Gefitinib is more effective in never-smokers with non-small-cell lung cancer: experience among Asian patients. Br J Cancer 2005; 93: 23–8.

248. Razis E, Skarlos D, Briascoulis E et al. Treatment of non-small cell lung cancer with gefitinib (Iressa, ZD1839): the Greek experience with a compassionate-use program. Anti-Cancer Drugs 2005; 16: 191–8.

249. Schuette W, Nagel S, Schaedlich S et al. Clinical benefit in NSCLC: advanced-stage patients require symptom-improving palliation. Experiences from the 'Iressa' expanded access program. Onkologie 2005; 28: 195–8.

250. Veronese ML, Algazy K, Bearn L et al. Gefitinib in patients with advanced non-small cell lung cancer (NSCLC): the expanded access protocol experience at the University of Pennsylvania. Cancer Invest. 2005; 23: 296–302.

251. Ho C, Murray N, Laskin J et al. Asian ethnicity and adenocarcinoma histology continues to predict response to gefitinib in patients treated for advanced non-small cell carcinoma of the lung in North America. Lung Cancer 2005; 49: 225–31.

252. Natale RB. Epidermal growth factor receptor-targeted therapy with ZD1839: symptom improvement in non-small-cell lung cancer. Int J Radiat Oncol Biol Phys 2004; 59(2 Suppl): 39–43.

253. Park J, Park B-B, Kin J-Y et al. Gefitinib (ZD1839) monotherapy as a salvage regimen for previously treated advanced non-small cell lung cancer. Clin Cancer Res 2004; 10: 4383–8.

254. Chang G-C, Chen K-C, Yang T-Y et al. Activity of gefitinib in advanced non-small-cell lung cancer with very poor performance status. Invest New Drugs 2005; 23: 73–7.

255. Cappuzzo F, Bartolini S, Ceresoli GL et al. Efficacy and tolerability of gefitinib in pretreated elderly patients with advanced non-small-cell lung cancer (NSCLC). Br J Cancer 2004; 90: 82–6.

256. Haringhuizen A, van Tinteren H, Vaessen HFR et al. Gefitinib as a last treatment option for non-small-cell lung cancer: durable disease control in a subset of patients. Ann Oncol 2004; 15: 786–92.

257. Santoro A, Cavina R, Latteri F et al. Activity of a specific inhibitor, gefitinib (Iressa™, ZD1839), of epidermal growth factor receptor in refractory non-small-cell lung cancer. Ann Oncol 2004; 15: 33–7.

258. Sandler AB, Gray R, Brahmer J et al. Randomized phase II/III trial of paclitaxel (P) plus carboplatin (C) with or without bevacizumab (NSC#704865) in patients with advanced non-squamous non-small cell lung cancer (NSCLC). An Eastern Cooperative Oncology Group (ECOG) trial – E4599. J Clin Oncol 2005; 23(16s) (abstract LBA4).

259. Herbst RS, Sandler AB. Non-small cell lung cancer and antiangiogenic therapy: what can be expected of bevacizumab? Oncologist 2004; 9 (Suppl 1): 19–26.

260. De Lena M, Ramlau R, Hansen O et al. Phase II trial of oral vinorelbine in combination with cisplatin followed by consolidation therapy with oral vinorelbine in advanced NSCLC. Lung Cancer 2005; 48: 129–35.

261. Westeel V, Quoix E, Moro-Sibilot D et al. Randomized study of maintenance vinorelbine in responders with advanced non-small-cell lung cancer. J Natl Cancer Inst 2005; 97: 499–506.

262. Socinski MA. Addressing the optimal duration of therapy in advanced, metastatic non-small-cell lung cancer. ASCO Educational Book 2003: 144–52.

263. Makrantonakis PD, Galani E, Harper PG. Non-small cell lung cancer in the elderly. Oncologist 2004; 9: 556–60.

264. Janssen-Heijnen ML, Smulders S, Lemmens VE et al. Effect of comorbidity on the treatment and prognosis of elderly patients with non-small cell lung cancer. Thorax 2004: 59: 602–7.

265. Chen Y-M, Perng R-P, Shih J-F et al. Chemotherapy for non-small cell lung cancer in elderly patients. Chest 2005; 128: 132–9.

266. Gridelli C, Maione P, Rossi A et al. Treatment of locally advanced non-small cell lung cancer in the elderly. Curr Opin Oncol 2005; 17: 130–4.

267. Blackhall FH, Bhosle J, Thatcher N. Chemotherapy for advanced non-small cell lung cancer patients with poor performance status 2. Curr Opin Oncol 2005; 17: 135–9.

268. Maione P, Perrone F, Gallo C et al. Pretreatment quality of life and functional status assessment significantly predict survival of elderly patients with advanced non-small-cell lung cancer receiving chemotherapy: a prognostic analysis of the multicenter Italian Lung Cancer in the Elderly Study. J Clin Oncol 2005; 23: 6865–72.

269. Gridelli C, Aapro M, Artizzoni A et al. Treatment of advanced non-small-cell lung cancer in the elderly: results of an international expert panel. J Clin Oncol 2005; 23: 3125–37.

270. Ramsey SD, Howlader N, Etzioni RD et al. Chemotherapy use, outcomes, and costs for older persons with advanced non-small-cell lung cancer: evidence from Surveillance, Epidemiology, and End Results–Medicare. J Clin Oncol 2004; 22: 4971–8.

271. Gridelli C, Manegold C, Mali P et al. Oral vinorelbine given as monotherapy to advanced, elderly NSCLC patients: a multicentre phase II trial. Eur J Cancer 2004; 40: 2424–31.

272. Quoix E, Breton J-L, Ducoloné A et al. First line chemotherapy with gemicitabine in advanced non-small cell lung cancer elderly patients: a randomized phase II study of 3-week versus 4-week schedule. Lung Cancer 2005; 47: 403–12.

273. Tibaldi C, Ricci S, Russo R et al. Increased dose-intensity of gemcitabine in advanced non small cell lung cancer (NSCLC): a multicenter phase II study in elderly patients from the 'Polmone Toscano Group' (POLTO). Lung Cancer 2005; 48: 121–7.

274. Pereira JR, Martins SJ, Nikaedo SM et al. Chemotherapy with cisplatin and vinorelbine for elderly patients with locally advanced or metastatic non-small-cell lung cancer (NSCLC). BMC Cancer 2004; 4: 69.

275. Ohe Y, Niho S, Kakinuma R et al. A phase II study of cisplatin and docetaxel administered as three consecutive weekly infusions for advanced non-small-cell lung cancer in elderly patients. Ann Oncol 2004; 15: 45–50.

276. Feliu J, Martin G, Madroñal C et al. Combination of low-dose cisplatin and gemcitabine for treatment of elderly patients with advanced non-small-cell lung cancer. Cancer Chemother Pharmacol 2003; 54: 247–52.

277. Hirsh V, Latreille J, Kreisman H et al. Sequential therapy with vinorelbine followed by gemcitabine in patients with metastatic non small cell lung cancer (NSCLC), performance status (PS) 2, or elderly with comorbidities – a multicenter phase II trial. Lung Cancer 2005; 49: 117–23.

278. Marsland TA, Garfield DH, Khan MM et al. Sequential versus concurrent paclitaxel and carboplatin for the treatment of advanced non-small cell lung cancer in elderly patients and patients with poor performance status: results of two phase II, multicenter trials. Lung Cancer 2005; 47: 111–20.

279. Comella P, Frasci G, Carnicelli P et al. Gemcitabine with either paclitaxel or vinorelbine vs paclitaxel or gemcitabine alone for elderly or unfit advanced non-small-cell lung cancer patients. Br J Cancer 2004; 91: 489–97.

280. Baka S, Ashcroft L, Anderson H et al. Randomized phase II study of two gemcitabine schedules for patients with impaired performance status (Karnofsky performance status ≤70) and advanced non-small-cell lung cancer. J Clin Oncol 2005; 23: 2136–44.

281. Belvedere O, Grossi F. To treat or not to treat advanced non-small-cell lung cancer patients with impaired performance status? J Clin Oncol 2005; 23: 7231–2.

282. Herbst RS, Kim ES. Novel therapeutic options for non-small-cell lung cancer (second-line and subsequent therapy). ASCO Educational Book 2003: 654–6.

283. Han J-Y, Lee DH, Kim HY et al. A phase II study of weekly irinotecan and capecitabine in patients with previously treated non-small cell lung cancer. Clin Cancer Res 2003; 9: 5909–14.

284. Chen Y-M, Perng RP, Lee C-S et al. Phase II study of gemcitabine and vinorelbine combination chemotherapy in patients with non-small-cell lung cancer not responding to

previous chemotherapy. Am J Clin Oncol 2003; 26: 567–70.

285. Koizumi T, Yoshiike F, Inou H et al. Phase I trial of bi-weekly paclitaxel and gemcitabine as second-line therapy for patients with non-small-cell lung cancer previously treated with platinum-based chemotherapy. Med Oncol 2004; 21: 133–8.

286. Kindwall-Keller T, Otterson GA, Young D et al. Phase II evaluation of docetaxel-modulated capecitabine in previously treated patients with non-small cell lung cancer. Clin Cancer Res 2005; 11: 1870–6.

287. Nugent FW, Mertens WC, Graziano S et al. Docetaxel and cyclooxygenase-2 inhibition with celecoxib for advanced non-small cell lung cancer progressing after platinum-based chemotherapy: a multicenter phase II trial. Lung Cancer 2005; 48: 267–73.

288. Gridelli C, Gallo C, Di Maio M et al. A randomised clinical trial of two docetaxel regimens (weekly vs 3 week) in the second-line treatment of non-small-cell lung cancer. The DISTAL 01 study. Br J Cancer 2004; 91: 1996–2004.

289. Gervais R, Ducolone A, Breton JL et al. Phase II randomised trial comparing doxetaxel given every 3 weeks with weekly schedule as second-line therapy in patients with advanced non-small-cell lung cancer (NSCLC). Ann Oncol 16: 90–6.

290. Esteban E, González de Sande L, Fernández Y et al. Prospective randomised phase II study of docetaxel versus paclitaxel administered weekly in patients with non-small-cell lung cancer previously treated with platinum-based chemotherapy. Ann Oncol 2003; 14: 1640–7.

291. Quoix E, Lebeau B, Depierre A et al. Randomised, multicentre phase II study assessing two doses of docetaxel (75 or 100 mg/m²) as second-line monotherapy for non-small-cell

lung cancer. Ann Oncol 2004; 15: 38–44.

292. Georgoulias V, Kouroussis C, Agelidou A et al. Irinotecan plus gemcitabine vs irinotecan for the second-line treatment of patients with advanced non-small-cell lung cancer pretreated with doxetaxel and cisplatin: a multicentre, randomised, phase II study. Br J Cancer 2004; 91: 482–8.

293. Pectasides D, Pectasides M, Farmakis D et al. Comparison of docetaxel and docetaxel–irinotecan combination as second-line chemotherapy in advanced non-small-cell lung cancer: a randomized phase II trial. Ann Oncol 2005; 16: 294–9.

294. Shepherd FA, Dancey J, Ramlau R et al. Prospective randomized trial of docetaxel versus best supportive care in patients with non-small-cell lung cancer previously treated with platinum-based chemotherapy. J Clin Oncol 2000; 18: 2095–103.

295. Dancey J, Shepherd FA, Gralla RJ et al. Quality of life assessment of second-line docetaxel versus best supportive care in patients with non-small-cell lung cancer previously treated with platinum-based chemotherapy: results of a prospective, randomized phase III trial. Lung Cancer 2004; 43: 183–94.

296. Hanna N, Shepherd FA, Fossella FV et al. Randomized phase III trial of pemetrexed versus docetaxel in patients with non-small-cell lung cancer previously treated with chemotherapy. J Clin Oncol 2004; 22: 1589–97.

297. Di Maio M, Perrone F, Gallo C et al. Supportive care in patients with advanced non-small-cell lung cancer. Br J Cancer 2003; 89: 1013–21.

298. Yarbro JW, Mastrangelo MJ (eds). Symptoms and quality of life in advanced non-small cell lung cancer. Semin Oncol 2004; 31(Suppl 9).

299. Morère J-F. Role of epoetin in the management of anaemia in patients with lung cancer. Lung Cancer 2004; 46: 149–56.

300. Vansteenkiste J, Tomita D, Rossi G et al. Darbepoetin alfa in lung cancer patients on chemotherapy: a retrospective comparison of outcomes in patients with mild versus moderate-to-severe anaemia at baseline. Support Care Cancer 2004; 12: 253–62.

301. Rosen LS, Gordon D, Tshekmedyian NS et al. Long-term efficacy and safety of zoledronic acid in the treatment of skeletal metastases in patients with nonsmall cell lung carcinoma and other solid tumors. Cancer 2004; 100: 2613–21.

302. Macbeth F, Toy E, Coles B et al. Palliative radiotherapy regimens for non-small-cell lung cancer. The Cochrane Database Syst Rev 2006; (1).

303. Kramer GW, Wanders SL, Noordokl E et al. Results of the Dutch national study of the palliative effect of irradiation using two different treatment schemes for non-small-cell lung cancer. J Clin Oncol 2005; 23: 2962–70.

304. Erridge SC, Gaze MN, Price A et al. Symptom control and quality of life in people with lung cancer: a randomised trial of two palliative radiotherapy fractionation schedules. Clin Oncol (R Coll Radiol) 2005; 17: 61–7.

305. Hoskin PJ. Palliative radiotherapy for non-small-cell lung cancer: which dose? Clin Oncol (R Coll Radiol) 2005; 17: 59–60.

306. Sundstrøm S, Bremnes R, Brunsvig P et al. Immediate or delayed radiotherapy in advanced non-small cell lung cancer (NSCLC)? Data from a prospective randomised study. Radiother Oncol 2005; 75: 141–8.

307. Kramer GW, Gans S, Ullmann E et al. Hypofractionated external beam radiotherapy as retreatment for symptomatic non-small-cell lung carcinoma: an effective treatment? Int J Radiat Oncol Biol Phys 2004; 58: 1388–93.

308. Chen S, Yu L, Jiang C et al. Pivotal study of iodine-131-labeled chimeric tumor necrosis treatment radioimmunotherapy in patients with advanced lung cancer. J Clin Oncol 2005; 23: 1538–47.

309. Escobar-Sacristán JA, Granda-Orive JI, Gutiérrez Jiménez T et al. Endobronchial brachytherapy in the treatment of malignant lung tumours. Eur Respir J 2004; 24: 348–52.

310. Maziak DE, Markman BR, MacKay JA. Photodynamic therapy in nonsmall cell lung cancer: a systematic review. Ann Thorac Surg 2004; 77: 1484–91.

311. Freitag L, Ernst A, Thomas M et al. Sequential photodynamic therapy (PDT) and high dose brachytherapy for endobronchial tumour control in patients with limited bronchogenic carcinoma. Thorax 2004; 59: 790–3.

312. Thanos L, Mylona S, Pomoni M et al. Primary lung cancer: treatment with radio-frequency thermal ablation. Eur Radiol 2004; 14: 897–901.

313. Jin GY, Lee JM, Lee YC et al. Primary and secondary lung malignancies treated with percutaneous radiofrequency ablation: evaluation with follow-up helical CT. AJR Am J Roentgenol 2004; 183: 1013–20.

314. Lee JM, Jin GY, Goldberg SN et al. Percutaneous radiofrequency ablation for inoperable non-small cell lung cancer and metastases: preliminary report. Radiology 2004; 230: 125–34.

315. Yasui K, Kanazawa S, Sano Y et al. Thoracic tumors treated with CT-guided radiofrequency ablation: initial experience. Radiology 2004; 231: 850–7.

316. Belfiore G, Moggio G, Tedeschi E et al. CT-guided radiofrequency ablation: a potential complementary

therapy for patients with unresectable primary lung cancer – a preliminary report of 33 patients. AJR Am J Roentgenol 2004; 183: 1003–11.

317. Mamon HV, Yeap BY, Jänne PA et al. High risk of brain metastases in surgically staged IIIA non-small-cell lung cancer patients treated with surgery, chemotherapy, and radiation. J Clin Oncol 2005; 23: 1530–7.

318. Gaspar LE, Chansky K, Albain KS et al. Time from treatment to subsequent diagnosis of brain metastases in stage III non-small-cell lung cancer: a retrospective review by the Southwest Oncology Group. J Clin Oncol 2005; 23: 2955–61.

319. Carolan H, Sun AY, Bezjak A et al. Does the incidence and outcome of brain metastases in locally advanced non-small cell lung cancer justify prophylactic cranial irradiation or early detection? Lung Cancer 2005; 49: 109–15.

320. Furák J, Troján I, Szöke T et al. Lung cancer and its operable brain metastasis: survival rate and staging problems. Ann Thorac Surg 2005; 79: 241–7.

321. Getman V, Devyatko E, Dunkler D et al. Prognosis of patients with non-small cell lung cancer with isolated brain metastases undergoing combined surgical treatment. Eur J Cardiothorac Surg 2004; 25: 1107–13.

322. Iwasaki A, Shirakusa T, Yoshinaga Y et al. Evaluation of the treatment of non-small cell lung cancer with brain metastasis and the role of risk score as a survival predictor. Eur J Cardiothorac Surg 2004; 26: 488–93.

323. Datta R, Jawahar A, Ampil FL et al. Survival in relation to radiotherapeutic modality for brain metastasis. Am J Clin Oncol 2004; 27: 420–4.

324. Hotta K, Kiura K, Ueoka H et al. Effect of gefitinib (Iressa, ZD1839) on brain metastases in patients with advanced non-small-cell lung cancer. Lung Cancer 2004; 46: 255–61.

325. Chiu C-H, Tsai C-M, Chen Y-M et al. Gefitinib is active in patients with brain metastases from non-small cell lung cancer and response is related to skin toxicity. Lung Cancer 2005; 47: 129–38.

326. Lucchi M, Dini P, Ambrogi MC et al. Metachronous adrenal masses in resected non-small cell lung cancer patients: therapeutic implications of laparoscopic adrenalectomy. Eur J Cardiothorac Surg 2005; 27: 753–6.

9
Mesothelioma

Rolf Stahel

Several factors have contributed to increasing awareness of mesothelioma, including the predicted rise in incidence over the next decade, the fact that the disease is almost entirely attributable to occupational asbestos exposure, and – perhaps most importantly – the recognition that patients can benefit from systemic chemotherapy and in earlier stages of disease might benefit from more aggressive multimodality approaches, including extrapleural pneumonectomy. Recently, several review articles in major journals have been published describing advances in the field.[1–4]

Although the commercial use of asbestos is forbidden in much of the developed world, consumption of asbestos is increasing in Asia, Latin America and the former Soviet Union.[5] In Europe, where commercial use of asbestos is banned, first analysis predicted that male mesothelioma deaths will continue to increase and peak in the year 2020.[6] More recent models suggest that the increase may be leveling off already and the peak should occur earlier, between 2010 and 2015.[7,8]

MOLECULAR PATHOLOGY

Cytogenetic studies have revealed high complex karyotypic changes involving all chromosomes, with chromosomal losses being more frequent than chromosomal gains.[8a] A number of recurrent abnormalities have been found, including deletion of chromosomes 9p21 and 22q12. Deletion of the 9p21 region results in loss of the tumor suppressor gene *CDKN2A* (also known as *INK4A* and *MTS1*), which encodes two proteins: p16[INK4A] and (through an alternative reading frame) p14[ARF] (also, confusingly, known as p19[ARF] and p16β). The p16[INK4A] protein inhibits cyclin-dependent kinases, and thus the phosphorylation of the retinoblastoma protein (pRb), and leads to cell-cycle arrest, whereas p14[ARF] promotes p53 stability by inhibiting MDM2. There is loss of p16[INK4A] in most mesothelioma cell lines and many mesothelioma tumors.[9] Often, a codeletion of the methylthioadenosine phosphorylase gene is also present,[10] and loss of this gene renders cells dependent on de novo synthesis of purine derivatives. The neurofibromatosis type 2 gene (*NF2*) at the 22q12 locus is mutated or inactivated in a high proportion of mesothelioma cell lines and a smaller proportion of tumors.[11,12] The *NF2* gene product merlin inhibits cell proliferation, decreases the expression of cyclin D1 and arrests cells at G_1 phase of the cell cycle.[13] *NF2*-knockout mice exposed to asbestos developed mesothelioma more frequently than wild-type mice and the tumors have frequent homologous deletions of *CDKN2A* and *CDKN2B* (also known as *INK4B* and *MTS2*).[14] The similarities in alteration of these genes between asbestos-induced mesotheliomas in mice and human mesotheliomas have been corroborated in another study.[15]

The growth of mesothelioma cells can be stimulated by a series of different growth factors, including platelet-derived growth factor A and B (PDGF A and B), transforming growth factor α (TGF-α), insulin-like growth factor I (IGF-I) and vascular endodothelial growth factor (VEGF).[16–19] A recent series of studies also demonstrated the role of the Wnt signaling pathway in mesothelioma, including the activation of Wnt signaling through overexpression of Disheveled and β-catenin,[20] and apoptosis induction by blocking the Wnt pathway,[21,22] Mesotheliomas express the Met receptor and its ligand, hepatocyte growth factor, and it has recently been shown that inhibition of the Met receptor resulted in growth inhibition.[23]

Receptor tyrosine kinases signal through the phosphatidylinositol 3-kinase (PI3K)/Akt survival pathway. Malignant mesothelioma tumor specimens demonstrate high levels of phosphorylated Akt expression.[24] The PI3K signaling pathway is implicated in the development of malignancy and promotes cell cycle progression and resistance to apoptosis. Activated PI3K generates a lipid second messenger, which is essential for translocation of Akt to the plasma membrane, where it is phosphorylated and activated by phosphoinositide-dependent kinase 1. Phosphorylated Akt then conveys downstream signals, promoting cellular proliferation and survival over apoptosis. Activity of the PI3K/Akt pathway is negatively regulated by the *PTEN* ('phosphatase and tensin homologue deleted on chromosome 10') tumor suppressor gene, and overexpression of *PTEN* in mesothelioma cells induced hypophosphorylation of Akt and apoptosis.[25] Exposure of mesothelioma cell lines to LY294002, a PI3K inhibitor, results in decreased phosphorylated Akt and apoptotic cell death in vitro, and tumor burden reduction in vivo.[24]

Several ways to interfere with apoptotic pathways in mesothelioma have been elaborated in mesothelioma cell lines and tumor models. Antisense oligonucleotides directed at *bcl-x*$_L$ and *survivin* induce apoptosis in mesothelioma cell lines,[26,27] and the activity of tumor necrosis factor apoptosis-inducing ligand (TRAIL) has been the subject of several reports.[28–31]

DNA microarrays have been used as diagnostic tools to differentiate between pleural mesothelioma and lung adenocarcinomas,[32] and to compare mesothelioma cell lines or tissue with primary pleural mesothelial cells or tissue. In this way, genes such as *JAGGED1*, the serine/threonine protein kinase *NIK*, *CCND2* (cyclin D2), *fra-1*, *cIAP-2/IAP-1* and *survivin* have been shown to be differentially expressed in malignant pleural mesothelioma (MPM).[33–35] Results from two centers demonstrated that DNA microarrays of mesothelioma could identify gene expression profiles that predicted treatment-related outcome.[36–38] Investigators hope to identify genes of importance for tumorigenesis in mesothelioma by large-scale transcriptional profiling. A first extensive report from the Boston group identified three potential new candidate oncogenes and one candidate tumor suppressor gene.[39]

Correlative studies examining biologic properties of mesothelioma in association with outcome have led to the identification of factors associated with poor prognosis, including Ki-76 expression,[40] cyclooxygenase-2 (COX-2) expression,[41,42] matrix metalloproteinase-2 (MMP-2),[43] VEGF[44] and loss of p16^{ARF}.[45] Most of these studies are based on small patient sets, and confirmation of the results in larger studies are required before definitive conclusions can be drawn.

DIAGNOSIS

The morphologic diagnosis of pleural mesothelioma is generally made by a pleural biopsy. A recent study examined the accuracy of pleural biopsy in identifying the subtype of mesothelioma – epithelial, sarcomatous or mixed – by comparing the results to the morphologic diagnosis at extrapleural pneumonectomy.[46] Of 192 patients with epithelial mesothelioma at final diagnosis, 91% were correctly identified at pleural biopsy. In contrast, only 44% of 101 patients with mixed subtype and 70% of 10 patients with sarcomatoid subtype were correctly identified..

Immunohistochemistry is of great importance in the differential diagnosis between mesothelioma and adenocarcinoma. The Wilms's tumor susceptibility gene 1 (WT1) product is overexpressed in mesothelioma, demonstrating a strong nuclear staining on immunohistochemistry.[47] An update of the utility of immunohistochemical markers has been published by Ordonez.[48] The most recent addition to the markers useful for positively identifying mesothelioma is the monoclonal antibody D2-40 directed at the oncofetal M2A antigen expressed in germ cells, germ cell tumors and the lymphatic endothelium. This marker has been described as being as sensitive as calretinin[49] and more sensitive than cytokeratin 5/6 and WT1.[50] Another marker recently identified as staining epithelial mesothelioma, but not adenocarcinoma, is podoplanin, which is also expressed in tumors of lymphatic origin and Kaposi's sarcoma.[51] Mesothelin is highly sensitive but less specific for mesothelioma, as it is also strongly expressed in non-mucinous carcinomas of the ovary and in pancreatic adenocarcinomas.[52] The distinction between malignant mesothelioma and reactive mesothelial cells in cytologic specimens from effusions is difficult. A recent study has demonstrated that antibody clone E29 against the epithelial membrane antigen (EMA), but not clone Mc5, is negative on reactive mesothelial cells and positive on a large proportion of mesothelioma cells, and thus might help in this distinction.[53]

The identification of mesothelin-related proteins as serum markers of mesothelioma[54] has raised great hopes for their potential to monitor disease under therapy and these markers are being investigated for screening of individuals exposed to asbestos.[55,56]

MULTIMODALITY THERAPY, INCLUDING EXTRAPLEURAL PNEUMONECTOMY

The role of surgery in pleural mesothelioma continues to be a matter of debate.[56] The procedures used for the treatment of mesothelioma are thoracoscopy and pleurodesis, pleurectomy and decortication, and extrapleural pneumonectomy. A recent systematic review based on the literature from 1985 to 2004 did not allow us to determine whether the use of extrapleural pneumonectomy improves survival or effectively palliates symptoms of pleural mesothelioma.[57] However, extrapleural pneumonectomy is the only procedure that has been associated with long-term survival and cure in selected patients, usually in conjunction with chemotherapy and/or radiotherapy. The largest published experience with extrapleural pneumonectomy in conjunction with adjuvant chemotherapy and radiotherapy has come from the Boston group. A update from this group included 183 patients intended for the trimodality approach.[58] The median survival in the 176 patients alive after surgery was 19 months, and the estimated 2- and 5-year survival rates were 38% and 15%, respectively. This group also reported recently on the complications of extrapleural pneumonectomy in 328 consecutive patients operated on between 1980 and 2000.[59,60] Minor and major complications were noted in 60% of the patients, and the overall mortality rate was 3.4%. The incidence and management of complications of extrapleural pneumonectomy have also been analyzed by the surgical group in Leicester, UK.[61] Their postoperative mortality rate was 6.7% of 79 patients. Risk factors for perioperative morbidity were induction chemotherapy for acute lung injury and symptomatic mediastinal shift, right-sided procedures for pneumonia, and admission to the intensive care unit and prolonged operations for technical complications such as dehiscence of the diaphragmatic patch, chylothorax or fistulae and for gastrointestinal complications. The work of both groups demonstrates that the procedure should only be performed by an experienced team.

The availability of more effective chemotherapy regimens and the experience of neoadjuvant chemotherapy in stage IIIA non-small cell lung cancer prompted investigators to explore the role of neoadjuvant chemotherapy and extrapleural pneumonectomy in pleural mesothelioma. In a pilot study on 19 patients treated at the University Hospital of Zürich, the response rate to neoadjuvant cisplatin and gemcitabine was 31%, and 16 patients underwent extrapleural pneumonectomy with no perioperative mortality.[62] The median survival of all patients was 23 months, and 2 of these patients continue to remain disease-free now >5 years after surgery. These results were confirmed in a prospective multicenter phase II trial, whose preliminary results have been communicated.[63] Following the demonstration of the superiority of the combination of pemetrexed and cisplatin over cisplatin alone in advanced pleural mesothelioma, several groups are further exploring a neoadjuvant approach with the new combination. Although the published results so far are suggestive that radical surgery may indeed be associated with a longer survival than chemotherapy alone, final proof of this concept will only come from a randomized study. These data will hopefully be forthcoming from the Mesothelioma and Radical Surgery (MARS) trial initiated in the UK.

After extrapleural pneumonectomy, most patients have tumor recurrence in the ipsilateral chest. The rate of local relapse reported earlier from the Boston group was 35%.[64] A phase II trial of postoperative radiotherapy in high doses from the Memorial Sloan-Kettering Cancer Center suggested a decrease in the local failure rate to 6%.[65] In contrast to these findings, hemithoracic radiation after pleurectomy and decortication was not found to be a effective treatment option.[66] Intensity-modulated radiotherapy after extrapleural pneumonectomy has been intensively investigated by the MD Anderson group[67,68] and appears promising in reducing the rate of local relapse. Whether high doses of intensity-modulated or conformal radiotherapy are feasible and provide better local control after extrapleural pneumonectomy in a neoadjuvant setting is the topic of a Swiss phase II multicenter study.

Patient selection for radical surgery remains an important topic of investigation. Whereas most centers relay on computed tomography (CT) scanning and mediastinoscopy for patient selection,[69] other groups advocate more extensive surgical staging, including laparoscopy and peritoneal lavage. In a series from Houston, 9 out of 41 patients mediastinoscopically negative for contralateral mediastinal lymph nodes had lymph node involvement documented after surgery.[60] Laparoscopic evidence of transdiaphragmatic or peritoneal involvement was identified in 9% of 109 patients and peritoneal fluid lavage was positive in 2% of 78 patients.

The role of positron emission tomography (PET) and PET–CT for staging and selection of patients for surgery is under investigation. A first report on PET demonstrated increased uptake of pleural mesothelioma in 62 of 63 patients examined and identification of 6 patients with N3 or M1 disease, subsequently confirmed by other means. However, the sensitivity of PET in identifying the 21 patients with surgical T4 status was only 19%, and for the 9 patients with surgical N2 it was only 11%.[70] In a first publication on the role of integrated PET–CT for the staging of potentially resectable pleural mesothelioma, extrathoracic disease – which was not identified by conventional staging – was found in 7 of 29, but tumor stage was correctly identified in only 15 of 24 and nodal stage in only 6 of 17 patients.[71] Thus, based on these studies, the major role of PET and PET–CT lies in the identification of extrathoracic disease and not in the determination of T and N stage.

SYSTEMIC THERAPY

Several studies have now demonstrated the beneficial effect of chemotherapy in pleural mesothelioma, in terms of survival and/or palliation of symptoms. The role of cisplatin as the most active agent has been elucidated, based on literature overview. Two recent large randomized trials have proven the benefit of the addition of a folate antagonist. Based on the activity of pemetrexed and cisplatin or carboplatin observed in two phase I studies, a large prospective trial comprising 456 patients compared cisplatin alone versus cisplatin and pemetrexed.[72] The response was evaluated by measuring the thickness of the pleural rim at three different levels, as initially proposed by Byrne and Nowak.[73] Response and survival were significantly improved with combination therapy, with response rates of 17% versus 41%, and a median survivals of 9.3 versus 12.1 months favoring the combination of cisplatin and pemetrexed. Pemetrexed has since been registered for mesothelioma in many countries. Based on the single-agent activity of raltitrexed and the activity of raltitrexed in combination with oxaliplatin,[74] the European Organization for Research and Treatment of Cancer (EORTC) Lung Cancer Group examined whether the addition of raltitrexed to cisplatin would improve the outcome in patients with pleural mesothelioma.[75,76] Two hundred and fifty patients were randomized. The response rate was examined by RECIST (response evaluation criteria in solid tumors) criteria and was 13.6% with cisplatin and 23.6% with cisplatin and raltitrexed. The median survival was significantly improved: 8.8 months for cisplatin versus 11.4 months for cisplatin and raltitrexed. There was no significant difference in health-related quality-of-life measurements. These two trials established the combination of cisplatin and a folate antagonist as the current standard for chemotherapy of malignant mesothelioma.

Two other studies from the UK made an important contribution to establishing the role of chemotherapy for palliation of symptoms in malignant mesothelioma. An update of the experience from the Royal Marsden Hospital, London, focuses on the palliative benefits of mitomycin, vinblastine and cisplatin (MVP) in patients with malignant mesothelioma, including 43 patients with a performance score of ≥ 2.[76] Although the rate of objective responses was only 13.5% and the median survival only 7 months, 69% of patients reported an improvement of symptoms. The symptoms best responding to treatment were pain in 71%, cough in 62% and dyspnea in 50% of patients. Another study from the same institution examined the effect of early or delayed chemotherapy in symptomatically stable patients in a randomized trial that also used MVP chemotherapy.[77] Twenty patients were in the early-chemotherapy group, and 22 patients in the delayed-chemotherapy group, of whom 17 eventually received chemotherapy. The median time to symptomatic progression was significantly better in the early-chemotherapy group than in the late-chemotherapy group, at 25 weeks compared with 11 weeks. There was also a trend to better survival in the early-chemotherapy group, at 14 months compared with 10 months.

With the role of cisplatin combination chemotherapy (preferably with a folate antagonist) firmly established, an increasing number of patients now receive the benefits of chemotherapy, either as neoadjuvant treatment before extrapleural pneumonectomy or as palliative treatment for inoperable or advanced disease. Consequently, in many of these patients, questions about second-line chemotherapy will arise. Manegold et al[78] examined the use of second-line chemotherapy in patients treated in the phase III pemetrexed study. Thirty-seven percent of patients treated with cisplatin and pemetrexed and 47% of patients treated with pemetrexed received second-line chemotherapy. Multiple regression analysis showed that second-line chemotherapy was significantly associated with prolonged survival, after adjusting for prognostic factors and treatment group. The most commonly used agents were cisplatin and gemcitabine combinations, followed by single-agent anthracyclines and vinorelbine.

New agents for the treatment of mesothelioma are under investigation. In a phase I study with the histone deacetylase inhibitor suberoylanilide hydroxamic acid in advanced cancer, unconfirmed responses have been reported in 3 of 13 patients with mesothelioma, prompting further investigations in this disease.[79] Growing knowledge of the molecular pathologic properties of mesothelioma, the limited effect of current therapies and the increasing number of new agents targeting molecular tumor characteristics offer the opportunity to investigate new therapeutic approaches. Only a few final reports of these investigations have been fully published so far. Despite the high expression of epidermal growth factor receptor (EGFR) and promising preclinical data, the EGFR tyrosine kinase inhibitor gefitinib was found to be inactive in malignant mesothelioma.[80] Because PDGF was thought to be an important factor in the pathogenesis of mesothelioma and KIT expression was reported to be present in one-third of mesotheliomas in one small series, the activity of imatinib has been examined in a phase II study.[81] No responses were observed. Several investigators examined the effect of thalidomide. One study on 40 patients, 50% of them with no previous form of therapy, was reported in full.[82] No responses were observed, but disease stabilization of 6 months or more was documented in 27% of patients.

Response assessment in malignant mesothelioma remains difficult. WHO criteria for response are based on bidimensional measurable disease; this not suitable for most patients with pleural mesothelioma, whose disease can only be assessed by unidimensional measurements. RECIST are better suited to mesothelioma, since they specify the use of unidimensional measurements. Here, a partial remission is defined by a decrease in 30% of the sum of the longest diameter in all target lesions. Because the nature of pleural mesothelioma is to grow as a rind, modified RECIST criteria were developed using – instead of the longest diameter – the sum of two measurements perpendicular to the chest wall at three different levels. Response according to these criteria predicted for survival and forced vital capacity.[73,83,84] Whereas modified RECIST is the standard currently used in assessing response in pleural mesothelioma, more sophisticated methods such as computerized analysis of CT scans[85] and total lesion glycolysis determined in PET–CT[86] have been developed and await clinical validation.

Quality-of-life measurements are of increasing importance for judging the effect of systemic therapy. Several quality-of-life measurements have been validated recently for pleural mesothelioma, including the EORTC Core Quality of

Life Questionnaire (QLQ-C30) and the Lung Cancer Module (QLQ-LC13), as well as the Lung Cancer Symptom Scale (LCSS-Meso).[87,88]

Several studies have been published on prognostic factors for pleural mesothelioma, and scoring systems have been developed. The most commonly used scoring system have been developed by the Cancer and Leukemia Group B (CALGB) and the EORTC.[89,90] The EORTC prognostic score allows assignment of patients to low- or high-risk subgroups. Its validity has recently been re-examined on patients treated in three phase II studies at St Bartholomew's Hospital in London. Assignment to low- and high-risk groups according to the EORTC prognostic score stratified for overall survival in all three studies, thus confirming its value for patient selection or for comparison between clinical trials.[91]

REFERENCES

1. Treasure T, Sedrakyan A. Pleural mesothelioma: little evidence, still time to do trials. Lancet 2004; 364: 1183–5.

2. Robinson BW, Lake RA. Advances in malignant mesothelioma. N Engl J Med 2005; 353: 1591–603.

3. Robinson BW, Musk AW, Lake RA. Malignant mesothelioma. Lancet 2005; 366: 397–408.

4. Steele JP, Klabatsa A. Chemotherapy options and new advances in malignant pleural mesothelioma. Ann Oncol 2005; 16: 345–51.

5. Kazan-Allen L. Asbestos and mesothelioma: worldwide trends. Lung Cancer 2005; 49(Suppl 1): S3–8.

6. Peto J, Decarli A, La Vecchia C et al. The European mesothelioma epidemic. Br J Cancer 1999; 79: 666–72.

7. Pelucchi C, Malvezzi M, La Vecchia C et al. The mesothelioma epidemic in Western Europe: an update. Br J Cancer 2004; 90: 1022–4.

8. Hodgson JT, McElvenny DM, Darnton AJ et al. The expected burden of mesothelioma mortality in Great Britain from 2002 to 2050. Br J Cancer 2005; 92: 587–93.

8a Sandberg AA, Bridge JA. Updates on the cytogenetics and molecular genetics of bone and soft tissue tumors. Mesothelioma. Cancer Genet Cytogenet 2001; 127: 93–110.

9. Cheng JQ, Jhanwar SC, Klein WM et al. p16 alterations and deletion mapping of 9p21-p22 in malignant mesothelioma. Cancer Res 1994; 54: 5547–51.

10. Illei PB, Zakowski MF, Ladanyi M et al. Homozygous deletion of CDKN2A and codeletion of the methylthioadenosine phosphorylase gene in the majority of pleural mesotheliomas. Clin Cancer Res 2003; 9: 2108–113.

11. Sekido Y, Pass HI, Bader S et al. Neurofibromatosis type 2 (NF2) gene is somatically mutated in mesothelioma but not in lung cancer. Cancer Res 1995; 55: 1227–31.

12. Cheng JQ, Lee WC, Klein MA et al. Frequent mutations of NF2 and allelic loss from chromosome band 22q12 in malignant mesothelioma: evidence for a two-hit mechanism of NF2 inactivation. Genes Chromosomes Cancer 1999; 24: 238–42.

13. Xiao GH, Gallagher R, Shetler J et al. The NF2 tumor suppressor gene product, merlin, inhibits cell proliferation and cell cycle progression by repressing cyclin D1 expression. Mol Cell Biol 2005; 25: 2384–94.

14. Altomare DA, Vaslet CA, Skele KL et al. A mouse model recapitulating molecular features of human mesothelioma. Cancer Res 2005; 65: 8090–5.

15. Lecomte C, Andujar P, Renier A et al. Similar tumor suppressor gene alteration profiles in asbestos-induced murine and human mesothelioma. Cell Cycle 2005; 4: 1862–9.

16. Versnel MA, Claesson-Welsh L, Hammacher A et al. Human malignant mesothelioma cell lines express PDGF β-receptors whereas cultured normal mesothelial cells express predominantly PDGF α-receptors. Oncogene 1991; 6: 2005–11.

17. Lee TC, Zhang Y, Aston C et al. Normal human mesothelial cells and mesothelioma cell lines express insulin-like growth factor I and associated molecules. Cancer Res 1993; 53: 2858–64.

18. Morocz IA, Schmitter D, Lauber B et al. Autocrine stimulation of a human lung mesothelioma cell line is mediated through the transforming growth factor α/epidermal growth factor receptor mitogenic pathway. Br J Cancer 1994; 70: 850–6.

19. Strizzi L, Catalano A, Vianale G et al. Vascular endothelial growth factor is an autocrine growth factor in human malignant mesothelioma. J Pathol 2001; 193: 468–75.

20. Uematsu K, Kanazawa S, You L et al. Wnt pathway activation in mesothelioma: evidence of Dishevelled overexpression and transcriptional activity of β-catenin. Cancer Res 2003; 63: 4547–51.

21. You L, He B, Xu Z et al. An anti-Wnt-2 monoclonal antibody induces apoptosis in malignant melanoma cells and inhibits tumor growth. Cancer Res 2004; 64: 5385–9.

22. You L, He B, Xu Z et al. Inhibition of Wnt-2-mediated signaling induces programmed cell death in non-small-cell lung cancer cells. Oncogene 2004; 23: 6170–4.

23. Mukohara T, Civiello G, Davis IJ et al. Inhibition of the met receptor in mesothelioma. Clin Cancer Res 2005; 11: 8122–30.

24. Altomare DA, You H, Xiao GH et al. Human and mouse mesotheliomas exhibit elevated AKT/PKB activity, which can be targeted pharmacologically to inhibit tumor cell growth. Oncogene 2005; 24: 6080–9.

25. Mohiuddin I, Cao X, Ozvaran MK et al. Phosphatase and tensin analog gene overexpression engenders cellular death in human malignant mesothelioma cells via inhibition of AKT phosphorylation. Ann Surg Oncol 2002; 9: 310–16.

26. Hopkins-Donaldson S, Cathomas R, Simoes-Wust AP et al. Induction of apoptosis and chemosensitization of mesothelioma cells by Bcl-2 and Bcl-x_L antisense treatment. Int J Cancer 2003; 106: 160–6.

27. Xia C, Xu Z, Yuan X et al. Induction of apoptosis in mesothelioma cells by antisurvivin oligonucleotides. Mol Cancer Ther 2002; 1: 687–94.

28. Broaddus VC, Dansen TB, Abayasiriwardana KS et al. Bid mediates apoptotic synergy between tumor necrosis factor-related apoptosis-inducing ligand (TRAIL) and DNA damage. J Biol Chem 2005; 280: 12486–93.

29. Rippo MR, Moretti S, Vescovi S et al. FLIP overexpression inhibits death receptor-induced apoptosis in malignant mesothelial cells. Oncogene 2004; 23: 7753–60.

30. Liu W, Bodle E, Chen JY et al. Tumor necrosis factor-related apoptosis-inducing ligand and chemotherapy cooperate to induce apoptosis in mesothelioma cell lines. Am J Respir Cell Mol Biol 2001; 25: 111–18.

31. Stewart JH, Nguyen DM, Chen GA et al. Induction of apoptosis in malignant pleural mesothelioma cells by activation of the Fas (Apo-1/CD95) death-signal pathway. J Thorac Cardiovasc Surg 2002; 123: 295–302.

32. Gordon GJ, Jensen RV, Hsiao LL et

al. Translation of microarray data into clinically relevant cancer diagnostic tests using gene expression ratios in lung cancer and mesothelioma. Cancer Res 2002; 62: 4963–7.

33. Kettunen E, Nissen AM, Ollikainen T et al. Gene expression profiling of malignant mesothelioma cell lines: cDNA array study. Int J Cancer 2001; 91: 492–6.

34. Singhal S, Wiewrodt R, Maiden LD et al. Gene expression profiling of malignant mesothelioma. Clin Cancer Res 2003; 9: 3080–97.

35. Ramos-Nino ME, Scapoli L, Martinelli M et al. Microarray analysis and RNA silencing link fra-1 to cd44 and c-met expression in mesothelioma. Cancer Res 2003; 63: 3539–45.

36. Gordon GJ, Jensen RV, Hsiao LL et al. Using gene expression ratios to predict outcome among patients with mesothelioma. J Natl Cancer Inst 2003; 95: 598–605.

37. Pass HI, Liu Z, Wali A et al. Gene expression profiles predict survival and progression of pleural mesothelioma. Clin Cancer Res 2004; 10: 849–59.

38. Gordon GJ, Rockwell GN, Godfrey PA et al. Validation of genomics-based prognostic tests in malignant pleural mesothelioma. Clin Cancer Res 2005; 11: 4406–14.

39. Gordon GJ, Rockwell GN, Jensen RV et al. Identification of novel candidate oncogenes and tumor suppressors in malignant pleural mesothelioma using large-scale transcriptional profiling. Am J Pathol 2005; 166: 1827–40.

40. Beer TW, Buchanan R, Matthews AW et al. Prognosis in malignant mesothelioma related to MIB 1 proliferation index and histological subtype. Hum Pathol 1998; 29: 246–51.

41. Edwards JG, Faux SP, Plummer SM et al. Cyclooxygenase-2 expression is a novel prognostic factor in malig-

nant mesothelioma. Clin Cancer Res 2002; 8: 1857–62.

42. O'Kane SL, Cawkwell L, Campbell A et al. Cyclooxygenase-2 expression predicts survival in malignant pleural mesothelioma. Eur J Cancer 2005; 41: 1645–8.

43. Edwards JG, McLaren J, Jones JL et al. Matrix metalloproteinases 2 and 9 (gelatinases A and B) expression in malignant mesothelioma and benign pleura. Br J Cancer 2003; 88: 1553–9.

44. Demirag F, Unsal E, Yilmaz A et al. Prognostic significance of vascular endothelial growth factor, tumor necrosis, and mitotic activity index in malignant pleural mesothelioma. Chest 2005; 128: 3382–7.

45. Borczuk AC, Taub RN, Hesdorffer M et al. p16 loss and mitotic activity predict poor survival in patients with peritoneal malignant mesothelioma. Clin Cancer Res 2005; 11: 3303–8.

46. Bueno R, Reblando J, Glickman J et al. Pleural biopsy: a reliable method for determining the diagnosis but not subtype in mesothelioma. Ann Thorac Surg 2004; 78: 1774–6.

47. Kumar-Singh S, Segers K, Rodeck U et al. WT1 mutation in malignant mesothelioma and WT1 immunoreactivity in relation to p53 and growth factor receptor expression, cell-type transition, and prognosis. J Pathol 1997; 181: 67–74.

48. Ordonez NG. Immunohistochemical diagnosis of epithelioid mesothelioma: an update. Arch Pathol Lab Med 2005; 129: 1407–14.

49. Granville LA, Younes M, Churg A et al. Comparison of monoclonal versus polyclonal calretinin antibodies for immunohistochemical diagnosis of malignant mesothelioma. Appl Immunohistochem Mol Morphol 2005; 13: 75–9.

50. Chu AY, Litzky LA, Pasha TL et al. Utility of D2-40, a novel mesothelial marker, in the diagnosis of malignant

mesothelioma. Mod Pathol 2005; 18: 105–10.

51. Kimura N, Kimura I. Podoplanin as a marker for mesothelioma. Pathol Int 2005; 55: 83–6.

52. Ordonez NG. Value of mesothelin immunostaining in the diagnosis of mesothelioma. Mod Pathol 2003; 16: 192–7.

53. Saad RS, Cho P, Liu YL et al. The value of epithelial membrane antigen expression in separating benign mesothelial proliferation from malignant mesothelioma: a comparative study. Diagn Cytopathol 2005; 32: 156–9.

54. Robinson BW, Creaney J, Lake R et al. Mesothelin-family proteins and diagnosis of mesothelioma. Lancet 2003; 362: 1612–16.

55. Creaney J, Robinson BW. Detection of malignant mesothelioma in asbestos-exposed individuals: the potential role of soluble mesothelin-related protein. Hematol Oncol Clin North Am 2005; 19: 1025–40.

56. Treasure T, Waller D, Swift S et al. Radical surgery for mesothelioma. BMJ 2004; 328: 237–8.

57. Maziak DE, Gagliardi A, Haynes AE et al. Surgical management of malignant pleural mesothelioma: a systematic review and evidence summary. Lung Cancer 2005; 48: 157–69.

58. Sugarbaker DJ, Flores RM, Jaklitsch MT et al. Resection margins, extrapleural nodal status, and cell type determine postoperative long-term survival in trimodality therapy of malignant pleural mesothelioma: results in 183 patients. J Thorac Cardiovasc Surg 1999; 117: 54–63; discussion 63–5.

59. Sugarbaker DJ, Jaklitsch MT, Bueno R et al. Prevention, early detection, and management of complications after 328 consecutive extrapleural pneumonectomies. J Thorac Cardiovasc Surg 2004; 128: 138–46.

60. Rice DC, Erasmus JJ, Stevens CW et al. Extended surgical staging for potentially resectable malignant pleural mesothelioma. Ann Thorac Surg 2005; 80: 1988–92; discussion 1992–3.

61. Stewart DJ, Martin-Ucar AE, Edwards JG et al. Extra-pleural pneumonectomy for malignant pleural mesothelioma: the risks of induction chemotherapy, right-sided procedures and prolonged operations. Eur J Cardiothorac Surg 2005; 27: 373–8.

62. Weder W, Kestenholz P, Taverna C et al. Neoadjuvant chemotherapy followed by extrapleural pneumonectomy in malignant pleural mesothelioma. J Clin Oncol 2004; 22: 3451–7.

63. Stahel R, Weder W. Neoadjuvant chemotherapy in malignant pleural mesothelioma. Lung Cancer 2005; 49(Suppl 1): S69–70.

64. Baldini EH, Recht A, Strauss GM et al. Patterns of failure after trimodality therapy for malignant pleural mesothelioma. Ann Thorac Surg 1997; 63: 334–8.

65. Rusch VW, Rosenzweig K, Venkatraman E et al. A phase II trial of surgical resection and adjuvant high-dose hemithoracic radiation for malignant pleural mesothelioma. J Thorac Cardiovasc Surg 2001; 122: 788–95.

66. Gupta V, Mychalczak B, Krug L et al. Hemithoracic radiation therapy after pleurectomy/decortication for malignant pleural mesothelioma. Int J Radiat Oncol Biol Phys 2005; 63: 1045–52.

67. Stevens CW, Forster KM, Smythe WR et al. Radiotherapy for mesothelioma. Hematol Oncol Clin North Am 2005; 19: 1099–115.

68. Forster KM, Smythe WR, Starkschall G et al. Intensity-modulated radiotherapy following extrapleural pneumonectomy for the treatment of malignant mesothelioma: clinical implementation. Int J Radiat Oncol Biol Phys 2003; 55: 606–16.

69. Schouwink JH, Kool LS, Rutgers EJ et al. The value of chest computer tomography and cervical mediastinoscopy in the preoperative assessment of patients with malignant pleural mesothelioma. Ann Thorac Surg 2003; 75: 1715–18; discussion 1718–19.

70. Flores RM, Akhurst T, Gonen M et al. Positron emission tomography defines metastatic disease but not locoregional disease in patients with malignant pleural mesothelioma. J Thorac Cardiovasc Surg 2003; 126: 11–16.

71. Erasmus JJ, Truong MT, Smythe WR et al. Integrated computed tomography–positron emission tomography in patients with potentially resectable malignant pleural mesothelioma: staging implications. J Thorac Cardiovasc Surg 2005; 129: 1364–70.

72. Vogelzang NJ, Rusthoven JJ, Symanowski J et al. Phase III study of pemetrexed in combination with cisplatin vs cisplatin alone in patients with malignant pleural mesothelioma. J Clin Oncol 2003; 21: 2636–44.

73. Byrne MJ, Nowak AK. Modified RECIST criteria for assessment of response in malignant pleural mesothelioma. Ann Oncol 2004; 15: 257–60.

74. Fizazi K, Doubre H, Le Chevalier T et al. Combination of raltitrexed and oxaliplatin is an active regimen in malignant mesothelioma: results of a phase II study. J Clin Oncol 2003; 21: 349–54.

75. van Meerbeeck JP, Gaafar R, Manegold C et al. Randomized phase III study of cisplatin with or without raltitrexed in patients with malignant pleural mesothelioma: an intergroup study of the European Organisation for Research and Treatment of Cancer Lung Cancer Group and the National Cancer Institute of Canada. J Clin Oncol 2005; 23: 6881–9.

76. Andreopoulou E, Ross PJ, O'Brien ME et al. The palliative benefits of MVP (mitomycin C, vinblastine and cisplatin) chemotherapy in patients with malignant mesothelioma. Ann Oncol 2004; 15: 1406–12.

77. O'Brien ME, Watkins D, Ryan C et al. A randomised trial in malignant mesothelioma (M) of early (E) versus delayed (D) chemotherapy in symptomatically stable patients: the MED trial. Ann Oncol 2006; 17: 270–5.

78. Manegold C, Symanowski J, Gatzemeier U et al. Second-line (post-study) chemotherapy received by patients treated in the phase III trial of pemetrexed plus cisplatin versus cisplatin alone in malignant pleural mesothelioma. Ann Oncol 2005; 16: 923–7.

79. Kelly WK, O'Connor OA, Krug LM et al. Phase I study of an oral histone deacetylase inhibitor, suberoylanilide hydroxamic acid, in patients with advanced cancer. J Clin Oncol 2005; 23: 3923–31.

80. Govindan R, Kratzke RA, Herndon JE 2nd et al. Gefitinib in patients with malignant mesothelioma: a phase II study by the Cancer and Leukemia Group B. Clin Cancer Res 2005; 11: 2300–4.

81. Mathy A, Baas P, Dalesio O, et al. Limited efficacy of imatinib mesylate in malignant mesothelioma: a phase II trial. Lung Cancer 2005; 50: 83–6.

82. Baas P, Boogerd W, Dalesio O et al. Thalidomide in patients with malignant pleural mesothelioma. Lung Cancer 2005; 48: 291–6.

83. Byrne MJ, Davidson JA, Musk AW et al. Cisplatin and gemcitabine treatment for malignant mesothelioma: a phase II study. J Clin Oncol 1999; 17: 25–30.

84. van Klaveren RJ, Aerts JG, de Bruin H et al. Inadequacy of the RECIST criteria for response evaluation in patients with malignant pleural mesothelioma. Lung Cancer 2004; 43: 63–9.

85. Armato SG 3rd. Computerized analy-

sis of mesothelioma on CT scans. Lung Cancer 2005; 49(Suppl 1): S41–4.

86. Steinert HC, Santos Dellea MM, Burger C et al. Therapy response evaluation in malignant pleural mesothelioma with integrated PET–CT imaging. Lung Cancer 2005; 49(Suppl 1): S33–5.

87. Hollen PJ, Gralla RJ, Liepa AM et al. Adapting the Lung Cancer Symptom Scale (LCSS) to mesothelioma: using the LCSS-Meso conceptual model for validation. Cancer 2004; 101: 587–95.

88. Nowak AK, Stockler MR, Byrne MJ. Assessing quality of life during chemotherapy for pleural mesothelioma: feasibility, validity, and results of using the European Organization for Research and Treatment of Cancer Core Quality of Life Questionnaire and Lung Cancer Module. J Clin Oncol 2004; 22: 3172–80.

89. Herndon JE, Green MR, Chahinian AP et al. Factors predictive of survival among 337 patients with mesothelioma treated between 1984 and 1994 by the Cancer and Leukemia Group B. Chest 1998; 113: 723–31.

90. Curran D, Sahmoud T, Therasse P et al. Prognostic factors in patients with pleural mesothelioma: the European Organization for Research and Treatment of Cancer experience. J Clin Oncol 1998; 16: 145–52.

91. Fennell DA, Parmar A, Shamash J et al. Statistical validation of the EORTC prognostic model for malignant pleural mesothelioma based on three consecutive phase II trials. J Clin Oncol 2005; 23: 184–9.

10
Summary

Heine H Hansen

A short summary of the management of small cell lung cancer (SCLC), non-small cell lung cancer (NSCLC) and mesothelioma is given in this chapter based on the evidence from randomized trials, even though it should be realized that patients included in clinical trials are not representative of the patient population as a whole. Additional information on the management of lung cancer can be found in recent review articles.[1–5] Reviews of abstracts presented at the 2005 American Society of Clinical Oncology (ASCO) meeting have also been published.[6,7]

SMALL CELL LUNG CANCER

Limited disease

Surgical resection, followed by postoperative chemotherapy, is the treatment of choice for the rare patient who presents with stage I or II disease. The results for SCLC are equivalent to the treatment of stage I and II NSCLC. For the more typical SCLC patient who presents with bulky limited disease, combination chemotherapy is the mainstay of treatment, in conjunction with radiotherapy. For chemotherapy, the combination of etoposide and cisplatin (EP) has become the most commonly recommended regimen. The combination of carboplatin and etoposide produces similar results to cisplatin and etoposide and has a more favorable toxicity profile.

Based on meta-analyses, chest irradiation has shown superior results in patients receiving combination chemotherapy and radiotherapy compared with those receiving chemotherapy alone. The optimal timing and dosing of chest irradiation are still uncertain, but there is a tendency to initiate radiotherapy early during the first two courses at total doses of at least 50 Gy. Hyperfractionated radiotherapy given twice a day has yielded superior survival data in one randomized trial compared with conventional radiotherapy when combined with cisplatin and etoposide.

Prophylactic cranial irradiation (PCI) has also been demonstrated to have a statistically significant impact on survival in patients with limited disease who achieve a complete remission, whereas no such data exist for patients with extensive disease achieving a complete remission. The optimal dose and timing of radiotherapy are again uncertain; most frequently, the total dose does not exceed 30 Gy given in fractions of 2.5 Gy daily.

Extensive disease

A combination of etoposide and cisplatin is the preferred standard treatment. The replacement of etoposide by irinotecan given together with cisplatin has resulted in significantly better median and 1-year survival in one randomized trial, whereas no difference was observed in a subsequent trial. Again, carboplatin can be substituted for cisplatin because of similar activity and fewer side effects, even though myelosuppression is greater. Recent results have indicated that a four-drug combination of etoposide, cisplatin, epirubicin and cyclophosphamide may be superior to etoposide and cisplatin alone.

With regard to maintenance therapy, the hypothesis has been tested of adding either oral etoposide or topotecan to the treatment regimen in patients demonstrating a response to initial therapy. The results showed a slight improvement with etoposide in terms of median progression-free survival, whereas topotecan did not show any significant difference. The impact of dose intensification remains uncertain.

None of the phase III trials incorporating new agents has shown superior results compared with classical combinations such as cisplatin/carboplatin and etoposide.

In patients presenting with poor prognostic factors, such as performance status 3–4, involvement of the liver and bone marrow, or severe comorbid diseases, the initial dose of chemotherapy should be reduced, and careful monitoring is recommended over the first weeks.

Elderly patients with poor performance status and widespread disease have a substantially higher risk of incurring treatment-related complications, and generally have a poor outcome. Supportive measures alone are often the best option for some of these patients.

Recurrent disease

The treatment options depend on the anatomic site of relapse, symptomatology and previous treatment. Local relapse in patients without prior chest irradiation is best treated with palliative radiotherapy. Late relapse in patients who initially responded to a platinum-containing regimen should receive the same regimen again. Otherwise, single-agent chemotherapy with topotecan or combination chemotherapy with cyclophosphamide, doxorubicin and vincristine is the treatment of choice. Newer agents are being tested in this group of patients, either as single agents or in combinations, but are yielding response rates of <20%.

NON-SMALL CELL LUNG CANCER

A short summary of the management of NSCLC is given in this section. Chapter 8 provides detailed information on the current treatment options for patients with this disease.

Stages I, II and resectable IIIA

Stage I

The standard therapy for stage I NSCLC continues to be complete surgical resection when possible. This should include lobectomy plus sampling of all mediastinal nodal stations or complete lymph node dissection. However, the surgical technique to perform a lobectomy or pneumonectomy and mediastinal exploration may change as experience with minimally invasive surgery grows. Recent data have revealed encouraging results with video-assisted thoracic surgery (VATS) lobectomy and mediastinal sampling or dissection. With minimally invasive surgery becoming more popular, the efficacy of minimal resections such as segmentectomy and wedge resection is also being readdressed as smaller tumors (<1–2 cm) are being identified with spiral computed tomography (CT) scans. Another critical question is the relationship of tumor size to nodal metastasis. Data have been presented suggesting that histology and size may be beneficial in determining nodal risk.

For patients who are medically inoperable, advances in radiotherapy such as three-dimensional (3D) conformal and stereotactic radiosurgery are producing more durable results with decreased toxicity.

Stage IB–IIIA

The results of several large randomized trials of postoperative chemotherapy have been published, but these results differ and are therefore difficult to interpret. It appears that the weight of evidence suggests that postoperative cisplatin-based chemotherapy improves survival after surgery in patients with stage IB–IIIA NSCLC, resulting in an absolute survival advantage of 5 years. Similar results have been obtained by Japanese investigators using an oral drug combination of uracil and tegafur (UFT), both in individual trials and when meta-analysis of the results was performed. The results were most impressive in patients with adenocarcinomas.

Alternatively, neoadjuvant therapies are increasingly being used. Although large randomized trials investigating this important topic continue to enroll patients, recent experience has indicated that neoadjuvant chemotherapy does not significantly increase surgical morbidity or mortality.

For patients with operable stage III (N2) disease, the number of lymph nodes involved and the ability to eradicate tumor from the lymph nodes with neoadjuvant therapy have been found to be important prognostic factors. The pivotal question about the role of surgery in the treatment of stage IIIA (N2) disease is still open and awaits the results from several ongoing trials.

As multimodality therapy leads to improved survival for patients with operable NSCLC, an increased frequency of isolated brain metastases has been observed, and the potential value of PCI is being tested in selected subgroups.

Inoperable stage III

Current chemotherapy/radiotherapy is the standard of care for patients with inoperable stage III NSCLC. However, numerous questions remain regarding the optimal means to combine these two modalities and whether there is a benefit of additional therapy before or after chemotherapy/radiotherapy. Randomized phase II trials with newer cytotoxic agents given with concurrent radiation or trials incorporating an induction or consolidation chemotherapy approach have failed to show median survivals beyond the standard 16–18 months in most instances. Trials evaluating altered radiotherapy fractions have also not improved survival. Important areas of future research include the roles of 3D conformal radiotherapy, intensity-modulated radiotherapy (IMRT), hyperfractionated radiotherapy and the addition of targeted agents, with several of the latter demonstrating radiosensitization.

Stage IV (and IIIB with pleural effusion)

Doublet chemotherapy for stage IIIB with pleural effusion and stage IV NSCLC patients with adequate performance status has been shown in multiple randomized studies to improve survival and quality of life, and remains the standard of care. Numerous randomized trials have been performed during the last decade in order to identify the best platinum-based regimen; no major differences have been observed with respect to efficacy – only with regard to toxicity and cost. Current trials have continued to support this finding. Furthermore, randomized trials that included a non-platinum regimen showed such regimens to the equivalent in efficacy to platinum regimens, but with a more favorable toxicity profile. Controversy continues over the number of cycles of chemotherapy to be administered in the first-line setting. Several guidelines suggest a maximum of 6 cycles, but there is an accumulation of data indicating that 3–4 cycles are sufficient. Although numerous phase II cytotoxic regimens have been evaluated, none has produced amazing results. The major focus has therefore switched to targeted therapies.

A variety of targeted agents are currently being evaluated. Among these, the most promising are the epidermal growth factor receptor (EGFR) inhibitors gefitinib (Iressa) and erlotonib (Tarceva) and a monoclonal antibody against the vascular endothelial growth factor receptor (VEGFR), bevacizumab (Avastin). Among these, gefitinib and erlotinib have been approved by health authorities in various countries as second- or third-line treatment for NSCLC patients resistant to conventional combination chemotherapy.

A host of targeted agents are at earlier stages of clinical evaluation, such as cyclooxygenase-2 (COX-2) inhibitors, the preapoptotic inhibitor exisulind, proteasome inhibitors, bexarotene (Targretin) and vaccines.

Improving upon the efficacy of second-line docetaxel, investigators have focused on the addition of a second cytotoxic agent or on giving taxanes in a weekly schedule. Among the targeted agents, erlotinib has resulted in improved survival and quality of life in a large randomized trial comparing erlotinib with placebo. When added to paclitaxel and carboplatin chemotherapy, bevacizumab has also yielded higher response rate, progression-free survival and median survival in advanced NSCLC, with the majority of patients having adenocarcinoma.

Several small studies showed a favorable survival improvement for doublet therapy, but further investigation is needed. Pemetrexed (Alimta), a novel multitargeted antifolate, has in a randomized trial resulted in similar response rates, median survival and overall survival as docetaxel, but toxicity favored the pemetrexed arm, with significantly less neutropenia.

For the elderly population or patients with poor performance status, two-drug cytotoxic combinations, single-agent chemotherapy with vinorelbine or gemcitabine, and targeted therapy with gefitinib or erlotinib have proved to be of therapeutic value.

MESOTHELIOMA

Surgery should be considered when mesothelioma remains localized, usually as extrapleural pneumonectomy. Chemotherapy and/or radiotherapy have not yet proved to be effective in preventing local recurrence, nor has the use of photodynamic therapy or intracavitary chemotherapy.

With respect to chemotherapy, quantitative and qualitative overviews of the literature have suggested that cisplatin may play an important role in combination therapy. It is also emerging that response rates of 30–40% can be obtained when combining cisplatin with other agents, e.g. raltitrexed and pemetrexed. A combination of cisplatin and pemetrexed has in one randomized trial been superior to cisplatin alone, resulting in superior response rate, duration of response and quality of life.

REFERENCES

1. Laskin JJ, Sandler AB. State of the art in therapy for non-small cell lung cancer. Cancer Invest 2005; 23: 427–42.

2. Grunenwald DH. The role of surgery in non-small-cell lung cancer. Ann Oncol 2005; 16(Suppl 2); ii220–2.

3. Buter J, Giaccone G. Medical treatment of non-small-cell lung cancer. Ann Oncol 2005; 16(Suppl 2): ii229–32.

4. Giaccone G. Twenty-five years of treating advanced NSCLC: what have we achieved? Ann Oncol 2004; 15 (Suppl 4): iv81–3.

5. Movsas B. Will future progress in non-small-cell lung cancer be step by step … or by leaps and bounds? J Clin Oncol 2005; 23: 5859–61.

6. Bonomi P. Lung Cancer I. ASCO Annual Meeting Summaries 2005; 154–9.

7. Bonomi P. Lung Cancer II. ASCO Annual Meeting Summaries 2005; 164–9.

Index

N.B. Combination drugs are shown with components in alphabetical order.